SOTHIS PRESS

Sothis Press aims to completely reimagine the public domain book with an emphasis on universal access to captivatingly designed print editions. We believe that technology will enable every single book ever published to be perpetually accessible in beautiful print form. Sothis is beauty in ubiquity.

www.sothis.press
1 Waterhouse Square, London, ECIN 2ST

Gunn's Domestic Medicine, or Poor Man's Friend

John C. Gunn

SOTHIS PRESS

ISBN 978-1-83548-157-8

Gunn's Domestic Medicine,
or Poor Man's Friend
is in the public domain.

This edition is published by
Sothis Press © 2023. The company
is registered in England and Wales.
The Company Number is 14900389.

GUNN'S

DOMESTIC MEDICINE,

OR

POOR MAN'S FRIEND,

IN THE HOURS OF AFFLICTION PAIN AND SICKNESS,

THIS BOOK

POINTS OUT IN PLAIN LANGUAGE FREE FROM DOCTOR'S TERMS,

THE DISEASES OF

MEN, WOMEN AND CHILDREN,

AND THE LATEST AND MOST APPROVED MEANS USED IN THEIR CURE, AND IS EXPRESSLY WRITTEN FOR THE BENEFIT OF

FAMILIES,

IN THE WESTERN AND SOUTHERN STATES.

IT ALSO CONTAINS

DESCRIPTIONS OF MEDICAL ROOTS AND HERBS OF THE WESTERN AND SOUTHERN COUNTRY, AND HOW THEY ARE TO BE USED IN TDE CURE OF

DISEASES;

ARRANGED ON A NEW AND SIMPLE PLAN,

BY WHICH THE PRACTICE OF MEDICINE IS REDUCED TO PRINCIPLES OF COMMON SENSE.

Why should we conceal from mankind,
That which relieves the distresses of our fellow-beings?

EIGHTH EDITION.

PUMPKINTOWN, TEN;
S. M. JOHNSTON, PUBLISHER.

1839.

INDEX.

INTRODUCTION.

Man, in the early days of nature, lived in a state of health, both in body and in mind. The earth produced its fruits for him without culture; there were neither irregularities nor inclemencies of the seasons. In a state of innocency, and under a mild and clement sky, there was nothing to produce disease; spring was perpetual. Protected by the immediate presence of the Almighty, and as yet innocent of any violations of his law, he was happy in the enjoyments which the spontaneous benevolence of nature afforded him. But he has been the artificer of his own untoward destinies! He has transgressed the sacred laws of his Creator—and incurred the penalties annexed to his own transgressions! *His days are now shortened, and encumbered with disease;* spring is no longer perpetual; for him now, "*the earth brings forth thorns and briers,*" and for him the world has been visited with earthquakes, sterility, storms, and variations of the seasons, which blight the fruits of his labors, and bring mortal diseases and fatal maladies on their wings.

Among the moral causes that have abridged the life of man, there is one which merits the attention of the philosopher—it is civilization! Civilization, by polishing man, and depriving him of his primitive rudeness, seems to have enervated him:—it seems to have made him purchase the advantage, at the expense of a multitude of diseases and miseries to which the first inhabitants of the world were strangers—and with which the savages who only give way to the impulses of nature are still unacquainted. Man in associating with his fellow beings in large assemblages, seems in some measures to have relaxed the strong ties on his earthly existence; society—by extending the circle of his wants, by giving greater energy, to his passions and by generating those that are unknown to the man of nature,

A

seems to have become a frightful and inexhaustible source of calamities. But was not man born for society; did not his individual weakness, and his severe and pressing wants, make him abandon at an early period the wandering life he had led in the forests in persuit of game—and associate with his fellow man? Could he not by associating with his fellow beings, the better protect his existence, secure his happiness, and expand his truly astonishing faculties! There exists no country, in which men are not found in a social state; this is the case even in the most remote and frightful solitudes, from the Arabian deserts to the Polar regions. But cannot the social ties of men be drawn too close! Witness our large and opulent cities, where the population is immense, and where assembled multitudes seem to be crowded on each other; where, although the comforts and luxuries of life are to be found in abundance, the horrors of want are extreme! Are not these extremes always hostile to the social nature of man; are not these large cities continually the seats of mortal diseases; the abodes of crime and immorality; and, are not physical and moral depravity, always the consequences of such enormous accumulations of people?

When men first united, it was in small bodies; and they passed their days in innocence and simplicity. We should not then be astonished if they were robust, and if they then arrived to a great age. They were exempt from the greater part of the diseases which affect us, because they had none but natural wants, which they could always satisfy without excess. The beverage of nature quenched their thirst without the aid of spiritous liquors—and the friendly hand of nature gave them sustenance; but, in proportion to the increase of associations, they generated a multitude of factitious wants, which continually torment us their offspring, and render us unhappy; whence, instead of those simple foods which always prolonged life, man has the poisons of every chemical and foreign luxury served upon his table: and what are the results? Why—prematurely borne down with infirmities, and devoured with remorse, he dies disgusted and exhaused with excesses—refleeting on innocent nature whom he has outraged! The greatest number of diseases and infirmities are of our own begetting; because we have infringed the healthy laws of nature. Fifteen out of tewnty cases of sickness, are produced by ourselves; it is by luxury and scandalous excesses, that we render our existence unhappy, and abridge its length.

Man is a creature of habit; urged on by the propensities of his nature, he not only abridges the period of his life, but inflicts on himself the displeasure of his CREATOR. The rising morn, the radient noon, the shadowy eve, all tell him as they pass, that his temporal existence is short—his advance to eternity rapid!

When we view man in all his bearings and dependencies, we find, and the profoundest philosophers have done no more, that he is involved in mystery. The greatest philosophers have only discovered that they live; but from whence they came, and whither they are going, are by *nature* altogether hidden: that impenetrable gloom surrounds us on every side, and that we can seek in *Revelation* alone, the only source of comfort and explanation. The seasons are a memento of life. *Spring*, breathing into life the new-born flowers; *Summer*, with his genial warmth, ripening his luscious fruits; *Autumn*, with her golden harvest, bestowing plenty on man:—and *Winter*, with her icy mantle, sounding the requiem of the departed seasons. First comes creeping infancy; next, merry boyhood and aspiring youth; then resolute and industrious manhood:—and last of all, decripid, cold, and declining age; emblematic of the winter of existence. the shortness of human life.

Behold the changes that have taken place in Tennessee and, in the whole western country, within the lapse of a few short years! Look for the wigwam of the poor Indian, who was once lord of the soil you now possess:—it is gone—and his bones mingle with the dust of his habitation. The storm of enterprising civilization has wrecked its fury on the poor Indian; his land has passed into the hands of the white man:—whose splendid mansion now rests on the graves of his ancestors. His peaceful forests, once the abodes of solitude and savage life, in which he unmolested traced his game, now resound with the festivities of civilization, and the business hum of labor. Those innocent and forlorn people, who received our fore-fathers in the spirit of friendship, instead of being fostered by the genial hand of civilization, have been driven to the feet of the Rocky or Oregon Mountains, and present a sad and solitary spectacle of their former greatness! In a few more years, the race of the poor Indian will be forever extinguished, and his council fires blaze no more;—the wilderness has been subdued, and the house of God has been built, where once ascended the smoke of warlike and idolatious sacrifice; cultivated fields and gardens extend over a thousand valleys in the west, never before since the creation reclaimed to the use of civilized man; in the enjoyment of civil and religious liberty, institutions of learning are hourly springing forth, diffusing the light of knowledge, and establishing the enjoyments and happiness of the WESTERN WORLD. A few years since, even within the memory of many of the prosent inhabitants, this immense region was a perfect wilderness:—the darkened intellect of the savage knew God but in the winds and thunders; on every side, the dark foilage of the shadowy forest waved in the silent majesty of nature, and her noble rivers moved on in silence, with no other commerce than the peltry of the hunter savage. Most of these rivers are now navigated by steamers, affording the quickest facility of transportation, and the most lucrative commerce; supplying the remote interior of our country with the rich products of every foreign climate; our public roads are covered every year with the advance guard of civilization, and demonstrate what must in a short period be the result, under our *wise, equitable*, and *potlitic institutions* of government. The tree of peace spreads its broad branches from the Atlantic to the Pacific; a thousand villages are reflected from the waves of almost every lake and river; and the west now echoes with the song of the reaper, until the wilderness and "the solitary place has been glad for us, and the desert has rejoiced and blossomed as the rose."—God in the infinitude of his mercy, has stored our mountains, fields, and meadows, with simples for healing our diseases, and for furnishing us with medicines of our own, without the use of foreign articles; and the discoveries of each succeeding day convince us that he has graciously furnished man with the means of curing his own diseases, in all the different countries and climates of which he is an inhabitant. There is not a day, a month, a year, which does not exhibit to us the surprising cures made by roots, herbs and simples, found in our kingdom of nature, when all foreign articles have utterly failed:—and the day will come, when calomel and mercurial medicines will be used no longer, and when we will be independent of foreign medicines, which are often difficult to be obtained, frequently adulterated, and always command a price which the poor are unable to pay. The yet uncultivated wilds of our country, abound in herbs and plants possessing medicinal virtues—and probably thousands of them, whose virtues and qualities remain unknown. The travels of Lewis and Clarke, led to high expectations in every branch of science:—the observations and inquiries of these gentlemen, particularly of Lewis, were directed, among other things, to the diseases and medical remedies of our Indians; and they have given a large portion of interesting information on these points. Much, however is left to be done by the wisdom of our Legislative bodies on these points:—for the time is rapidly approaching, when the beautiful temple of medical science, will stand divested of all *quackeries* and *superstitions*, and its rebuilders be rewarded by the blessings, the gratitude, and the admiration of mankind.

Professional pride and native cupidity, contrary to the true spirit of justice and christianity, have, in all ages and countries, from sentiments of self interest and want of liberality, delighted in concealing the divine art of healing diseases, under complicated names, and difficult or unmeaning technical phrases. Why make a mystery of things which relieve the distresses and sufferings of our fellow beings! Let it be distinctly understood, when I speak of professional pride and avarice, that I do not intend to cast an imputation on all my proffession, for want of that heaven born principle, *charity* to our fellow beings. On the contrary, we are furnished by history, with many prominent examples of this divine form of humanity. Hippocrates dispensed health and joy wherever he went, and often yielded to the solicitations of neighboring princes, and extended the blessings of his skill to foreign nations. The great Boerhaave did a great deal for the poor, and always discovered more solicitude and punctuality in his attendance on them, than on the rich and powerful:—on being asked his reasons for this, he promptly replied—"God is their pay-master."—Heberdens liberality to the poor was so great, that he was once told by a friend, he would exhaust his fortune: "no," said he, "I am afraid that after all my charities, I shall die shamefully rich." Fothergill once heard of the death of a citizen of London, who had left his family in indigent circumstances,—the doctor immediately called on the widow, and informed her he had received *thirty guineas* from her husband, while he was in prosperous circumstances, for as many visits; "I have heard of his reverse of fortune—take this purse—which contains all I received from him—it will do thy family more good than it will do me." Similar occurrences of the liberality of this great and good man, might be given almost without end: indeed it is said, that he gave away one half of the income of his extensive and profitable business, to the needy and afflicted—amounting, in the course of his life, to more than one hundred thousand pounds. What an immense interest, in celestial honor and happiness, must this sum not produce at the great day of accounts—the general judgment! With what unspeakable gratitude and delight, may we not suppose the many hundreds—perhaps thousands, whom he has fed, clothed, and relieved in sickness, by his charities, will gaze on their benefactor in that solemn day, while the Supreme Judge accredits those acts as done to himself, in the presence of an assembled Universe.

But—these good and great men, have gone where we must all shortly follow—and are now receiving the rich reward of all their virtues, in that kingdom where pain and affliction cease. When we trace the powers of human intellect, and the monuments of human greatness, and all that genius has instituted and labor accomplished, when we trace these things through all their grades of advancement and decline—where is the pride of man? Behold in each successive moment, the monuments of the rich, the great, and the powerful—tumbling into their native dust—and the hand of time mingling the proud man's ashes with those of the menial slave, so that their posterity cannot distinguish them from each other! When the sable curtain of death is drawn, where is the bright intellect of genius—and where are those we have loved and honored? At the threshold of eternity, reason leaves us and we sink, notwithstanding all our precautions, and the aid of distinguished physicians. Yet, such is the course of nature, that those who live long, must outlive those they love and honor. Such, indeed, is the course of nature, and the condition of our present existence, that life must sooner or later *lose its associations*, and those who remain a little longer, be doomed to walk downward to the grave *alone* and *unregarded* without a single interested witness of their joys or griefs! It is evident that the decays of age *must* terminate in death;—yet where is the man who does not believe he may survive another year?

Piety toward God, should characterise every one who has any thing to do with the administering of medicine; nor should any individual ever administer medicine, without first imploring the Almighty for success on his prescriptions—for where is the man, who can anticipate success, without the aid and blessing of heaven? Galen vanquished Atheism, for a considerable time, by proving the existence of a God, from the wise and curious structure of the human body. Botallus, the illustrious father of blood-letting in Europe, earnestly advises a physician never to leave his house, without preferring a prayer to God to aid and enlighten him. Cheselden, the famous English anatomist, always implored the aid and blessing of heaven on his hand, whenever he laid hold of an instrument to perform a surgical operation. Sydenham, the great luminary and reformer of medicine, was a religious man; and, Boerhaave spent an hour every morning in his closet, in reading and commenting on the *Scriptures*, before he entered on the duties of his profession. Hoffman and Stahl, were not ashamed of the *Gospel of*

Christ; and, Waller has left behind him, a most eloquent defence of its doctrines. Doctor Fathergill's long life, resembled au altar from which incense of adoration and praise ascended daily to heaven; and Hartley, whose works will probably only perish with time itself, was a devout christian. To this record of these great medical men, I shall add but one remark—which is, that the authoritative weight of their names alone, in favor of the truth of *revealed religion,* is sufficient to turn the scale against all the *infidelity* that has ever disgraced the science of medieine, sinee its earliest discoveries.

I have seen the flower of life fade, and all its freshness wither; I have seen the bright eye of beauty loose its lustre and my last and best friends, close their eyes in the cold and tranquil slumbers of death—and have said, "where are the boasted powers of medicine, the pride of skill, the vain boast of *science?*"—How humiliating to the pride of man! Let every physician put this solemn question to himself:—what will avail all the means I can use, without the aid of the Almighty? All efforts, founded on years of experience and study, vanish at the touch of death; and, the hold on life proffessed by the physician, is as brittle and slender as that possessed by his patient:—the next moment may be his—and those remedies so often used with success, in the cases of others, will assuredly fail him in his own case at last. In some unexpected moment, a wave in the agitated sea of life will baffle all his struggles; and he, in his turn, will be compelled to pay that *debt,* which *nature* has claimed from thousands of his patients. When on the couch of death, and whilst perusing the works of Rousseau, the last words of the great Napoleon were, in the language of that author, "it is vain to shrink from what cannot be avoided; why hide that from ourselves, which must at some period be found; *the certainty of death,* is a truth which man knows—but which he willingly *conceals from himself.*"—We shall all shortly finish our allotted time on earth, if even unusually prolonged, leaving behind us all that is now familiar and beloved. Numerous races of men will succeed us, entirely ignorant that we once lived, and who will retain of our existence, not even the vestage of a vague and empty remembrance!

OF THE PASSIONS.

All the passions of man, seem to have been bestowed on him by an all-wise Creator, for wise and beneficent purposes; and it is certainly the province of human wisdom, to keep them under due regulation. In a moral point of view, when the passions run counter to reason and religion, *nationally*, and *individually* they produce the most frightful catastrophes. Among nations if suffered to transcend the bounds of political justice, they always lead to anarchy, war, misrule and oppression: and among individuals, do we not easily trace the same dreadful and disasterous consequences? With monarchial and despotic governments, we frequently see the unruly and ungoverned passions of *one man*, destroying and laying waste, whole empires in a single campaign: and with democratical or republican institutions of government, have we not frequently witnessed the turrific cousequences, to moral and political justice, which arises from the disorganizing and tribulent passions of the *sovereign people*. Individually and nationally, then, the consequences of misdirected and uncontrolled passions are precisely the same, as regards every thing connected with political, legislative, and moral justice.

But, as it is not my intention to enter into a dissertation on the passions, farther than as they relate to man as an individual, and to their influence on the state of his physical system. I will first observe, that it is of the very highest importance to the healthy action of the human system, that the passions should be held in due subjection. If you give way to the passions, you destroy the finest of the vital powers: you destroy digestion and assimilation; you weaken the strength and energies of the heart, and of the whole nervous system. The stomach is the *workshop* of the whole human frame, and all its derangements are immediately felt in the extremities: and to prove how strongly the connexion exists, between the stomach and the heart, the latter immediately ceases to beat, when the powers of the former sink and are destroyed. Distress of mind is always a predisposing cause of disease; while on the other hand, a calm and contented disposition, and a proper command over our passions and affections, are certain to produce consequences which operate against all predisposing causes of disease. Any complaint arising from great agitation of mind, is more obstinate than any occasioned by violent corporeal agitations. For instance, eating and drinking, and particularly the case of drinking, disease may be combatted by *rest, sleep* and *temperance:* but neither temperance, rest, nor even sleep itself, as every one knows, can much affect those diseases which have their seat in the passions of the mind. I shall not enter into the subject of the passions at full length.

FEAR.

Fear is a base passion, and beneath the dignity of man. It takes from him reflection, power, resolution and judgment; and in short, all that dignity and greatness of soul, which properly appertain to humanity. It has great influence in *occasioning, aggravating,* and *producing* disease. It has been a matter of much speculation with me, whether any man is born *constitutionally* a coward.—and my decided opinion is, that cowardice and courage are generally the ffects of habit and *moral influence** I have frequently

**Immediately preceding the great battle of Waterloo, on which were about to be suspended the great political and military destinies of Europe, Napoleon employed a guide who was well acquainted with the country, to accompany him in reconnoitering the field of battle, and the relative positions of the hostile armies. When the battle commenced, his peasant guide, who had never before been exposed to the tumultuous shock of hostile armies, manifested strong and decided indications of fear—by dodging from side to side at the sound of the shot. Napoleon observed it and taxed him with* seen brave men, acknowledged to be such on great and important occasions during the late war, who trembled at the mere approach of danger, and acknowledged their want of firmness. The great duke of Marlboro' was once seen to tremble on the eve of battle; being asked by a soldier, the cause of it—the Duk made the following reply—"my body trembles at the danger my soul is about exposing it to?' And does it not appear surprisingly singular, but no less true, that a man shall be one day, brave, and the next a coward. That there is a close affinity between the condition of the physical system and the passions there can be little doubt: the same man, who under the influence of opium, would brave danger in its most giant form, is seen to shrink like a *sensative plant,* when deprived of that influence. There seems to be a reciprocal exercise of influence between the body and the mind, which by man is absolutely inexplicable; but of this we are certain, that cowardice disorders and impeads the circulation of the blood: hinders breathing with freedom; puts the stomach out of order, as well as the bowels: affects the kidneys and skin, and produces bad effects on the whole body—and it may be for these and similar reasons; that the ancients elevated courage into a *moral virtue.* Many persons have fallen down dead, from the influence of cowardice or fear; and can it then be doubtful, that this passion has much influence in producing and modifying diseases? I feel assured from practical

---

cowardice, which he acknowledged. He then reasoned with him on the absurdity of his conduct. "Do you not know," said he, "that there is a power infinitely superior to man, who rules and governs all, and who holds in his hands all our destinies! If this be true of which there can be no doubt, you cannot die until your time arrives; why then dodge the sound of a ball; when you hear it, it has passed you; and besides, when dodging the mere sound of one shot, you may throw yourself in the way of another." This reasoning had the effect; it banished all suggestions of fear, and the guide afterwards rode erect and steady, and manifested no indications of fear. I mention this circumstance to show how much we are under the influence of mortal power, or the force of reason, respecting both cowardice and courage.

experience, that in disorders that are epidemical or catching, the timid, cowardly and fearful, take them much oftener than those who are remarkable for fortitude and courage. Napoleon was so well convinced of these facts, that when his army of Egypt was suffering dreadfully from the ravages of the plague, in order to inspire his souldiers with courage, and to ward off those dangers which might arise from the fears of his army, frequently touched the bodies of those infected, with his own hands. Fear weakens the energy or strength of the heart, and of the whole nervous system; the infectious matter has greater power on the frame at this time—consequently the system being deranged, losses its healthy action, and cannot resist and throw off the epidemical disease.

HOPE.

Hope! what a source of human happiness rests in the pleasures of hope. Man cherishes it to his very *tomb.* Take from him hope, and life itself would be a burthen. How wisely has our Heavenly Father blended in our cup of *misery*, soft whispers of our future exemption from its influence. Without hope, how wretched, how miserable our existence: what a powerful effect it has, when laboring under pain and bodily disorder! It raises the spirits; it increases the action and power of the heart, and nervous system; moderates the pulse: causes the breathing to be freer and fuller—and quickens all the secretions. It is therefore proper and advisable in all disorders, to produce hope in the mind, if you wish to have any chance to effect a cure. Is there a being who lives without this balm of consolation, this hope of heavenly birth, which tells of happier days in bright anticipation! If such are the advantages of hope, as to the things of this field of thorns and briers—this vale of tears—what may we expect from that emotion, when it embraces the *certainty* of enjoying felicity with God in eternity.

When in ordinary health and engaged in the pursuits of life, hope is attended with many favorable effects of a fortunate event, without possessing the physical disadvantges; the anticipation of happiness does not affect us so excessively as the actual enjoyment; yet it, has frequently produced more benefit by its influence on health, than fortune realized.

JOY.

This is a benificent passion; it produces an extraordinary effect, and is of infinite benefit to the constitution, when indulged in moderation; but if it should be excessive, or very sudden, it frequently does serious and lasting injury to persons in good health; and to those who are weak, or afflicted with disease, it sometimes terminates fatally. The following instance of the melancholy effects of the too sudden infiuence of joy, will fully exemplify the power of this passion on the physical system, even when in health. It may be relied on, as it came very nearly under my own observation. A gentleman in the State of Virginia, who had once been very wealthy, but whose pecuniary circumstances had become much depressed, not to say desperate, as a last hope of redeeming himself and his family from distressing embarrassments, purchased a lottery ticket, for which he gave the last hundred dollars he could command. The purchase was made, under a presentiment if such it may be called, that a certain number would draw the highest prize. All his property was then under execution. When the day of sale arrived, his father-in-law and himself took a walk into the fields, leaving his family much distressed with their misfortune. A gentleman on horse-back, immediately from Richmond, rode up to the house and asked for Mr. B——, and was directed by his wife where he would be found. When the gentleman rode up to Mr. B——, without exercising the least precaution, he announced the fact that the ticket had drawn one hundred thousand dollars! The effect was such as might have been expected; Mr. B——immediately fainted, and was with much difficulty and after many exertions, restored.—in the circumstance I have just related, the great influence of this passion will easily be seen; and I trust it will be distinctly inferred from it, that excesses of joy are frequently as dangerous to the constitution of humanity, as those of grief, if not more so. I need scarcely remark here, that to persons laboring under disease, as well as to those in merely delecate health, joyful intelligence ought always to be communicated with much caution.

ANGER.

"Next, anger rushed its eyes on fire!"—Of this most dreadful of the human passions, had I sufficient space to allot it, much might be said that would be of high importance. There is no passion incidental to humanity, an indulgence in which leads to so many dreadful, not to say horrid and frightful consequences:

> "To count them all would want a thousand tongues—
> A throat of brass and adamantine lungs!"

I have before remarked, that all our passions were intended by the God of nature, if kept under the control of reason and humanity, to be beneficial to the happiness of man. This position is demonstrable by reason, and sanctioned by the highest authority—the word of God himself, "*who never made any thing in vain.*". It is not the application of our passions to their natural, reasonable and legitimate objects, that constitutes crime, and ends in misery and misfortune: No—it is the abuse of those passions by unrestrained and intemperate indulgence—and the prostitution of them to ignoble and disgraceful purposes! Was a noble spirit of resentiment, for unprovoked and wanton injuries, ever intended by the God of nature, to degenerate into *senseless anger* and *brutal rage?* A noble spirit of resentiment, upon the strictest moral principles, was intended to punish wanton and unprovoked aggression, and by preventing a repetition of the deed, to *reform the offender.* I am perfectly aware that I here occupy a new, but by no means an untenable ground. Was the passion of *love*, the refined solacer of civilized life; the harbinger of successful procreative power, the nurse which ushurs into life successive millions of the human race, ever intended by the God of nature to degenerate into brutal *lust;* and to be followed by a train of *venereal diseases* which cankers life at its very core "and visits the iniquities of the fathers, upon the children to the third and fourth generations?" Was the deep seated and natural sentiment of *self preservation*, that essential safeguard of man in every stage of his moral existence, ever intended to degenerate into that childish superstitious, base, and ignoble passion called *fear?* Was the elevating and ennobling passion of *emulation*, that only seeks to rival superior excellence, so honorable to the pride of man, and so consonant to the native dignity of his soul, ever intended to degenerate into a dastardly passion of *envy* which seeks to destroy by slander, and defamation, the excellence it has not the honest virtue even to *attempt* to rival? Those who blindly decry the legitimate gratification of the human passions, although they may do so from what to them seems the best of motives, ought to be aware that they do not arraign the wisdom of *Providence*, for implanting them into the human bosom; and they ought also in all cases, to avoid confounding the natural and legitimate *uses* of the passions, with the abuses of their lofty, and powerful energies. The passions, confined to their native objects, and as I have said before, kept in due subjection to the restraints of reason and moderation, are essential to the enjoyments, the preservation, and the happiness of man; they only become dangerous and criminal, when permitted to produce misrule in the human breast, and are placed beyond the arbitrium and control of moral virtue, which is the true science of human wisdom. I remarked in the outset, that there was no passion known to humanity, an unrestrained indulgence in which was so fatal in its consequences to the peace of society, and the happiness of man, as ANGER. This deformer of the human countenance and character, is every where to be found; and its ravages seem co-extensive with its existence: in other words, it seems to live through all human life, and to extend through the whole extent of human society.

It is even sometimes seen to wrinkle and deform the maidden cheek of youthful beauty, with a frown! But do not my fair country-women know, that the passsions never fail to leave their impress on the countenance, and that hibitual anger will render them more disgusting than the witch of Endor? They may be assured and my remarks are not founded on cursory and superfiicial observations, that the more of native beauty there is to be found in the female countenance, the more easily will it be deformed by the vicious passion, and particularly by that demon Anger. The female countenance is more expressive of the finer, softer, and mere amiable passions, than that of man: in other words, the female face seems to be formed from finer materials, and to have been cast in a finer mold, and it is from these causes, that the female face is more expressive of the moral feelings, and sooner betrays indications of a depraved and vicious temper. The stern countenance of man, can assume and maintain a fixture of expression under any circumstances; and it is the consciousness of this power, that frequently tempts him to play the hypocrite and deluder:—for were he conscious that his face would always betray the emotions of his soul, he would never even attempt to deceive! To the practiced eye of phylosophical research and rigid scrutiny, no expression of the human countenance ever passes unobserved; to such an eye all the wiles of the human heart stand unrevealed; nor can any subterfuge, of counterfeit expression, conceal the reality from its observation. The scripture itself sanetiens this doctrine. "*A man shall be known by his loo*—and a proud man by his gait." If my fair country-women would reflect well on the doctrine I have just laid down, they would always cultivate the softer and more benevolent feelings of the heart; and always endeavor to *be in reality*, what they would wish to appear; for they may receive it as a valuable truth, not to be controverted by any of the artifices of self deception, that they were never formed hy the God of nature for deception and hypocrisy; and that the purity and elevation of their moral feelings, or the corruptions and depravity of their real characters, are as easily distinguished from each other, as is the surface of the ocean in a settled *calm*, from that same ocean, when lashed into mountain billows by the winds of heaven.

Do we not see the ravages of this moral curse called anger in every department of society? We see it beneath the domestic roof, embittering the enjoyments of the rich and poor; laying waste the harmonious sanctity of connubial life, and often entailing misery and misfortune on a helpless and unoffending offspring. But this is not all. We see it manifesting itself in its most horrid forms, in our halls of legislation; in our seats of legal justice; and even in our elections, in which every man ought to be permitted to act with perfect freedom, and without the least accountability to another. In all our electioneering conflicts, at least of late years, we can see the old and disgraceful maxim revived and fully acted on:— "those who are not for us are against us,"—as if a man could not exercise a right of selection, and prefer one man to another, without forfeiting the friendship, and incurring the enmity of all the opposite parties. If we would reflect correctly on this subject, we would soon discover, that personal friendship, and personal enmity, ought to have nothing to do with the matter: we would soon distinguish, that a real statesman, or enlightened legislator, ought to be the mere tool, for factional purposes, of no party whatever. The noble and devoted patriotism, which gave birth to our truly great political institutions, emphatically, forbids, that the *American people* should ever sacrifice to the narrow views of *party spirit*, what was destined by the God of nature, for the *benefit of the human race!* This government presents to Europe, a spectacle of no ordinary character; in which their statesmen read the future destinies of man, and the political fate of nations. We are the only people of any age or country, who have organized a truly *representative government*, whose experiments in legislation—diplomacy and arms, are to settle the important question yet undecided, whether the mass of mankind can bear the *wide tolerations of political freedom;* and whether man, under any circumstances, is capable of assuming and exercising the *high prerogative of self government.* For what a stake then, against all the monarchies and despotisms of Europe and Asia, are this people and this government contending;—a stake as I before remarked, in which the whole human race are interested! Before this view of the subject, my reader, how do our party squabbles and brawls at elections, dwindle down to nothing: to less than nothing. God forbid, that I should ever seem to turn censure of the age: or assume a *dictatorial tone* even in the cause of truth and moderation. I have been led into a slight notice of the preceding subjects, by their strong connexion with the moral condition of man, and his too frequent subjection to the ravages of a most devastating, and I had almost said, a most *damnable passion*, which it seems is scarcely controlable, by all the energies of reason and moral sentiment combined. Anger was never yet an evidence of justice, a proof of virtue, or a demonstration of superior intellect; a mind of elevated endowments, will always endeavor to correct its sanguinary impulses and to expel its influence.. The man of cool reflection. sees in its unrestrained dominion, a thousand evils which escape common observation.—He sees that it frequently fills our prisons with delinquents; that it is sometimes the cause of endless remorse; and that it often loads the gallows with a melancholy victim? To speak of other than moral and religious remedies, for this dreadful malady, would be idle and nugatory. I might tell you as a physician, to deluge your heads with water as cold as the snows of Zembla; I might tell you to open every vain in your bodies, to calm the raging and ungovernable impulses of anger; I might tell you, that an emetic would curb the tumultuous fever of rage, and restore you to yourselves: all these remedies would produce a temporary cure; they would be but clipping the twigs from the *Bohon upas*, and leaving the root untouched! The only sovereign powers, or remedies if you please, which can be efficient in correcting the evils of anger, must be sought for in early education, aud in moral and religious principles, instilled into the mind at an early period of life.

JEALOUSY.

This is a passion, the causes of which have seldom been investigated, although the effects of it are every where to be found. The causes of it have generally something to do with love; but not always. The *coxcomb* and *coquett*, both of whom are incapable of genuine love, may be powerfully effected by *jealousy;* yet in both these cases, the lady and gentleman have only experienced a *slight mortification of their vanity*, and love of general admiration. The wound here is not deep; and is generally healed by the consolatory admiration of some other jilt or jackpudding, as the case may be. I am not going to speak of the jealousy of the *warrior*, which is sanguinary and daring; of that of the *diplomatist*, which is politic, cunning and circumventive; or of that of the statesman, which is embittered by spectres and phantoms of future glory?—Nor will I trouble myself with noticing the jealousy of the *poet*, which is harmless though vindictive:—of the *historian*, which is longwinded and untiring in the pursuit of fame:—or of the *philosopher* and *man of general science*, which is learnedly dull, and heavily investigative, in the pursuit of truths which eternally elude human researches! I shall confine myself to the single subject, of that jealousy which sometimes subsists between *Husband and Wife*, and which generally renders both the objects of public curiosity, compassion or contempt.

Marriages are contracted upon various principles: such as the love of person, the love of fame, the love of money, &c. So soon as the rites and ceremonies of marriage are duly solemnised, and rendered matter of legal record, the parties individually acquire certain *rights* and *privileges*, of which it is a breach of the municipal law to deprive them as well as a violation of the law of God. If the love of money induced the lady to marry the gentleman, or the gentleman the lady, any deviation of conduct however indecent and immoral on the one part, ought never to be complained of on the other, provided the true intent and meaning of the compact be complied with, in relation to the *cash itself!* The same doctrines apply, in the case of a marriage contracted on any other principles. If the *fame* of either of the parties, induces the other to enter into the marriage bonds, and there be no other stipulation expressed or implied, infidelity to the nuptial bed, profligacy of conduct, and even the most indecent deviations from moral rectitude, ought never to make a breach between the parties; the tenor and spirit of the compact being complied with, there is nothing more to be said. Nor would there be in nine cases out of ten, if married persons who are induced to captiousness and disagreement, would only be particular in calling to mind, the *real motive* which operated in inducing them to marry. If the mere love of *person,* without any considerations relating to temper, moral excellence, and intellectual elevation of character, were the leading principle which induced the parties to bear the yoke of life together, surely neither of them have a right to complain of the want of excellencies, which were overlooked, disregarded and absolutely undervalued in the stipulations of the compact. I think this reasoning is fair; and absolutely too logical to be refuted; and as I intend this book as a family museum of useful instruction and advice, I trust that what I have so fare said on the subject of jealousy, and other causes of domestic discontent, will have its due weight. What right have parties who have been improperly matched or rather those who have improperly matched themselves, to disturb the peace of whole neighborhoods and communities, with their whinings, scoldings, and recriminations of each other: Will these proceedings benefit the parties themselves? Will these bickerings and brawls, divorce them from each other? Will their domestic disagreements, and their "*fisticuff combats;*" if they should happen to be so far advanced in the "*sweets of connubial love,* reflect any respectability or honor, on their innocent and unoffending offspring? Will their neighbors endeavor to compose their strifes, and hush them into peace with a soothing lullaby? No: they will in ten cases out of eleven, be gratifyed at finding out, that there are others more miserable than themselves; and do every thing they possibly can, to inflame the contest, by taking sides. 'Some will take the part of the husband; these are generally the *gentlemen* of the little body politic: some will take the part of the wife; these are generally the lady peace-makers of the neighborhood: and before six months pass around, the whole country will be roused to a war of words—and resemble a puddle in a storm." &c &c.

But to conclude the subject of this species of *jealousy*, with as much seriousness as it seems to deserve; it may be remarked, that the passion is generally founded on the tales and hints of servants, the surmises of tale-bearing gossips, and the malignant innuendoes of those who delight in the diffusion of slander and defamation. There is a class of people in all societies, who are seriously afflicted with a disease called by physicians "*cacoethes loquendi*." It is a disease that is generated between *ignorance, petty malignity* and *restlessness* of *tongue*, which forbids the repose of society; in English, it is the "disease of talking." These people have considerable powers of invention; but from their ignorance of the common topics of enlightened and manly conversation, they seem to be absolutely compelled to *lie their way into notice!* The education of these people, commences at an early period of life. When very young, just perhaps able to go on an errand to a neighboring house, they are immediately asked on their return home, as to every thing they saw or heard there: their answers are such as might he expected, a mixture of truths and lies. Finding at length, that their parents are interested in such tales—they commence with telling *fibs*,—and end, *confirmed* and *malignant liars!* Parents, this is especially addressed to you: it is worthy of your most serious consideration.

But there is a species of *jealousy* of a most malignant and terrible character, such as that delineated by Shakespear in his Moore of Venice, which sometimes takes possession of the human bosom, and shakes the threne of reason to its very centre. This *passion*, or rather this *insanity*, seems to me to be founded on almost speechless and unbounded *love;* a love bordering on absolute veneration and idolatry. This is an abstruse and intricate subject, and I freely confess that I approach it with unfeigned diffidence.

There certainly does exist, in the very nature of man, certain strong *sympathies* and *antipathies*, for which he is absolutely unable to account on reasoning principles: and which, therefore, must be referred to the *native inspirations of human instinct*. These sympathies and antipathies are every where to be found; nor do I believe there exists, on earth, one single individual, male or female, arrived at mature age, who has not strongly felt the influences of these *instinctive*, I will not say *unerring principles*. They are discoverable in our choices of dogs, of horses, of farms; in fact, they are discoverable in all cases, where the biasses of self interest and ambition have no voice: and where nature herself rules the empire of election. Doctor Fell once asked Dean Swift, what was the reason, after all the advances he had made to conciliate his friendship, that he could not gain him over; and received the following reply, which speaks a volumn on the subject.

"I do not like you Doctor Fell,
The reason why I cannot tell,
I do not like you Doctor Fell."

These attractive and repulsive principles have been felt by every individual; and the probability is, that their influence is *stronger* or *weaker*, in proportion to the warmth or coldness of the human temperament: for I hold it to be impossible, that so *sensative* a being as man, can ever behold an object possessed of any strength of character, and feel perfectly *indifferent* respecting it. If these sentiments of attraction or disgust, existed only in cases where the character of the object portended *benefit* or *injury* to the beholder, the matter might easily be explained, upon the rational principle of *self-interest* on the one hand, or of *self-preservation* on the other. Such however is not the fact; every man knows, from his own experience, that the first view of an object is pleasing or displeasing, attractive or repulsive; and in fact, an object of *attachment* or *disgust* in some degree, without the least relation to the sentiments of self-interest or self-preservation.—How much stronger, then, must be our feelings of attachment or disgust for an object, when we know or believe that the character of that object is to determine, under certain circumstances, happiness or misery of our whole lives!' Parents and guardians of the destinies of youth, if you can for one moment suspend the delusions which fascinate you, respecting wealth and aggrandizement, I wish you to remember:—that the closer in contact you bring those who have no natural affinity for each other, the *greater* and *more distant will be the rebound!* Have you never experienced an emotion of loathing and disgust, merely by being in the presence of an object, whose native and unalterable character was repugnant to yours? In other words, have you never experienced a *moral nausea* of all the sensibilities of your nature, by being compelled to an association with a being whose feelings, whose sensibilities, whose very modes of thinking, spoke a language abhorrent to your souls! If you have, you can form some idea of the irresistible repulsions, which sometimes influence the conduct of persons in the married state; freeze the few and cold affections which habits of enforced associations may have produced; and which seldom fail, sooner or later,—either to make them unfaithful to each other, or to seperate them forever. This is not a thread bare dream of the imagination, a mere chimera of the fancy; the affections of mankind are absolutely beyond their control. How often have you seen instances in which the purest and strongest sentiments of parental duty, and all the efforts of reason herself, have been unable to overcome a repugnance to the marriage bond. Was this apparent contumaciousness, the offspring of wilful disobedience, and a fixed design to thwart your intentions of bestowing connubial happiness on your child? no:—it was the struggle of nature herself in deep distress: it was the last effort she could make, to prevent the violation of one of the most sacred of her laws!

Seeing then, as I think has been clearly demonstrated, that human affections are not under our control, at least so far as to be influenced by sentiments of duty, or admonitions of reason, are we not to presume, from the great variety of motives which influence many to enter the marriage bond, that thousands are badly paired and worse matched? I think so; and those who doubt the fact, for their own satisfactory conviction of error, will do well to investigate the real causes, of so much domestic discontent as is every where to be found; of so many quarrels and connubial bickerings, and finally, of so many *divorçes*. I assert it to be the fact; and it will be supported by the experience of thousands, that wedlock is a perfect hell, and the worst one we know of on earth, even when surrounded by all the splendors of wealth and trappings of power, if it is not hallowed by human affections––and I assert further, and am in no way apprehensive of *experimental contradiction* that where wedlock is consecrated by fixed and virtuous love, it is and must be a source of high enjoyment, even surrounded by the hardships, privations and daily sufferings of labor and drudgery. I have often been surprised, on going into some of our cabins on the frontiers; there was the meat hanging in the chimney; the bread-tray on the only table; the straw-bed on a rude frame; the blankets and counterpanes about the floor, from which perhaps a dozen or less of healthy, ruddy children had just risen; there was the corn in the crib, the cow standing with her head in at the door, and the meal-bag under the bed. Great God, I have said to myself, is it possible that weded love can exist in such a place as this! But I was soon undeceived; the whole enigma was solved satisfactorily; it had been a marriage of pure and virtuous love untrammeled by the calculations of avarice, the meanness of false pride, and the groveling aspirations of petty ambition.

On the other hand, I have frequented the mansions of the great, the wealthy and the powerful; where surrounded by luxury and wealth, and reclined at ease on a gilded sopha, love might have held a court superior in splendor and magnificence, to that said to have been held in the fabled mansions of Jove! What did I see? I saw discontent, suspicion and prying distrust, lowering in every eye. I saw that the hearts of the inhabitants of these splendid mansions were estranged from each other. I saw the servants in varied liveries, gliding in solemn silence from room to room; nor did one sound of cheerfulness or festivity, break the dull monotony of this splendid solitude, this gilded, carpeted, and festooned hell of *wedded misery!* I saw the owners of all this wealth and waste of luxury, take their solitary meal; for nature had denied them offspring, in revenge for a violation of her laws. They approached the festive board, which was loaded with luxuries of every climate, with eyes averted from each other. No social converse; no interchange of thought or sentiment, enlivened the cold and hollow splendor of the scene. The servants in attendance helped them; even the common forms of superficial politeness were unobserved; nor did they recognize the presence of each other, unless in stolen and hateful glances. They seemed to sit on thorns; and no sooner was their miserable repast ended, than the one betook himself to the *gaming table* and probably the other to her *paramour.*

These two delineations of life, are not mere visions of the fancy; they are to be met with in every country. They prove conclusively, that marriages contracted from improper motives, are always followed by consequences destructive to human happiness, and the best interests of mankind. All the conflicts, discontents and jealousies of the married state, may be traced to improper motives for marriage or improper conduct after it. Perhaps there is one exception which I shall name. The husband sometimes becomes jealous of the wife, and the wife of the husband, where there is no infidelity on either side, from the mere *consciousness of being unworthy of an attachment.* Cases of this character frequently occur; and it may generally, if not in every instance, be laid down as a fixed and settled principle in human nature that where there is no positive demonstration of *connubial delinquency*, the party disposed to suspicion & jealousy, derives these surmises of deviation, from the simple fact of a consciousness of being *too depraved to be an object of love!* I am aware that this is a severe, and degrading sentence, against those who entertain causeless suspicions: but the opinion is not less true than severe. The following is the routine of reasoning, usually observed by a man about becoming jealous of his wife. "This woman arrests much of the public attention. She is every where well spoken of. In all public assemblies where I am considered a mere shadow, she commands the most unbounded respect, and I view every compliment paid to *her* beauty and accomplishments, as an indirect satire on *myself.* I am undoubtedly her inferior in every thing; and partienlarly in sensibility and intelligence. I am conscious of my own meanness and depravity; she possesses too much perspicacity and penetration, not to have discovered my real character—*and cannot love me.*—I saw her bowed to in the street; she returned the compliment with a smile. Yesterday from my neglect and inattention, a gentleman of fine appearance and commanding manners and address, handed her to her carriage; she thanked him for his polite attentions—*by h——n she never did love me!* At Mrs. Fidget's ball the other night, she attracted general attention; her chair was continually surrounded by gentlemen of figure, compared with whom I felt myself a mere cipher; a gentleman bowed politely to her in passing:—angels and ministers defend me! It was the gentleman who handed her into her carriage—and I am no more thought of—I am a lost man forever." A man of *fancied miseries* and *imaginary cuckoldom,* behold your portrait! This is the light in which the world beholds you.

Having now in some measure accounted for the passion of jealousy, which is unfortunately too prevalent in this country, I will conclude the subject by some general remarks.

The marriage compact is entered into for two purposes. 1st. The happiness of the parties themselves;—2d. The rearing and educating properly, the offspring of the marriage contract. The principle of a genuine attachment, such as ought always to be found in wedded life, can never exist in any degree of perfection, unless there is a natural affinity between the parties—in temper, disposition, passions, tastes, habits and persuits of mind. When this congeniality is absolutely and entirely wanting, the parties will gradually and almost imperceptibly become estranged from each other, and finally experience the influence of indifference, and more probably of settled and confirmed hatred. In this event, if our laws would sanction the practice, and if there were no offspring to provide for, it would be much more consonant with justice and expediency, that the parties could separate and elsewhere form new and more agreeable engagements. It certainly is worse than useless, to compel persons to associate together, and that too in the most close and intimate manner, when they are mutually actuated in relation to each other, by sentiments of hatred and contempt. According to the present state of things, in relation to divorcement, the person wishing a releasment from the marriage bond, must first become *publicly* and *notoriously infamous;* or resort, as has been proved by the several late executions of malefactors, to the dreadful alternative of *murder*. What a terrible lesson do these late executions hold out to society, on the subject of marriage, and the absolute necessity of its being based on genuine love.

Many persons marry who only fancy themselves in love! A little master or miss, who would have been well employed in reading the fables in the spelling-book, gets hold of the "Sorrows of Werter," or Rosseau's "Eloisa"—or Pethrarch's "Laura," or some other work of the same character, in which unfortunate love is delineated in the colors of the rainbow, and leads its unfortunate and most melancholy victims of *whordom* and *suicide!* With a head full of such trash, and a heart as tender and susceptible, as a beef-steak, that has been well beaten for the gridiron, nothing will do the little gentleman or lady, but the very fact of falling in love; and that too, with the very first object w' ich presents itself. Papa and mamma are cruel; they will not assent to the match and the event is probably an elopement. Then comes the appalling discovery that the lady is not quite a goddes, nor the gentleman entirely a demigod; then comes the discovery; that they are badly paired, and infinitely worse matched; the gentleman becomes tired of the lady, and the lady of the gentleman; and finally their papas and mammas have to take them home and support them. I have known many instances of this kind, which clearly proves, in addition to what I have noticed above, that marriages ought to be predicated on natural congeniality of character, and as far as possible, sanctioned by the exercise of reason and reflective power.

I have mentioned the rearing and education of offspring, as duties annexed to the married state. How can such elevated and responsible duties, be performed by persons who are disqualified even from regulating their own conduct, so as to set a correct moral example? I am very willing to admit that teachers of much ability are every where to be found; but no influence can possibly act on the infant and youthful mind, in the formation of future character, with half the force, depth and durability of impression, as that derived from the precepts and example of parents: and I presume it will be admitted, that those who are destitute of the capacity to make a judicious selection of partners for life, are scarcely capable of forming the infant mind. The wives of the Greeks and Romans and their domestic regulations, were truly the nurses and nurseries of those two great races of statesmen and heroes. The best biographers of Washington, whose moral, political and military life, presents the noblest portrait of man to be found on the records of time, ascribe much of the purity, elevation and patriotism of his character, to the sound judgment and intellectual energies of his mother.—The influence which the manners, example and precepts of a mother, exercises over the intellectual dawnings of the youthful mind and passions, can scarcely be appreciated by men of the most acute and profound observation; a proof of which, in addition to the million of others which might be adduced, may be inferred from the remarks made by the illustrious and greatly unfortunate captive of St. Helena, on the moral and intellectual qualifications of his mother.

The truth is, and I mention it with no ordinary sentiments of regret, that the education of females in the United States, is not only viewed in too unimportant and contemptible a ligth, but that it is absolutely disgraceful to *the spirit of our institutions* and *the real genius of the people.*

LOVE.

This is one of the master passions of the human soul, and when experienced in the plenitude of its power, its devotions embrace with despotic energy and uncontrolled dominion, all the complicated and powerful faculties of man. It was implanted in the human bosom, for the noblest and most beneficent of purposes, and when restricted to its legitimate object, and restrained within due bounds by moral sentiment, may be called the great fountain of human happines. No passion incidental to humanity embraces so vast a space, and such an infinite multiplicity of objects:—it commences in the cradle with tender emotions of filial attachment and veneration for our parents; it animates and accompanies us through all the chequered vicissitudes of life, attaching itself to every object which can afford us enjoyment and happiness, and finally, in accompaning us to the last resort of the living, it concentrates all its pure and sublime energies at the great *fountain of existence,* the throne of the LIVING GOD.

Like all other elementary principles of human nature, its *essence* baffles the keenest researches of philosophy and science; and its *existence* can only be recognized by a *consciousness* of its presence, and the effects which are manifested in every department of life, by multiplied exhibitions of its energies. It attaches the infant to its parent, and the domicile of its earliest days of helplessness and dependence; it attaches the youth to the objects of his playful years, to the companions of his innocent and festive mirth, and to the first objects of his youthful fancy, Without its animating influence, as concentrated on objects of *true glory,* the hero would degenerate into a poltroon, the statesman into a political driveller, and the patriot into a mere citizen of the world, without friends—without home—and without those endearing and sacred ties, which bind us to our native land! The beneficent and heavenly aspirations of love, are every where to be found; they bind the solitary and warlike savage to his native forest; the Moor, the Arab and

C*

the Negro, to the burning plains of the torrid zone; the Russian, the Swede, the Norwegian and the Laplander to the snows and glaciers of the polar regions; and the courtly and civilized European and American, to the refinements and comforts of the more temperate regions of the globe. Without local, relative and personal attachments, man would be eternally discontented with his condition; he would become, like Cain, a fugitive and a vagabond upon the face of the globe; in fact, the deep foundations of domestic and national society would soon be broken up, and scattered to the winds of heaven, were it not for the strong attachments of man for the objects among which he is placed.

If you require proofs of the truth of this universal doctrine of love, ask the parent what price would induce him to part with his children; ask the husband of a woman of elevated and noble character, what sum in gold or jewels he would consider equivalent to her value; ask the savage what would induce him to abandon the dangers of the chase, and the deep and silent solitudes of nature, and to reside in your crowded cities, amidst the hum of business and the confusion of assembled multitudes. Ask the Samoiede and Laplander, what would induce them to exchange the fogs and snows of the north, for the mild and balmy temperature of countries presenting eternal spring and unfading verdure! They will tell you that they love their parents, their children, their friends, their country. Man, unlike the inferior animals of creation, is indeed the citizen of every climate; and, his capacities of forming local and relative attachments, are as varied and extensive as the powers by which he overcomes difficulties, and forces nature to yield him the comforts; conveniencies and positive enjoyments of existence.

Philanthropy, or love of our species, is founded on favorable perceptions of the purity, the beneficence, the elevation and the true dignity of the human character; nor did ever an individual, of any age or country, become a confirmed misanthrope but from contrary perceptions of human nature. A man who is naturally a hater of his species, without having had his character soured by the deceptions, frauds, and oppressions of mankind, is by nature cowardly, timid and selfish. Nothing great, patriotic, or disinterested, can be expected from such a man; he is cruel, vindictive, avaricious, fraudulent and roguish in the extreme; he only seems to have been placed among mankind as a sort of *standard of meanness and demerit*, by which we are enabled to measure and duly appreciate the *elevation of character* and *dignified virtues* of other men. There are various degrees of misanthropy, in a descending scale from that which characterised the mind and feelings of "Timon of Athens"—downward to the mean, sordid and exclusive *self-love*, which manifests itself in taking all possible advantages of mankind, for the hoarding and accumulation of ill-gotten wealth. These pigmy misanthropes, or haters of mankind on a petty scale, are every where to be found. They are the scoundrels who, in all societies, cheat and swindle on every occasion; they are the men who will sacrifice, or in other words, purchase at half its value, on an execution sale, the little property of the needy and who would not scruple to rob the widow and the orphan of the little that sickness and misfortune had spared them. You will see these swindling vagabonds, adding hypocricy to their petty villanies, by making an absolute mockery of religion itself, at the communion table. That insatiable avarice is a disease of the mind, there can be no doubt, and that this disease requires a moral treatment of cure, there can be as little question. If these men would reflect on the brevity of human life; if they would consider that their ill-acquired wealth must soon pass from their possession, and that death will unload them at the gates of eternity, surely they would soon discover the folly, impolicy and heuious immorality of such a course.

The passion of love, properly so called, or that strong and indissoluble attachment which frequently exists between the two sexes, is one of the noblest and most powerful emotions that ever animated the human bosom. As I remarked before, under the head of jealousy, this pure and elevated attachment, is the great solacer of human life; the harbinger of successful procreative power; the precursor and nurterer of successive millions of the human race; the great moral parent of all the numerous races of men to be found in every climate of the globe. It is the native of every country that has been invaded by the enterprize of man, and is found to bloom and flourish in perfection wherever man has fixed his habitation. It finds a congenial soil in the booth of the hunter, the hut of the savage, the tent of the wandering Arab, the leafy bower of the African of the Gambia, as well as in the haunts of civilization, and the palaces of kings.

As I have remarked under another head, there exists in the human bosom, certain *instinctive sympathies* and *antipathies*, which we are unable to control, either by the force of moral sentiment or the efforts of reason; and which are absolutely inexplicable by all the boasted powers of human genius. The existence of these instinctive principles, are only known by our own consciousness, and the powerful and decisive effects they are known to produce. No two human beings, especially of different sexes, and more especially if their affections were engaged by previons prepossessions, were ever yet in the presence of each other for any length of time, without experiencing the force, in a greater or less degree, of the sympathy or antipathy before noticed. When the attraction is mutally strong, the parties soon become conscious of a congeniality of temper, disposition, tastes, and sensibilities; this sympathetic attraction has by some writers on the subject, been denominated "*love at first sight*." When on the other hand, the physical, moral, and intellectual characters of the parties, are essentially and radically different from each other: in other words, and in more fashionable phraseology, when the natural character of the parties are the antipodes, or direct opposites of each other, the repulsive powers of natural antipathy are so strongly experienced, as to produce involuntary hatred, if not fixed and unalterable sentiments of contempt and detestation. I am thus particular in giving my opinions on these subjects, not only because I know that their correctness will be sanctioned by the actual experience of thousands, but because I trust they will be of service to many, in disclosing the extreme danger to human happiness, which invariably arises from uniting those to each other, by merely artificial and fictitious ties, whom God and nature have put assunder. By opposition of native character, I mean a plain and palpable dissimilitude of tempearaments, tastes, and intellectual and moral persuits. Can physical and moral beauty, be in love with physical deformity, and moral depravity of character? Can wisdom and intelligence be in love with folly and stupidity? Innocence and spotless purity, with guilt and corruption? Virtue with vice? No!

"Vice is a monster, of such frightful mien,
That to be hated, needs but to be seen."

I am willing to admit and believe it to be strictly true, that persons who are characterized by vice, corruption, guilt, stupidity, folly, moral depravity or personal deformity, may form strong attachments to persons of diametrically opposite characters:—this would but be admitting what every person knows; that vice and imperfection, under all their various forms and characters, if endowed with the common faculties of perception, must and always will pay involuntary tributes of respect, veneration, and such *love* as they are capable of experiencing, to virtue and moral purity wherever found. The love of the depraved and immoral portion of mankind, is precisely such as may always be expected from such characters: it is selfish, base and ignoble; utterly devoid of tenderness and consideration for the object beloved--it is precisely such love as the *wolf bears* for the *lamb;* or the *fox* for the *hen-roost!* It has always been a matter of much astonishment to me, that females of refined sensibilty, lofty sentiments of moral virtue, and high orders of intellectual power, should expect a reciprocation of pure and virtuous love, from the scum and dregs of society, the offscourings of brothels, and the hoary and depraved veterans of the gaming table! They might as well, I think, and with much better hopes of success, attempt to extract candor from confirmed hypocrites, honor from thieves, and humanity from highway robbers. There is no way of solving this enigma, that I know of, but by supposing that women of virtue and honor are incapable of distinguishing the *particular claims* which these gentlemen have to their *detestation* and *contempt*: or by presuming that they always, by the aid of their imaginations, invest the characters of such men with fictitious virtues, which have no existence: for I cannot suppose they can truly love them, and yet be fully acquainted with their intrinsic characters. The strength and quality of an attachment, must certainly depend, in a great measure, on the physical and moral qualities of the object beloved, and on the capacities of a lover to perceive and appreciate those qualities. I am perfectly convinced, and that too from experience, that a woman of moral purity of character, never excites the same impure sentiments and base passions, that are produced or excited by a female of a contrary character, and whose countenance and deportment betray indications of immoral habits and loose desires. There is something of immaculate purity; something of the very divinity of virtue, in the countenance and deportment of a woman of chaste desires, elevated moral sentiments, and cultivated intellectual powers, that represses the low-born suggestions of lust and depravity, and awes all the vicious passions, into cowardly submission to the dignity of female perfection. No man, however vicious and depraved in his habits and persuits ever yet had the impudence and audacity to contemplate the deliberate seduction of an accomplished and beautiful woman, unless he were under the influence of a species of *libidinous insanity;* had formed a contemptible opinion of the female character; or had discovered some vulnerable part in her armour of chastity and virtue.

Few women, and I mention the fact with much regret, are proof against the thrilling suggestions of *vanity*, the allurements of flattery, and the fascinations attendant on a passion for general admiration; they ought early to be taught by their parents and preceptors that *true pride*, which is in reality dignity of character, is always hostile to the foolish and dangerous suggestions of vanity; that *flattery*, called by an old and quaint writer, "*the oil of fool*," is a positive and direct insult; and that a female passion for universal admiration, especially in the married state, is hostile to domestic peace and absolutely at war with connubial enjoyment and happiness.

That flattery is an insult, is evident from the fact that no flatterer ever yet ventured upon the practice of his art, without first concluding that the object of his addresses was a fool; the truth is, that flattery is always addressed to our personal vanity, which in plain language means, a strong propensity to an over estimate of our own merits and perfections. Manly and dignified pride, has always been found a specific against the frivolous passion of vanity, and hence it has been frequently said, that a man or woman may be too proud to be vain: the fact is, that vanity is the false and empty pride of fools! Napoleon intended much when he expressed himself thus to some of his friends—"I had hoped and expected that the French were a proud nation; but I have found by experience that they are only vain." The passion for universal admiration is the distinguishing and strong characteristic of a *coquett;* it is the offspring of personal vanity, begotten upon coldness of temperament, ignorance and folly.—A coquett in the female world, is what a coxcomb is among men; a being void of sentiment, sensibility. and intelligence, and utterly incapable of genuine love.

The marriages of both coquetts and coxcombs, in conformity with the coldness and shallowness of their characters, are always predicated on other principles than those of attachment to the object. They are absolutely incapable of feeling the soft refinements, the elevated sentiments, or the deep-toned energies of real love: these people are never in danger of suffering the tortures of a *broken heart*, nor can they experience either much happiness or any considerable degree of misery in the married state. The love of general admiration is their master passion; and whenever this is the case, it is impossible that a *concentration of affections* can take place, and be *exclusively directed to a single object*; fire can never be produced from the separated and scattered sunbeams; they must be concentrated by a convex glass, called a lens, before they can be rendered sufficiently intense to produce warmth, heat and combustion. The love of general admiration, was wisely implanted in the human bosom, and for the best of purposes; but wherever it gains the full possession of the female breast, it freezes all the domestic and conjugal affections, and sometimes leads to jealousy and discontent, with all their dreadful train of consequences;—in other words, and I wish the sentiment to make a well-merited and indeliable impression, the married man who can prefer the admiration of other women to that of the wife of his bosom, is a traitor to all the hallowed solemnities of the marriage compact, and a cold and calculating violator of the laws of God! Nor on the other hand, is the married woman less a traitress to connubial love, to the honor and happiness of her husband and family, and to the best interests of society and domestic enjoyment, who can prefer the shallow and superficial admiration of fools and coxcombs, to the deep and devoted attachments of a husband, who would not scruple to make a sacrifice of life itself to ensure her happiness,—

"Woman alone was formed to bless
The life of man, and share his care:
To sooth his breast, when keen distress
Hath lodged a poisoned arrow there."—

I have mentioned that person's of diametrically opposite physical, moral and intellectual characters, could never assimilate with and become strongly attached to each other, notwithstanding the powerful attractions of the sexual instinct. By *opposite* natural and acquired characters. I do not mean mere *contrasts* of mental, and corporeal disposition and characteristics. I cannot otherwise disclose my precise meaning, respecting things which are direct *opposites*, and those which are only *contrasts* of each other; than by citing the example or colors. Black and white, for instance, are the *opposites* of each other, and when placed in juxtaposition always pain the eye; but, either of those colors, when compared with any other of the primitive colors or even shades, are only considered *contrasts.* St. Pierre in his studies of nature, has been explicit on this ingenious and novel subject, which is certainly worthy of much consideration. There seems to exist, between persons of opposite physical characters, a decided indifference as regards sexual communication; or if not a decided and entire indifference, there certainly does not obtain between them, that arduous and passionate sexual propensity, which is found between persons who are the contrasts of each other. I have remarked in innumerable instances the strong attachments which existed between persons of contrasted complexions, constrasted colors of the eyes and hair, and especially of strongly contrasted stature and dimensions; and I have no doubt, that the reader of this new, if not very interesting part of my reflections, will recollect very many instances, of the existence of marriages voluntarily entered into from the strongest of possible attachments, between persons who in point of stature and size, were perfect contrasts of each other. Ask a tall, robust and athletic man, what sort of a wife he would choose; and you will very soon ascertain, that his choice would fall on a female, the contrasted reverse of himself. In fact, you will always find on inquiry, that a lean man prefers a woman of size and rather large proportions—a short man, a woman of lofty stature—and so on, to the end of the chapter of contrasts in personal character. The gigantic and brawny Roman warrior, Mark Anthony, fell in love with the sylph-like and fairy form of Cleopatra the celebrated queen of Egypt, who was remarkable for being or very diminutive proportions, though very beautiful; in fact, thousands of such instances might be cited to from both ancient and modern history. This contrast of physical proportions and character, united in the marriage bond, seems to have been intended by **PROVIDENCE**, to equalize the breed of mankind, and to prevent them on the one hand, from running up into a race of *giants*, and on the other, from degenerating into a strain of diminutive and contemptible *pigmies*.

But on the subject of contrasts, this is not all: contrasts

in moral and intellectual qualities, seem to be equally favorable to love; and here again I am compelled to resort to figurative language to convey my meaning. There are concords and discords in music: perfect concords always fall on the ear with a dull and cold monotony; whilst perfect discords always grate harshly on the auditory nerves, producing exquisite sensations which are still more unharmonious and disagreeable. It will not be necessary to say much on this subject of moral and mental contrasts; I only suggest it, that the reader may make his own observations, respecting this singular anomaly in the human character. We know perfectly well, that persons of moderate intellectual powers, both male and female, provided their tempers and dispositions be gentle and amiable, are invariably the objects of love and the most tender regard, with those who possess uncommonly lofty and powerful characteristics of genius and intellect. This fact is even so notorious in all societies, as to have become a proverb; and, how often have we all seen instances in conjugal life, in which fortitude has been united to despondency—fickleness and inconsistency of resolution, with the most unshaken, and resolute tenaciousness of purpose—timidity, with consumate bravery, and the highest order of moral courage, with the shrinking cowardice of superstition and childish ignorance. We know these to be the facts, and can only account for it on the great scale of *divine wisdom* and *Providence*, by presuming them to be intended for equalizing the human species in wisdom and moral energy—and for forming additional and indissoluble bonds in the social compacts of mankind.

I have several times mentioned, and I think demonstrated, as far as the force of facts and moral reasoning will go, that the passion of love is measureably involuntary, and beyond the control of moral sentiment and reason; nor can there I think exist any doubt, not only that the *strength* of the passion depends on the peculiar temperaments of individuals, but that the *distinctive characteristics* of the passion or emotion called love, are essentially connected with the physical, moral and intellectual qualifications of the objects or persons beloved. If, then, the strength of the passion is in any proportion to the natural temperaments of individuals; and if its peculiar qualities or characteristics depend on the natural and acquired qualifications of the objects of attachment, how ridiculous, absurd and perfectly *irrational* it must be for any man or woman to expect, that he or she can possibly be an object of attachment, with any person of rational and scrutinizing mind, on account of qualifications which are not possessed, and which in fact are known and perceived to be entirely wanting. I mention the subject in this way, and place it in this light, in order to prevent the exercise of *hypocrisy* between the sexes, which is always dangerous in its consequences—and in order, also, that those whose happiness in life depends on their being objects of esteem, friendship, veneration, *attachment* and *love*, may see the absolute necessity of deserving the homage of such refined and virtuous sentiments; in other words, that they may be deeply impressed with the important and eternal truth, that candor, honor, and moral virtue, are the great passports to human happiness. I have often witnessed the tremulous solicitude of females, of the most amiable and exalted qualities of person and mind, respecting the public opinion of their merits and character, and frequently been interrogated by them on the subject. In these cases, I have uniformly answered, in the words of an old Grecian sage, "know yourself;" and your opinions of yourself, if correct and well founded, will be precisely such as are entertained for you, by those whose esteem and approbation are of any importance. Genuine and rational love, commences in the natural, and if I may be allowed the expression, as applicable to human nature, the instinctive sympathies of individuals for the society of each other; it is cemented and powerfully strengthened by the endearments of sexual enjoyment, of which I have before spoken; and it is crowned with both temporal and immortal duration, by the mild purity and unfading lustre of the moral virtues, and the imposing splendors of genius and intellectual power. As I said before it is confined to no particular climate, and to no exclusive region of the globe; its benign influence is experienced, as well among the polar snows of the North, as in the mild climates of the temperate zones. It is the exclusive guest of no particular rank in life: the rich, the poor, the exalted, the base, the brave are alike participant in its genial warmth, and heavenly influence. In the words of Lawrence Stern, "no tint of words can spot its snowy mantle, nor chemic power turn its sceptre into iron; with *love* to smile upon him as he eats his crust, the swain is happier than the monarch, from whose court it has been exiled by vice and immorality." This is that undebased and genuine love, which is founded in unlimited confidence, mutual esteem, and the mild sublimities of virtue and integrity of character. It illuminates the countenance with the sparkling brilliancy of soft desire; and is in fact, the safeguard of female virtue, and of chastity itselt whenever assailed by unprincipled and seductive fascination.

With respect to the passion of love, there is a common error of female education, which will also apply to the early instruction of males, of which I must speak in *plain terms* in the conclusion of this subject. Every human being, at a very early period of life, from peculiar modes of instruction, and the examples presented to the mind, form some idea of the qualifications which constitute *human excellence.* If for instance, at an early period, the parents and instructors of a female, impress upon her mind, that the mere decoration of the persou will render her an object of *tender regard,* without the cultivation of her moral and intellectual qualities, the result will be, and it cannot be avoided, that aiming at what she believes to be the great excellence of the human female character, both her moral and intellectual energies will retrograde into barrenness and insipidity: in other words, she will become what the world denominates a *pretty woman,* the idle of fools and coxcombs, but an object of compassion, indifference or contempt with men of lofty sentiments and distinguished characters. Peter, the great of Russia, on account of her superior intellectual endowments chose for a wife, and made her Empress of Russia, a woman of obscure and lowly origin. And in more modern times, I had the information from a person well acquainted with the facts, we find the spirit, discrimination and sound judgment of Peter the great, respecting the value of a woman of a cultivated mind, revived in the person and character of Lord Morgan. Sidney Owenson, his present wife, was the daughter of a Comedian on the Dublin stage. At an early period, this youthful female discovered strong traits of genius of a literary character, and Owenson though in impoverished circumstances, determined to educate his daughter. He did so; in consequence of which, she became an object of strong attachment with a man of distinguished mind, who preferred her to the titled and the rich, and she is now lady Morgan.

Mrs. Hamilton, a lady of some celebrity, who has written much on female education, makes the following remark on women: "where there is no intellect, there is no moral principle; and where there is no principle, there is no security for female virtue." This is the truth, but not the whole truth: had Mrs hamilton recognized religion as an essential requisite in preserving the moral virtues of women, she would probably have said all that was necessary on female education. The accomplishments of women, ought always to have some relation to their future duties in life; but it is evident, that the cultivation of their minds, cannot with justice to themselves and society be dispensed with, no matter what may be their future destinies. A cultivated mind is a never-failing passport to the best society; it always insures the extension of friendship and civility, when accompanied by correctness of conduct and a virtuous deportment: it prevents women from becoming the dupes of artifice, and the victims of seduction; it expands the heart to all the principles of sympathetic feeling for the distresses of others, and induces a commiseration for the misfortunes of mankind; it holds up to a distinct scrutinizing examination, the real characters of men, and enables a woman to make a judicious selection of worth, from a herd of coxcombs and fools, by which, if wealthy and distinguished by personal beauty, she may be *persecuted with addresses.* It fits her for the superintendence and regulation of a family, and enables her to make correct educational impressions on the minds of her offspring.

The want of mental culture, among fema'es of all ranks in life, has frequently lead to disastrous consequences. By mental culture, I do not mean those shallow and frivolous accomplishments which are sometimes taught at boarding schools; nor do I mean by a refinement of the female mind, a proficiency in drawing roses which resemble a copper coin, in thruming a waltz on the piano, or figeting through the lacivious gesticulations of an Italian or French fandango! I mean by mental culture, the acquisition of solid accomplishments; those which can be rendered useful to domestic policy; be an example to society in the correction of its morals, and reflect honor on the national character. Such an education always represses the waywardness of the fancy, and lops away the useless and often dangerous exuberance of a powerful imagination; it affords a never failing resource of comfort in solitude, and finds a healing balm for the wounds for a wayward and unfortunate destiny. In fine, no woman possessed of a judicious education, even under the pressure of the most trying misfortunes, ever yet lost the just equipoise between her strength and sensibility, or became the victim of a *broken heart!*

The exquisite miseries which spring from disappointed love, and sometimes terminate in a broken heart, for I am well persuaded there is really such a disease, always arise from visionary creations of the fancy, and disorders of the imagination: in other words, they are the offspring of overstrained and imaginary conceptions of the qualifications of the object of attachment; they are in fact, the melancholy results of an over-estimate of the virtues and perfections of human nature; of which the woman of a cultivated mind, and really philosophic acquisitions, stands in no possible danger. A woman who cultivates her imagination, by the unlimited perusal of novels and romances, at the expense of the soiid qualities of her understanding, is always in danger of becoming the victim of a wayward fancy; and should she live to have the errors of her imagination corrected by practical experience, will have nothing of the imagination left, but the *ashes of a consumed sensibility*, on which no future attachment can possibly be predicated. A woman of cultivated mind, sees objects as they really are—and not as they are clothed by an inflamed and disordered fancy; she knows that human nature is not perfection itself, and expects nothing from it, but what appertains to the natural character of man; she knows it to be a compound of weakness and strength, virtue and vice, wisdom and folly—and never over-estimating the virtues and perfections of an object of attachment, her desires are chastened by moderation, and her loves by the high-toned philosophy of true wisdom! Such a woman, unlike the melancholy victim of a morbid sensibility, and a high wrought and disordered imagination, is in no danger of sinking into the diseased apathy of disappointed love, and becoming the victim of partial or total insanity, or a disconsolate and broken heart; for which all the mere medical remedies known to human genius and science, are but miserable and inefficient palliatives. Religion, change of scenery, and attractive and interesting company, in some cases have considerable influence, in detaching the mind from the concentration of its reflections on an object of deep and vital love; but, in the more numerous instances, they have all been known to fail, and even to baffle all the efforts of friendship and parental attachment. In fact, it seems to me, and I have paid much attention to the subject, that judicious education, and a well cultivated mind, acting as preventatives to the disorders of the imagination, are almost the only and powerful specifics, against the occurrence of the miseries of disappointed love.

GRIEF.

This depressing affection of the mind, called a *passion*, when experienced in the extreme, sometimes degenerates into confirmed melancholy, despair and fatal insanity. It is the offspring of so many and such various causes, that it is next to impossible to enumerate them. It is sometimes caused by cheerless and gloomy presentiments of the future; sometimes by the heavy pressure of present evils and calamities; and not unfrequently, by strong and vivid recollections of losses which can never be retrieved. Against its inroads and often fatal effects on the health of the physical system, (which are varied according to the temperament and character of the individual,) neither the internal nor external exhibition of medical drugs can have much avail.

The force and effect which grief exercises and produces, in deranging the functions of the physical system, seem in a great degree to depend on the poignancy and accuteness of those sensibilities which characterize the nervous system. Where the nervous system is tremulously sensible, and easily susceptible of external impressions, which is generally the case with persons of distinguished genius, there is invariably found a constitutional melancholy, which delights in retrospections of the past, and serious if not cheerless anticipations of the future. At an early period of life, these persons are highly susceptible of the charms of nature, and also of her more gloomy and sombre scenery; and, being deeply sensible of the influence of what to other men would be *slight impressions*, their feelings always exhibit themselves in the extremes of animation or depression of spirits, for which they themselves are utterly unable to account. In fact it is not unusual to witness in the varying sensibilities of these persons, and that too in the lapse of a single day, the reflective calmness and profundity of the great southern Pacific ocean—the urbanity and cheerfulness attendant on anticipations of future prosperity and happiness—and those storms of ungovernable and unsubdued passions whose undulations resemble the mountain billows of the Atlantic, when lashed by the hurricanes and tarnadoes of the Torrid Zone! This is not only the constitutional temperament of true and unsophisticated genius, of which so much has been said and so little known, but it is also the soil which produces sensations of exquisite happiness and misery; distinguished principles of moral rectitude and depravity of conduct; *great virtues* and *great vices!*

Seriousness, depression of spirits, melancholy, GRIEF,

dispair, insanity, are but the different modifications of the same *passion*, or predisposition of the moral faculties, of whose essence we in reality know nothing abstractedly, only differing in degree of force and effect, in proportion to the strength and weakness of operating causes. For instance; *seriousness* and solemnity of feeling, are always produced in a mind of sensibility and reflection, by the sight of a dead body; of the human limbs lopped away in battle; of the human mind in ruins; and of human misery exhibited to us under any form: in these cases the effects produced are only temporary, and usually pass away with the removal of the objects which excited them. If, however serious and solemn feelings be often reproduced in the mind, by reiterated exhibitions of objects capable of exciting them, their impressions will become more durable, and soon produce a habitual tone of feeling, denominated *depression of spirits*. When this depression of spirits is habitually indulged in for any considerable lapse of time, it is apt to gain so great an aseendency over the *active* and *resolute* powers of the mind, as to dispose the person affected with its influence, to seek in solitud and retirement from society, and indulgence in inactivity, irresolution and gloomy reflections, which, becoming fixed and as it were immovable, settles down into melancholy. Seriousness, depression of spirits, and melancholy, sometimes produce mental derangements; but they are generally of a harmless, unobtrusive, silent and inoffensive character, where the nervous system is tremulous and exceedingly delecate—or where the temperament, if I may be allowed the phraseology, is characterized by weakness, irresolution, and timidity.

Compared with the above affections, which seem at first view to have their seat in the imagination, and by some are denominated hypochondria in men, and hysterics in women, *grief* and *despair* are certainly affections of a more active and powerful character, and much sooner ending in fatuity or mental exhaustion, and outrageous or confirmed insanity.

As I have somewhere mentioned, and the probability is, that the fact will be acknowledged by all well informed physicians, by which I mean those who have discovered how *little* can be *essentially* known on the subject of affections of the mind, the particular and direct influence which these and other strong passions have in deranging the organization of the brain, cannot well be ascertained. All we know about the matter is that we cannot, think with accuracy and profundity of research without a well-organized brain, and that any derangement of that organization and its natural functions, produces co-equal and co-extensive derangements of the intellectual or mental powers. The probability is, that refined, susceptible, and strong organizations of the brain, considered in the aggregate, have much influence in imparting to the mind, those refinements of taste, susceptibilities of feeling, and superior intellectual capacities which we call *genius*, for want of a term which can be more clearly understood. We are perfectly aware, that without a well-organized *eye*, no definite or accurate ideas can be formed of colors—forms—dimensions—distances; that without a well organized and susceptible *ear*, no clear and distinctively correct impressions can be made, by what we call sounds, or vibrations of the air, for want of a more expressive term, on the auditory nerves: that without a well constructed *nasal organ*, vulgarly denominated a nose, no clear and distinct impressions can be made on the olfactory nerves, or nerves of smelling, by the effluvia arising from bodies: that, unless the portions of the nervous system which are incorporated with the *tongue* and its appendages, be unobstructed by malconformation of the organs of taste, no distinctions of flavor could be recognized, between sugar, gall, and vinegar; and, that unless the nerves which are spread over the cutaneous surface of the body, and particularly that of the hands, be perfect both in organization and tone, no adequate or correct ideas could ever be formed of the shape, solidity, &c. of bodies, with which we come in immediate contact. The fact seems to be, and I consider the theoretical conjecture inferior to none which has been published by medical men, that whenever the affections of the mind derange the tone & susceptibility of the senses, these derangements always bring to the sensorium, or focal point of mental impression, incorrect and distorted ideas of external objects, which, as in hypochondria, make us believe in the existence of phantasmagoira of a most childish and superstitious character. This is a species of insanity, connected with unnatural and painful seriousness—habitual depression of spirits—and confirmed melancholy.

On the other hand, when afflictive impressions are made upon the mind, of an unusually active and powerful character, and sufficient to impair and partially destroy the organization itself, as in the cases of intense and poignant grief, or absolute and hopeless depsair, the partial dissolution of the physical structure and organization of the brain, it is not improbable, leads to offensive, mischievous, and terrific insanity, amounting to absolute phrensy, and finally terminating in dissolution. The fact is, and it is well known to physicians, that a dissolution of the organic structure of the frame, if that dissolution take place in any vital organ, particularly the brain or stomach, between which there exists a close and almost identical sympathy, decidedly morbid effects are produced to the whole system, physical—moral—and mental; in fact the BRAIN may be called the *father*, and the STOMACH the *mother* of the system.

I have only as yet spoken of the influence which is produced upon the physical functions and system, by the passion of grief, and other strong affections of the same or a similar character. The same effects as those produced by the passions above enumerated, are sometimes the offspring of other causes, not connected in the first instance with the passions, but which afterwards operate strongly upon them, and assist in destroying the nervous, vital and moral functions and organization of the system. We know perfectly well, for instance, that there are many substances which, when taken into the stomach, affect the passions strongly by irritation and excitement—produce morbid derangements of the physical functions—and not unfrequently, moral and mental alienations. The effect of tincture of cantharides on some of the passions, when taken into the stomach, is perfectly well known; nor do I believe, that if its application to the stomach were long continued, it would ever fail to produce morbid irritations and inflammations, which would terminate in functional derangement, and actual dissolution of organic structure in the brain. The effect which opium produces, where it is used in immoderate quantities, as among the Turks, is well known; and that it not unfrequently ends in derangements of the physical system, and absolute insanity with all its horrours. Nor is the intemperate use of spiritous liquors, used to such excess and in such immoderate quantities in our own country, far behind the use of opium, in producing the same deleterious effects on the brain, through the medium of the stomach. Every man who will tax his recollections, will find his memory furnished with inumerable instances, in which a long train of physical diseases has been followed by derangements of the intellects, which none of the boasted powers of science or medicine could relieve or rectify, merely from the immoderate use, or rather abuse of spiritous liquors. Have we not all witnessed instances in which the abuse of spiritous liquors has produced visceral obstructions of a most deadly character—and mental derangements which have been confirmed and rendered durable to the end of life? How is this fixed and confirmed mental alienation to be accounted for, but upon the presumption that those stimulants, long continued, affect not only the nerves but the organic structure of the brain? Do we not know that a fit of intoxication is a paroxism of mental derangement—and that impressions often reiterated will wear their channels in the brain, injure its unrivalled and delicate organization, and render those effects durable? What are the effects, which immediately follow a fit of excessive intoxication? Are they not the very same as those produced by the influence of the passions of which I have before spoken? Are they not seriousness, depression of spirits, melancholy, *grief* despair, insanity? This is the point at which I intended to arrive, I intended to demonstrate in a plain and simple manner, that disease, insanity and death, are produced as well by *moral* as by *physical* causes; and that a physician ought to ascertain both the state of the *body* and *mind*, if he really intends to effect a cure or removal of the class of diseases just mentioned. I know it to be a common practice with physicians to listen to long details of the physical symptoms of their patients, without the least inquiry as to the moral or mental causes of their diseases; when the fact is, that in five cases out of ten, arising among persons of sedentary—refined—luxurious—studious—and intellectual habits; and among delicate females, in seven cases of diseases out of eleven, particularly, those which are obstructional, the causes will be found seated in the mind and passions. I need not enlarge on this subject; every man possessed of any experience and common sense, must have observed, both on himself and others, the remarkable effects produced on the physical system by the mind and passions; nor can such an individual be ignorant of the facts, that deleterious substances when taken into the stomach, frequently operate with immense power on the passions, as well as on the organic structure of the physical system. The truth is, that although we are well convinced of the intimate connection of the mind and body, and also of the reciprocal influcence they always exercise alternately over each other. no man has ever yet been able fully to develop the mysteries of that connexion, or the natural mediums by, and through which they operate on and influence each other; in other words, all we certainly know respecting the matters under consideration, must be confined to the *effects*, daily and hourly witnessed, in the reciprocal and varied action of the mind and its passions, and the body and its affections, on each other.

When morbid derangements of the system are derived from the action of the mind and passions, the consolations of religion and philosophy are of great importance; because they teach mankind, in a language not to be misunderstood, that cheerless and gloomy presentiments of the future, only unfit us for combating and vanquishing present difficulties: that the heavy pressure of present evils, and calamities which are irremovable, are lightened of half their ponderous and depressing influence, by that masculine fortitude which is derived from the inspirations of wisdom, and that celestial hope of relief which springs from genuine religion: and, that it is the height of human folly and weakness, unavailingly, to mourn over losses which can never be retrieved!

When the causes of our diseases and miseries are connected with physical principles, in some degree under our control, it becomes a moral duty, so far as it be possible, to remove them, and that too by physical means; and, I am decidedly of opinion, generally speaking, and a few individual cases which might be enumerated left out of view, that moral causes of disease and misery, are to be combated by moral means—and, that physical causes of functional derangement, and violations of organic structure derived from such causes, are to be combated and overcome by physical means. I am perfectly willing to admit, that the influences of the imagination, and of the animating passions, are very considerable in preventing disease, and removing obstructions when firmly seated; but I am not willing to allow, that either the imagination or animating passions, can render flexible the coats of an ossified artery, or remove a stone from the bladder! The fact is, that the line of demarkation, where moral causes cease to operate, and where the influence of physical ones commence, is a mystery hitherto too profound and inscrutable for the boldest efforts of human genius. We are well aware, that many malconformations of the human fetus take place previous to birth, such as in cases of hare-lip. external impressions on the skin, &c. But at what period of gestation such malconformations and external impressions cease to be made, it is absolutely impossible to conjecture, with even a probability of truth.

The following case of the powerful effects of imagination, put by Doctor Cypricanus, is recorded in this work, to place pregnant females on their guard, and to exemplify the effects of the imagination on highly susceptible materials. "A female child," says this distinguished man, "was born with a wound in her breast above four inches in length. It penetrated to the *musculi intercostales*, and was an inch broad, and hollow under the flesh round about the wound; besides which, there was a contusion with some swelling. at the lower part of the wound inside. The child came into the world without any violence; and consequently it did not receive the wound in its birth; it was caused by the strength of the imagination: for, about two months before, the mother had by chance, heard a report that a man had murdered his wife, and with his knife had given her a great wound in the breast—at which relation she changed, but not excessively. It is not merely probable but absolutely certain, that the child received the wound in its mother's body, at the very moment she was affrighted; because the wound was very sordid, and the inside as well as the outside beset with slime, proceeding from the water in which the child lies in its mother's womb—besides which, it had every appearance of an *old wound*."

The effects of grief, which is an extremely depressing passion, and its morbid influences on the body or physical system, are very remarkable. It diminishes bodily strength in general, and also the action of the heart in particular. It impedes the circulation of the fluids, stagnates the bile invariably, and occasions induration of the liver; or by throwing the bile into the circulation of the blood, it produces jaundice or dropsy. Grief allso diminishes the perspiration, renders the skin sallow, aggravates the scurvey; and is particularly effective in producing and aggravating putrid fevers; it also disposes persons to being easily affected with fever, arising from excessive irritability, or constipation or costiveness of the bowels. Its effects in changing the color of the hair are well known; and many instances have occurred, in which the hair has been turned from a deep black to gray in a few hours. From grief, blindness—gangrene—and even sudden death, or as it is emphatically called a *broken heart*, have not unfrequently resulted. From the excess of this passion, persons who indulge in melancholy reflections, for any length of time, become peevish and fretful. and so extremely irritable, that their minds find new food for sorrow in every object presented to them. Thus, the whole imagination becomes seriously affected with confirmed melancholy, sometimes producing nervous fevers, or what is still more dreadful, *total insanity*. The remedies usually resorted to with salutary effects, are gentle opiates taken with caution; exercise on horse-back; change of scene; the use of the *swing*, which has in very many instances, produced signally beneficial effects; friction of the body and limbs with flannel or a flesh-brush—this friction ought to be frequently resorted to and continued, to give impetus to the blood, when the extremities become cold; washing the body with strong vinegar, &c.—Mild wines temperately administered, may be given, and should they produce acidity of the stomach and loss of appetite, exercise and other tonics ought to be resorted to—change of climate is often in desperate cases found beneficial, also a diversion of the mind from its original imaginations, and particularly the frequent use of the tepid bath is recommended: and in cases of suppressions of the menstrual discharge occasioned by grief, the tepid bath has invariably been found beneficial. The powerful influence of the mind upon the womb, when affected by grief, can scarcely be computed by the best observers, who generally attribute to merely physical causes, effects which are to be sought for in the mind. But more will be developed on this important subject, as regards female diseases, under another and more appropriate head.

RELIGION.

This passion or affection of the human mind, properly defined and well understood, is *a deeply devotional sentiment of awe, veneration and love, for that inscrutable* BEING *who created the universe in his wisdom; supports it by his almighty power; and regulates the machinery of nature, in beneficence and love to his creatures.*

Considered merely in relation to his vital and animal functions, man seems to occupy the highest point in the scale of animated nature; but notwithstanding this distinguishing elevation, with some grand and distinctive exceptions to the general principles of existence, and those of a strong and decided character, he seems in many respects to be allied to the inferior orders of creation. Like the merely animal orders of nature inferior to himself, he is animated by loves and friendships, hatreds and enmities,—and by all the other passions and propensities, incidental to the merely animal creation. In common with the elephant, the lion, the dog and the fox, his heart seems to be the seat of life or vitality, and his brain the censorium of intellectual existence. Like them, he is furnished with a stomach to digest his food—and a heart to propel the vital fluid through the arterial and venous systems.. Like the inferior orders of creation, man is susceptible of the influence of heat and cold, and all the variations of temperature incidental to the changes of the seasons; like them, he can be deluged by rains, frozen by the snows of winter, and melted by the heats of summer. Like them, he is subjected to physical diseases, which can be mitigated or removed by the same means, and like them, he is animated by strong sentiments of self-preservation, and entertains an instinctive and powerful dread of both pain and dissolution! But here, the parallel between man, and the inferior orders of creation terminates; and he begins to take his departure from their earth born level, which they can never emulate, or even follow.

Man is the only animal in creation, who can raise his contemplations to the Deity, and experience a sublime sentiment of awe and veneration, for the unknown Author of his existence. The only animal in creation, capable of experiencing a strong solicitude for a knowledge of his origin, or who can direct his views and anticipations to a future existence, beyond the boundaries of time! He is the only being absolutely known to himself, who can form a conceptiou of space, which is an abstract idea of *infinity*—of time, which is an abstract conception of *eternity*—or of plastic and creative power, which leads to an abstract, but infinitely inadequate conception of the OMNIPOTENCE OF GOD! Man seems to unite in his moral and intellectual composition, the human extremes of strength and weakness, wisdom and folly. In infancy, or when not associated with his fellow-beings, he is a naked, defenceless, dependent and timid animal, exposed to diseases of every multiplied character—to dangers beyond arithmetical computation—and

E*

to death in all its varied and gigantic forms: yet, with all these incipient weaknesses, and seeming imperfections of his nature, in the plenitude of life and intellectual power, and when associated with his fellow-beings in social compact, he has satisfied his natural wants; rendered himself independent of every thing but his *Creator*; driven from his presence, enslaved to his purposes, or destroyed by the machinery and chemical power of his warlike inventions, all animals hostile to his life and preservation; and compelled the earth, the air, the waters and the woods, to yield him the sustenance, and even luxuries of life, and to furnish him with the means of constructing his habitation. He has done more. By referring his knowledge of particular facts, to the discovery of abstract and general principles, he has measureably unfolded the elements of science, by which he measures the earth, and discloses the laws which regulate the solar system—ascertains the distances and relative positions of the heavenly bodies; and determines the location of his own globe among them:—discloses the component parts of which the substratum of the earth itself is compounded, and by an effort of microscopic vision and profound sagacity, gives you a satisfactory analysis of a physical atom! Nor is this all; from obscure and imperfect original discoveries in nautical science, he has converted the bark canoes of the wandering savage into vehicles of burthen for international commerce, and imposing engines of war; and, instead of the petty barks of the ancients, by which they prosecuted an insignificant traffick along the shores and inlets of the Mediterranean, he has constructed ships of bulk and strength sufficient to master the winds of heaven and the waves of the ocean:—to discover and colonize new continents:—and to make his way in security, through trackless, unknown and almost shoreless oceans, to countries so remote as not even to be found in delineation on the mariners chart! Nor do the greatness of his discoveries, nor the sublime elevations of his character terminate here. The progressive improvements of man in *literature*, from *hieroglyphics*, which are the signs of things, to the use of *letters*, which are the signs or symbols of sounds, afford new and astonishing demonstrations of his powers.—We have proofs before us, if we will advert for a moment to the present state of mankind, of all the progressive stages of improvement through which he has passed, in arriving at his present state of moral and intellectual civilization, and scientific and literary refinements—nor need we recur to the empire of fable, nor the fictions of his early history, to arrive at the truth. A collective view of the present inhabitants of the globe, will furnish ample demonstrations of the following facts. In a state of savage and illiterate nature, *tradition*, as among the Indians of our own forests, afforded the only means of communication, between the present and future races of mankind. But, in proportion as man began to progress in discoveries relating to the arts and sciences; he became disgusted and dissatisfied with the errors and misrepresentations of *oral* tradition. and sought various expedients to perpetuate to his posterity, authentic testimonials of his sagacity, and durable monuments of his intellectual powers. *Hieroglyphics* and *pyramids* were resorted to in some countries, and pillars and public edifices in others; but, knowing all these to be liable to decay, and that their true meaning might be easily misunderstood or forgotten, he was not satisfied with a medium of intelligence, which would revive and perpetuate his knowledge and discoveries to future times until *literature* arose to record in unfading characters; the intelligence, the improvements in science and the fate of past generations. The discovery of, and progressive improvements in letters, have enabled man to trace his species through all anterior ages since the creation; nor would he now, were it not for *literature*, and the *discovery* of the *Art of Printing*, be enabled to profit at this advanced period of the world—by the records of history, and the divine inspirations of religion, virtue and pure morality, which are breathed forth in love and mercy to fallen man, by *holy writ!* It is from this divine and inspired work, that he derives a knowledge of all the attributes of his Creator; of the immortality of his own soul; and of all the duties he owes to God—his fellow-creatures—and himself. The reveries of all the sages & philosophers of antiquity, with the immortal Plato at their head, sink into cold insignificance, when compared with the divine consolations afforded to man, by that pure and unsophisticated religion, which is derived from the word of God; and while speaking of the pure and undefiled religion of Jesus Christ, I will first show what it is not; second—the abuses of its doctrines; third what it really is; and fourth—its benefits and consolations, in health and prosperity, sickness and misfortune.

The virtues and the boasted wisdom of man, purified and improved by the highest efforts of human reason, would be nothing without the support and consolations of the doctrines of the Scripture. The magnificence, splendor and sublimity of the great works of nature, from which alone, without the divine inspirations to be found in the word of God, he is enabled to form but an inadequate and finite conception of the attributes of an *Almighty Creator*, dazzle and confound the feeble efforts of man, in all his attempts to grasp at the divine perfections of his Maker—baffle all the high-toned energies of his reason and intelligence—and throw him to an infinite distance below, even an *imaginary conception* of the Deity. Thus circumstanced—thus surrounded by mysteries, which he cannot explain to himself—feeling a strong and deep-seated natural sentiment of immortality: and yet dreading the cold and silent horrours of the grave—the word of God, and faith in Christ alone, can afford him support and consolation in the hour of death; solve the otherwise inscrutable and sublime mysteries of his own existence; and reveal to him the dreadful enigmas of eternity! In fact, when man surveys with an attentive and philosophic eye, the vast and complicated machinery of the Universe;—when he discovers that all this complicated and boundless machinery is subject to the irresistable influence of laws infinitely beyond his conception:—when he essays to embody his own conceptions, of the attributes of that Being who created, and who rules and governs all:—and in fine, when he makes the feeble attempt, unaided by divine revelation, to identify his hopes of immortality and future happiness with the unchangeable laws of created nature, so vast, so boundless, and so complicated as they must be, he shrinks back upon his own insignificance, and involuntarily asks himself, "am I not a stranger to the eternal laws of my own destiny?—am I not a stranger to this God, the supreme creator of the Universe?—am I not lost in the immensity of his works, and the boundlessness of his power?"

Mere *opinions*, deduced from the boldest efforts of the reasoning faculties of man, never yet produced that *genuine religion* which absorbs his affections, concentrates his love and gratitude on his divine Creator, regulates his moral and intellectual energies for the production of his present and future happiness, and makes him satisfied with his own prospects of futurity. These are the reasons in all probability, why the ancient sages, who hoped for and partially believed in immortality, were unable to satisfy themselves, with rational and conclusive proofs of the future existence of the human soul: these are probably also the reasons, and they are founded in the wisdom and providence of God himself, why the great truths of immortality were veiled, in all ages, anterior to the true gospel dispensation, from the boasted sagacity and reasoning powers of the philosophers, and sages of antiquity:—for, could these men have arrived at any definite and certain conclusions on the future destinies of the human race, without the moral *purifications of true cristianity*, the consequences would have been dreadful to society and mankind, as can be easily demonstrated.

Suppose a man were enabled by the *unaided* efforts of reason, to demonstrate conclusively to himself, that anihilation, or an absolute and entire negation of existence, was his future and irrevocable doom:—what would be the immediate consequences of this appalling and dreadful discovery! Would he not feel that every affection of his soul was dissoived; and that existence itself was valueless? Would it not loosen every strong tie he feels on life—and sicken him with that lapse of time which must so soon reduce him to nothing? Where, under this gloomy and horrid anticipation, would be his affections for his parents, his wife, his family, his country:—what would become of the performance of his duties as a parent, a husband, a citizen, and a patriot:—where would be the endearing suggestions of his own self-love and insatiable desires of his present and future happiness, under the certain conviction that the elevated and noble energies of his soul would explode and be lost forever, when his carcass would become a clod of the valley!

But, let it be supposed that the powers of reason, *unaided* by the holy inspirations of Scripture were capable of arriving at the certain conviction of man's future happiness in eternity; and that the decree of the Almighty which awarded to him so auspicious a destiny, was absolutely irrevocable by his own conduct: and what would then be the consequences? With so brilliant a career of future happiness and celestial glory in full view, would not all the poor enjoyments of this life fade away—and even all the splendors of the visible creation become to him a blank? Would he take upon himself the cares of a family; assume the laborious duties of providing for a numerous offspring; or feel an interest in the common affairs of mankind? Would he experience any of those affections and friendships, which, under the present predicaments of life, are of such vast importance to the enjoyments of man? Can the eye which is accustomed to gazing at the sun, distinguish the darker and more sombre colorings of earthly objects! But with unalloyed and interminable happiness beyond the grave in full view, what in this life would be the feelings, emotions and conduct of a man subjected to the pains of disease, the evils attendant on poverty and want, and all the great aggregate of miseries and misfortunes, with which man in the present state of things is destined to agonize through life. Would he feel disposed to encounter gratuitously, evils and sufferings from which he could escape with impunity to happier regions.

And now let us suppose, that a man were enabled to distinguish nothing in his future destinies, but a submission throughout eternity to the *sufferings and speechless agonies of the damned;* that noting he could do would alleviate so dreadful, disasterous and horrible a destiny! and what would be the immediate results? Where, to the eye of such a man, would then be all the charms and fascinations of nature:

where all the varied and imposing splendors of the visible creation? What delight could he possibly experience in the performance of his moral duties, or in the practice of virtues which must terminate in a future condition infinitely worse than anihilation itself? Would not these dark and dreadful anticipations of a period, which *must soon arrive*, be eternally present to his imagination, with all their attendant horrours? Would they not haunt his waking dreams of future misery, and disturb his midnight slumbers with spectral phantoms of the sufferings of the damned, too frightful and tremendous for delination! But, what, under these awful and afflicting expectations, from which there were no distant hopes of exemption, would be the character and conduct of this unfortunate and miserable victim! Would he not say to himself;—"What to me are all the ties of parentage, of offspring, or of kindred; what interest have I in the affairs of life, the peace and happiness of society, or the moral conduct and regulations of mankind! Before the setting of to-morrow's sun my eyes may close forever on the light of day, on all the objects which once were dear to my infancy and youth, and on all the varied and sublime beauties, which characterize with magnificence and splendor, the mystic wonders of created nature! For me no morning sun will ever again arise; for me no vernal music of the grove will ever again awake; on my benighted soul, *predestined to endless torments*, no distant ray of feeble hope can ever dawn?"———Sectarians, remorseless fanatics, purblind bigots—you who deal with unsparing hand and intolerant zeal, the ineffable and everlasting miseries of deep damnation to your fellow beings, merely for differing from you in opinion respecting modes of faith and divine worship, behold in this faithful picture, the condition to which your narrow and selfish doctrines would consign the great mass of mankind! Approach and behold a picture, which might make you shudder for your blasphemous presumptions, in judging between erring and feeble man and his Maker, and wresting the high prerogative of divine and eternal justice, from the hands of the Almighty! If you can for a moment suspend the fiery and vindictive delusions of your intolerance and presumption, I wish you to contemplate with a dispassionate and discriminating eye, some farther results to which your infuriated and intolerant doctrines inevitably tend. If you alone are right, and if all other religious creeds are the offspring of error, which must of necessity terminate in future misery—what allurements to religion and morality do you hold out, to those who you say are predestined from all eternity to the inflictions of divine wrath: and to what a penury of beneficence and love, do you reduce the mercy and affections of the Deity to man. Do you suppose that the doctrines of particular and exclusive faith, are within the arbitrium or control of the voluntary powers of human intellect? In other words, do you presume that man can believe what he wishes, without divine assistance sought with purity of heart! And that he can ever be the voluntary devotee of religious errors, thereby sinning against light and knowledge, and dooming himself to endless and indescribable torments? To speak in plain terms, and without any courtly affectations of language detrimental to the interests of truth, can you suppose that any *rational being* since the creation of man, ever yet voluntarily consigned his soul to everlasting misery, by the *entertainment of religous opinions*, which he *knew to be wrong:* the truth is that the supposition implies, not only a contradiction in language, but an absolute and positive contradiction in the facts themselves!

But let us suppose for a moment, that your sect or persuasion alone are right in their faith and religious opinions, & that all others professing different modes of faith, and different opinions in religion, are in the entertainment of errors which must inevitably end in eternal punishments. Have you ever contemplated the absurdity of this intolerant and exclusive doctrine; have you ever viewed it with an unprejudiced and dispassionate eye and traced its malignant and desolating spirit, on the *past*, on the *present*, and on *future times*? If you have not, I will make the laudable attempt to burst your narrow and intolerant preujdices asunder; and to exhibit these disgraceful and dogmatical doctrines in all their native deformities.

By the Mosaical account of the creation, which we are

bound to believe authentic, the world is now nearly six thousand years old; but of the antideluvian races of men, and also of those who existed anterior to the gospel dispensation, I will malte none but the following simple and plain remark; that it would hardly comport with the common principles of justice, to consign all those numerous races of men to eternal perdition, for not believing in doctrines which had never been announced to them, and to which they were utter strangers! Since the first announcement of the gospel dispensation under our Saveiour, until the present time, a period of nearly *two thousand years* has elapsed; every *half minute* of which long period, according to the most authentic calculations which can be made, has witnessed the *birth* and *death* of TEN HUMAN BEINGS! There are, as nearly as the facts can be ascertained, about *eleven hundred millions human beings composing the population on the globe:* now—if you will ascertain the number of half minutes which have elapsed in two thousand years, and multiply that number by *ten*, you will have something like the number of deaths which have occurred since the coming of Christ. Under this strong, and new, and most important view of the subject; and considering likewise, that the immense and measureably unknown population of bot Africa and Asia have never embraced the christian dispensation; that the aboriginal inhabitants of both North and South America have ever been in the same uncivilized and unchristian condition; I wish you to inform me, ye bigots—ye fanatics—ye fiery and intolerant zealots, in the cause of a God autocratical, supreme, and infinitely *merciful* to feeble and erring man, how many human beings, out of the *countless myriads* who have sunk into the tomb in the long lapse of *two thousand years*, belonged to those *little sects* which doom all mankind to the horrours of deep and irrevocable damnation but themselves! But this is not all, according to the narrow and exclusive principles of your religious doctrines, which we will bring nearer to ourselves by an application of them to the present age, how many human beings out of *eleven hundred millions* which are now in existence, according to the purblind and intolerant dogmas of any *one* of your *exclusive professions of faith*, will be doomed never to reach the goal of infinite mercy, even through the merits of that *Saveiour* who died for the salvation of *all mankind!* These are views of the absurdity of some of your doctrines, and of the dreadful consequences they would have in their applications to mankind, too stubborn for the subterfuges of sophistry, too authentic in point of fact for refutation, and too plain for either denial or evasion.—But, let us advance a step farther; let us contemplate the appalling spectacle, which your wild, speculative and visionary theories of religion, would present to an assembled Universe at the end of time! Let us suppose, a period, the great day of accounts between man and his Maker, when an aggregation of all the various races of men, and of all the countless myriads who have existed between the commencement and the termination of time, would take place; here all arithmetical computations fail:—and the human imagination itself expires, in attempting to grasp at so vast, so unbounded a spectacle! Suppose also, that your paltry and disputacious conflicts here, and your narrow conceptions of divine justice, anlways inadequate and contradictory, because the offspring of ignorance, were to be made the irrevocable standard of adjudication by which countless and innumerable millions of the human race, were to be consigned to endless misery, ruin and despair? Would not so dreadful an exhibition of the consequences of your bigotry and intolerance, destroy your holy zeal and vindictive rage in the cause of religious and intolerant prejudices? Would not your sensibilites as men, weep tears of blood and forgiveness over the miseries of your fellow men? Would you not wish to revoke those prejudices against manking, which would populate the regions of the damned with myriads of your fellow-beings—disclose to you an *abortive* though *divine* scheme of redemption for fallen man—and torture your intellectual vision, with the spectacle of a *ruined creation* and an *almost solitary God!*

I have now shown, and I think conclusively, that the efforts of human reason, unaided by scriptural divinity, are, utterly incompetent to disclosing to mankind the great truths connected with the immortality of man:—that without the moral purifications of true christianity and genuine religion, such disclosures would have been fraught with dreadful consequences to mankind, instanced in the cases of future certainty as to *anihilation*, *future happiness* and *future misery*. I think I have done more; I think I have shown, as far as the moral reasoning powers of man can be applied to incontrovertible facts, that very many of the intolerant and sectarian *abuses* which have crept into the christian religion, from the bigotry and misdirected zeal of many of its belligerant and inflammatory champions, are utterly inconsistent with christian charity, truly divine worship, and the principles of *eternal justice:* in fine, I think I have shown conclusively, what pure and genuine religion *is not!*

As connected and incorporated with dangerous and intolerant *opinions in religion*, the abusive consequences which always flow from such opinions, especially when under the influence of the vindictive passions of men, require dispassionate consideration. I have said in another part of this work, when speaking of the moral philosophy of the passions, that when restrained within due bounds, and exercised only in relation to their native and legitimate objects, they were essential not only to the existence, but to the happiness of man. I now assert that the reverse of this proposition is equally true; in other words, that the passions when indulged in to excess, and suffered to produce anarchy and wide misrule in the human bosom, are fraught with innumerable miseries and misfortunes to mankind, in every department of life.

In sectarian doctrines, which relate to the entertainment of opinions connected with the temporal self-interests of mankind, it is to be expected that the passions in all their excesses, will always have considerable influence. The profossors of all the sciences which relate to the present state of man, are passionately influenced to the conversion of proselytes to their respective systems, because on the number of their converts depend not only their *wealth* and *fame;* but in numerous instances, the very *bread* which themselves and their families require for daily support. The same may be remarked, in relation to the leaders of all political partizans—and to all other zealots in political science. In these cases, and many others which might be enumerated, the stimulation of the passions, and all their disorganizing and dangerous excesses, are proportioned to the real or imaginary *self-interests* of man, and to the acute and energetic pressure of his immediately real or imaginary *wants*. In all these cases, we can account on rational principles, or more properly speaking on logical ones, for the slander and defamation with which scientifiic men of all professions usually load each other—and for all the personal enmity, envy and malignity, with which the low-lived spirit of grovelling ambition, usually persecutes a dangerous and aspiring rival! In all cases where we can connect the excesses of the passions, and the practice of intoleration and injustice, with the wants and immediate self-interests of men, there seems to be some colorable mitigation for their deviations from virtue, justice and moderation: but in cases where *Religion* alone is concerned: where all the temporal interests and conflictions of self-love are entirely out of the question, where the religious faith and opinions of men are accounts only to be referred to the lofty and unerring *tribunal of God himself*; the gratuitous persecutions of men, and their sanguinary zeal in the cause of an Almighty power, who needs not their assistance, can only be accounted for upon principles of wanton depravity, native cruelty of temper, and inate vindictiveness of soul! Does the Almighty require the sacrifice of the peace of society, and of all the affections of man for his fellow-beings, in the diffusion of an immaculate and benevolent religion, which expressly inculcates—"*peace on earth, and good will towards men?*" If my faith in the rectitude and purity of my own doctrines of salvation be perfect, will the persecution and destruction of the religious doctrines of other men, add any further demonstrations of truth to the support of my own creed? You may as well tell me, ye *bigots* and persecutors of mankind for the love of God, that the sun requires a lamp for the diffusion of his meridian rays—or that by conflagrating the habitation of a fellow being, you will build or repair your own! Why then consign to everlasting destruction, and that too without attempting their reformation, all those who may chance to differ from you in religious faith and opinion? Are not those who dissent from you in religious doctrines and opinions as *rational* as yourselves? Are they less interested in *knowing* the truths of genuine christian divinity, and in *practising* on the precepts which they inculcate, than you yourselves are? Do you suppose that any human being ever existed, who was endowed with ordinary principles of rationality, and common sentiments of self-love, who could voluntarily entertain errors of opinion in religion, knowing that the profession of such opinions would eventually consign their immortal souls, to deep and irredeemable misery! Why, then, persecute men for the entertainment of opinions, which are *misfortunes* and not *crimes!* Why, in other words, do you punish and persecute erring and feeble man, for involuntary errors of opinion, which, according to your own creeds, will be punished in a future life! Where are the credentials, from which you derive authority to sit in judgment between *man* and his MAKER: and to *assist* an OMNIPOTENT GOD, in the execution of *those laws* which his own *infinite wisdom*, AT THE CREATION, imposed on the UNIVERSE! Under this view of your conduct, which I place in a strong and correct light for your own contemplations, with the hope that you may be induced to abandon your *abuses* of the religion of the Saviour of mankind, and to treat your fellow-men with more lenity and compassion. I must confess myself utterly at a loss, which most to be astonished at your ignorance—presumption—or fanaticism. How ye biggotted and fanatical zealots—how do you reconcile your *inquisitions*, your *burnings* your *persecutions*, and your *intolerance in opinion*, with the mildly compassionate and humane example of the Saviour of the world; he who exclaimed amidst the protracted agonies of the CROSS, and whilst sweating drops of blood to wash out the crimsoned iniquities of mankind—"Father forgive them, for they know not what they do!" You are mistaken in attributing to pure and holy zeal in the cause of religion, your persecutions of those who differ from you in sectarian faith and doctrines: your worldly minded pride of making proselytes—your ambition to become conspicuous among men, as the defenders of the *true faith*—your secret aspirations after exaltations to high clerical offices—your love of worldly distinctions and temporal power—and not unfrequently, your cupidity and avarice, respecting good round *salaries* for the discharge of your official functions; these are the energetic and inflammatory motives, which urge you to your vindictive persecutions of mankind for *opinion's sake;* these are the real causes of your want of *charity* to each other, and to mankind in the aggregate.

I think I have now shown, in a tolerable clear and strong point of view, not only what religion *is not*—but also many of the *abuses* of its doctrines: let us now endeavor to understand something respecting what it *really is.*

"Feeble work of my hand," says the Almighty to his creature man, "I owe you nothing, but I give you existence. I place you in the midst of a Universe which bespeaks my wisdom and glory, and I surround you with blessings and enjoyments, which ought to excite in your bosom, pure and elevated sentiments of *love, admiration* and *gratitude*, to that inscrutable Being who made you for the enjoyment of happiness—and placed the objects of those enjoyments within your reach. Your love can add nothing to my felicity, your admiration to my power, nor your sentiments of gratitude to my glory; and I make you susceptible of these exalted and divine emotions, that you may render yourself happy both here and hereafter. The fidelity of your obedience to my laws will be the test of your own happiness; and, when you cease to '*love me, and keep my commandments,*' your breach of my precepts will offend me, and render yourself unhappy."

Such—according to our feeble and inadequate conceptions of a God of *love* and *mercy*, are the mild and benevolent sentiments entertained by him for his erring and dependant creature *man*—for he expressly announces in his holy word, "that he delights not in the death of a sinner."—These are some of the consolations of true religion, which, when fully merited by man, by a strict obedience to the words of the Scripture, and a full and entire faith in the merits of a blest Redeemer, nothing earthly can destroy. I do not intend to enter into a critical dissertation on the subject of religion, further than its divine spirit is connected with the moral condition of man, and his physical health and enjoyments. We know perfectly well, from our own consciousness, that the mere pleasures and enjoyments of this world, are insufficient to satisfy the moral desires of the human mind, when deeply impressed with an unerring sentiment of immortality. Give a man wealth and luxury unbounded; load him with titles and worldly honors; even clothe him with what Doctor Young calls "*a mortal immortality*"—and, like *Cæsar* when crowned emperor, and invested with the imperial purple, he will exclaim—"*and is this all!*" With respect to the enjoyments of this world, I mean those which are not connected with a future state of existence, and sentiments of pure and undefiled religion, it is a truth that has been recognized by the experience of all ages, that their satiation always produces indifference, and not unfrequently disgust. This circumstance alone ought to convince us. that the *desires* of man and his *capacities* for enjoyment, are not limited to this earthly sphere; and that there must be a future and more exalted state of being, where his capacities for moral and intellectual enjoyment will meet with objects suited to their elevation—and where the boundless desires which he is conscious of in this life, will meet with scenes of enjoyment as unlimited as those desires. It was from this view of the subject under consideration. and probably also from the strong impressions of the insufficiency of the enjoyments of this life, that the great Dr. Young exclaimed in his Night Thoughts—"*man must be immortal*, or heaven is unjust!" Do we not know perfectly well, that when the physical calls of nature are satisfied, lassitude and indifference succeed? Do we not also know, that when all the pleasures and enjoyments of this world are showered on us in profusion, there still exists in the human bosom, hopes and desires connected with sentiments of immortality, and objects of a more elevated and intellectual order of enjoyment than this world can afford? The fact is, that the desires, the capacities.

and the hopes of man as to futurity—when compared with the utter insufficiency of the objects of enjoyment actually under his control in this life, go very far to demonstrate satisfactorily the immortality of man. Do the affections of the brute for its offspring, like those of man for his relations and friends, survive the flight of time, and contemplate a reunion of those affections in another state of existence? The difference between the influence of reason and that of true religion, in relation to the future happiness and enjoyments of man, may be satisfactorily explained in a few words. *Reason* teaches man merely to *hope* for immortal existence and happiness, whilst pure *Religion*, supported by *faith in the Redeemer*, and by the *faithful practice of his precepts*, assures him of both future existence and future happiness. There is this further difference between reason and religion, and I think it a very palpable and plain one; reason cannot influence man's feeble hopes of immortality and future happiness, with sufficient motives for the practice of piety and virtue —whilst religion urges him imperiously to the performance of his duties to his God, to himself and to his fellow-beings, by the certainty of future *rewards* and *punishments*. These are the reasons why pure and genuine christians, I do not mean bigots, hypocrites or intolerant fanatics, are better citizens, better husbands, and better parents, than most other men; and these are the reasons also, why they are the happier classes of mankind. Reason may teach the existence of a great first cause, but it is utterly incompetent to disclosing his moral attributes of justice, love and mercy; or to defining for man his particular and indispensable duties in every department of life. The precepts of religion are plain and easy of comprehension; they can be understood and practiced by all ranks and grades of men. Reason, on the other hand, in attempting an explanation of the attributes of God, or the duties of man to that God, or his fellow-creatures, is eternally operating on imaginary and unknown principles, and making hair-breadth distinctions, which have no existence but in the sound of words without meaning: the errors of reason are founded in the ignorance of man, who knows nothing in reality of the essential or elementary principles of any one thing in heaven or on darth. The Scripture says, and any man can understand the denunciation, "whoso shedeth man's blood, by man shall his blood be shed." Now I would like to see the champion of reason, who can demonstrate satisfactorily that murder is a crime, and that it is punishable with death. But I will put another, and a more general and comprisive case, which will be quite sufficient. Municipal law is said to be founded on reason, which we call the mother of justice.—If reason be an unerring sentinal, and if law be the perfection of reason, as it is said to be by learned and profound civilians, why, have not *six thousand years* of reasoning been sufficient to reduce law to unerring principles of justice; and why, at this late and refined period of reason, do we so seldom find two persons of "counsel learned in the law," who agree in opinion respecting its real principles? The fact is, that in reasoning on all subjects involving morals, all we can possibly arrive at, is a high degree of probability, which amounts to little more than ingenious and plausible *conjecture.* If the mere exercise of reason be entirely sufficient to disclose to man his duties, to impel him to the performance of those duties, and to satisfy him respecting the all-important doctrines of futurity, why have the advocates of mere reason, so many doubts and difficulties on all these subjects:—the enigma is easily solved; the *ignorance* of man respecting the first principles, the *doubts* he always entertains of the infallibility of reasoning as a science, and the *consciousness* of being eternally liable to error in his rational deductions, involve him in labyrinths of confusion and dismay, from which no merely human powers of intellect or genius can possibly extricate him. While in the rise or day-spring of life; while enjoying uninterupted health and prosperity; and while indulging in anticipations of a protracted and fortunate term of existence here, the lordly and proud advocate of the all-sufficiency of reason, may indulge in *theorctical speculations* which he *imagines* he firmly believes in; but, let him become unfortunate in his adventures after earthly enjoyments, and infirm in his health; let his prospects of exemption from disease and misfortune darken around him:

and in this situation let him approach the unknown and mysterious confines of eternity. Where then will be his visionary and theoretical speculations respecting futurity; where the fortitude which ought to support him in his dissent to the cold and silent mansions of the dead; and where the celestial fire of hope and christian consolation that alone can light him to eternal happiness, relieve his gloomy apprehensions of anihilation—and shed even a splendor around the horrours of the grave!

Pure and vital religion, not that based on merely biggotted and sectarian prejudices, or on frivolous and childish distinctions respecting rites and ceremonies, is infinitely superior to reason, in *securing* to man all the moral enjoyments of this life, and in *assuring* him of those blessings which reason only *hopes* for in futurity. By pure and vital religion, I do not mean *hypocrisy* which is the religion of knaves, *fanaticism* which is the religion of madmen, *fear* which is the religion of cowardice, or *superstition* which is that of fools: I mean that pure and elevated sentiment of divine love and admiration for the DEITY, which leads us to *faith* in the great Redeemer of fallen and degraded man, and to the practice of benevolenc, virtue, toleration and charity for our fellow-beings. This divine and ennobling sentiment, when experienced in all its purity, banishes all the base, sordid, selfish, and ignoble passions from the human bosom, and elevates man as it were, to a communion with his Maker. It cultivates all the finer affections of man for his fellow-beings; makes him a provident and tender parent; a chast and faithful husband; a kind and benevolent master; and a useful, virtuous, and patriotic citizen: it makes him faithful in his friendships, virtuous in his loves, honest in his dealings, candid in his communications with mankind, moderate in his desires, unostentatious in his charities, and tolerant in his opinions. Fanatics, bigots, zealots, hypocrites: ye who practice fraud, violence, hypocrisy, and all the deceptions and mummery of *priestcraft* on the sons of men, and yet dare to call yourselves the disciples and followers of the immaculate Saviour of mankind, compare yourselves with this portrait of a ***real christian!*** There is a class of religionists in every christian country, who are impressed with the absurd opinion, that the *profession of faith* in particular sectarian creeds; and the *practice* of a few frivolous *rites and ceremonies*, are quite sufficient to entitle them to salvation. The probability is, that these people are deceiving themselves, or making the profession of religion a mere mask for iniquitous designs against the community; for, let their vicious passions or propensities be excited, and themselves thrown off their guard, and you immediately discover the true state of the case: in fact you soon discover them to be sensualists, swindlers and hypocrites. These people ought always to bear in mind, that those alone are genuine christians, who know the will of God, and practice its divine precepts: nor ought they ever to loose sight of the important and eternal truth—that it is *impossible* to *deceive the Almighty*. Compared with these hypocritical and unworthy *professors*, whose prayers are always on the "house tops," and whose devotions are *loud and emphatical* that they may be heard; the true christian exhibits an essentially different and greatly more elevated character.—He is modest, retiring and unobtrusive in his devotions; it is not the mere profession of piety and religion, that stimulates him in the performance of his duties—it is the heaven-born consciousness that his devotional exercises are acceptable to his Maker, and that they will render him serene amidst dangers and difficulties, animated and cheerful under the infliction of disease and sickness, and resigned to the will of his Creator. To such a man, diseases, infirmities and misfortunes in this life are nothing; he is above their influence: they can neither ruffle his passions, nor disturb the deep and settled serenity of his soul. The death-bed of such a man is not the death-bed of the Sinner: even the presence of the king of terrours cannot appal the resolutions, or shake the fortitude of the man whose reliance is on the love and mercy of his God. As a physician, I some years since, in Virginia, attended the couch of a devont christian, and a sincere believer in Christ; and was impressed with sentiments which can never be obliterated from my memory by the lapse of time. The patient was a poor methodist preacher: he had been seriously and dangerously indisposed nearly two years; and was evidently awaiting the summon to "that bourne from whence no traveller returns." Instead of seeing terrour and dismay depicted in his countenance, which I had often witnessed in the cases of those who were not christians, all was cheerful serenity and mild resignation; no ghastly expression of feature bespoke the terrour of death, no indications of mental distress told of remorse for an ill-spent life; nor did a single shade of gloomy anticipation, pass over the eye that was so soon to close in the cold and silent mansions of the dead! The last words of the innocent sufferer were, and they are deeply impressed on my memory,—"my life has been devoted to the service of my God, and to the benefit of my fellow-beings: I await with perfect resignation to his will, the call of my master." ———Here was an instance of the consolitary influence of true religion, which ought to prove conclusivly that it is connected with none of the gloomy and depressing passions. In truth, it has always been a matter of much astonishment to me, that the consolation which true religion promises mankind in a future state of existence, could ever have produced on the mind of any other impressions than those of cheerfulness fortitude and resignation. I never could conceive how genuine religion was connected, unless perverted to the excitement of the gloomy passions, by misconceptions of the attributes of God, with emotions of terrour and depressing apprehensions of futurity. Has man not assurences of an exemption from all the evils and calamities of this life, if he be a faithful and true christian, in a more perfect and elevated state of being, when his corruption shall put on incorruption—and when the mere mortal shall put on immortality? Are not the doctrines of true christianity, essentially connected with that *sunshine* of the breast, which we denominate *a good conscience*:—"and which nothing earthly can give, or can destroy!"—The christian religion was never intended by the Almighty, as a source of grief, mortification and suffering; it is a pure emenation of divine love and mercy towards feeble, erring and fallen mankind; and was surely intended by divine wisdom, as an unfailing source of joy, consolation and happiness, both here and hereafter, to the human race! I have been more particular on the subject of religion, than at first view might seem necessary to the interests of medical science; but I have been long convinced, that the sentiments we entertain of a future life, are not only essentially connected with the moral condition of mankind, but with the health and many of the diseases of the physical system, of which more will be said under the proper heads.

INTEMPERANCE.

Intemperance is the offspring of so many and such various causes, that it seems impossible to enumerate them, or ever to reduce them to any thing like scientific order. I will commence my remarks on intemperance, which in its broadest signification means *excess* in the gratification of our *propensities, passions*, and even intellectual *pursuits*, by emphatically observing, that it is generally found in strong and intimate connexion, when really traced to its origin, with the *pleasures* and *enjoyments* as well as with *miseries* and *misfortunes* of mankind. I have before remarked under another head, that with regard to the elementary principles of the passions, propensities, and intellectual powers of man we know absolutely nothing with certainty; and that all we can possibly understand with respect to them, is derived from our *consciousness* of their existence, and from the *effects* they daily and hourly produce for our observation.

Every capacity or power of the human system, physical and intellectual, when exercised in moderation, and with strict conformity to the laws of nature, is productive of enjoyment and happiness: this natural and moderate exercise of our propensities, passions, and mental energies, when matured into habits of life and character, we call *temperance;* and, it is the abusive degradation of those same intellectual powers, passions and propensities, by their unrestrained and excessive indulgence to the destruction of *health* and *happiness,* that we call *intemperance.* I will give some familiar examples of the application of these principles, in order that they may be fully comprehended by those for whom I write. We are all liable to *hunger* and *thirst:* and all of us require *sleep*, for the renovation of our bodily and mental powers when fatigued. These are natural wants; and their gratifications are always essential to health and happiness. We all know perfectly well, for instance, that when we satisfy our hunger and thirst in moderation, and renew the strength of our systems, of mind and body, by sleeping no more than the requisite time for producing those effects, the satisfaction of these natural wants invariably produces healthy action of body and mind, attended with enjoyment and pleasure. But on the other hand, when in eating or drinking, we overload and surcharge the stomach with meat and drink, and when in sleeping take more repose than is required for the renovation of our bodily and mental systems, our excesses are always productive of nausea, uneasiness, indigestion, and stupidity, and we habitually become *gluttons drunkards* and *sluggards*, and are a disgrace to ourselves and society. The same doctrine and mode of reasoning may be applied to the passions of mankind. When they are indulged in with natural moderation, and never suffered to run into riot and excess, they are always conducive to health. and productive of many of the enjoyments and pleasures of life; but. when they gain the ascendency of the moral feelings and rational powers, when they prostrate the bulwarks of religion and morality, and are indulged in all their debasing and destructive excesses, the progress of the passions proclaims the premature decay of health, strength, and happiness—and emphatically announces to the unfortunate victims of excess, that they are fallen indeed! In truth, what has just been remarked with regard to the natural *wants* and *passions* of men, may with strict justice be applied to the lofty and powerful energies of the *mind* itself. It has been truly remarked, by an accute and profound investigator of the faculties of the mind, that "he who thinks with great intenseness and profundity, will not continue to do so for many successive years,"—and in proof of this, I will note some instances which will have much weight in demonstrating the fact. Sir Isaac Newton, who was probably the greatest astronomer and mathematician of his own or any other age, several years previous to the close of his life, was utterly unable to comprehend the meaning of his own works: in addition to which I will notice as a well authenticated fact, that the celebrated Dean Swift, the energies of whose mind were inferior to those of no literary man of the same age; several years previous to his death became a driveller, and confirmed ediet. Whether it be true, that intense, subtile and powerful intellect, acts upon the mere carcass as a sharp sword does upon the scabbard, or whether the mind itself becomes exhausted and worn out, by an overstrained and continued excitement of its powers, I leave for metaphysicians to determine:—but we certainly do know, and the experience of all ages and generations proves the fact, that excessive mental exertion not only produces fatigue and lassitude in a few hours, but that if such exertion be continued for a few years in succesion, it invariably blunts and wears down the keenest and soundest intellectual energies of man. The broad and comprehensive view I have just given of *temperance* and *intemperance*, in regard to the physical wants, passions, and intellectual powers of man, I believe to be the only correct exposition on general principles that can be given; because it embraces all the destructive excesses to which man is prone, and refers all those excesses, to the *abuses* and *degradations* of his elevated and noble faculties.

I commenced with remarking, and I wish the principle to be kept in view by the reader, that the vices of intemperance when fairly traced to their origin, will always be found in connexion with the enjoyments and pleasures, as well as with the miseries and misfortunes of mankind.

Mankind may be distinguished into two great classes or divisions: *First*, those whose pleasures and enjoyments, and whose pains and miseries, partake so greatly of a physical character, as nearly always to be referable to corporeal or bodily functions and sensations: this class is composed of men who are properly denominated *sensualists;* in other words, they are individuals who can only be rendered happy or miserable through the medium of the senses. *Second*, those whose general characters partake more of the nature and habitual influence of the intellectual powers, and of the emotions and passions of the mind; and whose enjoyments, pleasures, sufferings, and miseries, are more intimately connected with the mind and imagination: these may with much propriety be denominated *mentalists*. Among the great aggregate of mankind, the reality of the distinction between *animal* and *intellectual* man, as regards the native bias of the human character towards one or the other extreme, is demonstrable from the following facts. Hunger and thirst, for instance, are corporeal wants; they are essential to the health, strength, and support of the physical or bodily system; and may be called corporeal or bodily passions, when they become so powerful as to impel men to gluttony and drunkenness: desires and propensities being nothing more, when considered in relation to the corporeal system, than slighter shades of the physical wants and passions of men. Love and ambition, on the contrary, are passions of the mind and imagination; they are the offspring of refined sensibility, and deep-toned energies of intellectual character; and when acting in their native sphere, are so far abstracted from all corporeal considerations, that they only occasionally act on the physical wants and passions, and then, only for the attainment of specific objects. When the passion of love, for instance, is directed to the perpetuation of the human species, which I will remark in passing, was not the ease in the love which existed between Jonathan and David, the intellectual passion of love only *acts* on the sexual and corporeal functions; but, I would ask any sceptic on this point, whether the love of literature, mathematics, astronomy, or any other science or intellectual pursuit, has any connection whatever with propensities, wants and passions, founded on the merely corporeal or bodily functions of mankind. And surely it will not be questioned, that the food and nourishment required for exercising, giving pleasure to, and strengthening the *mind*, are essentially different from those required for the sustenance, health, and strength of the *body*; and we all know perfectly well, in reference to the corporeal and intellectual functions and capacities of men, that the strong predominance of either class, operates unfavorably and sometimes destructively to the other. The fact is, that we oftentimes find the loftiest and strongest passions and mental energies, connected with delicate and sometimes feeble corporeal organization, debility of stomach, and prostration of strength: nor is it unusual to observe, that those who possess uncommonly high health and physical strength, are frequently in the other extreme, as regards the exercise of the mind and passions. But further, every man who has acquired any experience, respecting those states of the physical system when the mind and passions act with the greatest force, must know that a full stomach always blunts the mind and feelings; and that inanition or emptiness of the stomach, is favorable to intellectual operations. This fact is so well known, that the Creek Indians, in all their public deliberations on important national concerns, use what they call the *black drink*, made of the parched leaves of the spice-wood boiled, which vomits them copiously, and produces the inanition just mentioned; without which, they allege they are inadequate to deliberating on their national affairs. Some medical writer has remarked, that physical debility, and a diseased state of the system, impart as it were a preternatural excitement to the mind, and instances the cases of Boilieu, Erasmus, Pascal, Cicero, Galba, Pope, and several others, who were as remarkable for the feebleness of their physical constitutions, as they were for their gigantic energies of intellect: the same writer also remarks, that abortive, feeble, and sickly children, almost invariably display powerful characteristics of intellect when grown to maturity; and instances the cases of the great lord Littleton and Mrs. Ferguson, both of whom were seven months children; to which he might have added the case of Richard the Third, who according to Shakespear's account, was "deformed, unfinished, and sent into this breathing world scarce half made up." On the other hand, it has frequently been remarked, by men of acute and scrutinizing minds, that high health, great corporeal strength, and uncomnonmuscularity of frame, are seldom remarkable for subtile & profound genius, or for an attachment to purely intellectual pursuits. This is so notoriously true, that the opinions generally formed by the vulgar, of the *persons* of men who are conspicuous and renowned for great intellectual powers, are almost invariably the very reverse, of what may be called, the corporeally *contemptible* realities. In demonstration of this fact, innumerable instances might be given, in addition to those found in the persons of Alexander of Macedon, Frederic king of Prussia, John Philpot Curran, Aaron Burr, Alexander Hamilton. Thomas Jefferson, James Madison, Andrew Jackson, and lastly the late emperor Napoleon, who was nicknamed by his own soldiers, from his contemptible stature and proportions, the *little corporal.* I will here make an observation on this subject, which I do not recollect to have seen in any writer. We are always to presume, that the soundness and strength of the physical constitutions of men, lead to great longevity or length of days; and it is a fact as notorious as true, that such men are seldom or never possessed of much mind; in other words, the sword is not sufficiently sharp to cut the scabbard. I am acquainted with a man, a paupor of this country, who is said from good authority to be one hundred and ten years of age, who, I was informed on inquiry, never even in the meridian of life had more than a very ordinary mind: and Thomas Parre, who died in London on the 16th of November, 1635—aged one hundred and fifty two years, it is said was greatly noted for having been a man as remarkable, for his deficiency of mental energies, as for his lascivious and sensual propensities. "It was observed of him," says the London Medical Museum, "that he used to eat often, both by night and by day, taking up with old cheese, milk, coarse bread, small beer, and whey, and which is more remarkable; he ate at midnight, a little before he died. Being opened after his death, his body was still found very fleshy; his breast hairy, his genitals unimpaired, which served to confirm the report of his having undergone public censures for his incontenency," &c. &c. I would by no means wish to be understood, that there are no individuals, possessed of high health and great physical strength, who are remarkable for strong intellectual powers, Newton Johnston, Shakespear, and a thousand other instances might be given as exceptions to the general rule just noticed; but we are all well convinced, not only that high health and strength lead to corporeal amusements and pursuits, unfavorable to intellectual improvement—but that debility and disease act in various ways extremely favorable to accessions of mental strength! In the first place, debility and disease lower the tone of those passions, which impel us to active exertion and amusement; in other words, they impose a powerful restraint on the physical appetites and propensities—circumscribe us to amusements and pursuits connected with the operations of the mind—confine us to the company of our elders, whose superior experience and knowledge are beneficial to our intellectual improvement; and "by keeping up an action in the brain, in common with other parts of the body, they tend to impart vigour to the intellectual faculties."

From what has been said, I think it will appear evident, that from both natural and accidental circumstances, there is a distinction to be drawn between those men whose *pleasures* and *pains* are connected with physical or corporeal character, and those whose enjoyments and miseries are more intimately associated with the powers and passions of the mind: and it was for these reasons that I alleged in the outset, not only that *intemperance* was the offspring of various *physical* and *intellectual* causes, but that when traced to its origin, it would generally be found in strong and intimate connexion, as well with the *pleasures* and *enjoyments*, as with the *miseries* and *misfortunes* of mankind. This is a view of the subject of intemperance and its causes, which I presume has never before been taken by any writer; and although it must of necessity, like every thing else human, be subject to imperfections, both in data and conclusions, yet it may have some salutary tendencies. It may possibly invite the attention of the learned, to further and more satisfactory investigations of the subject; it may exhibit the necessity of seeking for the real causes of intemperance, in removing its habits and effects from the human system; and it may invite society to the exercise of more lenity and compassion, when laboring for the reformation of its unfortunate and melancholy victims.—Abuse and degradation were never yet influential in reforming the intemperate; for, what interest did any man ever yet feel, for the *preservation* of that which he has been convinced, by *abuse* and *degradation*, was of no estimation or value! Intemperance is confined to no rank in life; to no particular grade of genius and intellectual power, between a Socrates and an idiot; it is found in the hut of the savage, the haunts of the learned, the hovel of the beggar, and in the palaces of kings; its causes are as various as the the capacities of man for enjoyments and pleasures, and as multiplied as the various miseries and misfortunes, to which he is subjected through life: what a farce then it must be, for any physician to attempt to remove the different causes of intemperance, without knowing what those causes are, and by the application of one specific remedy to such an infinite variety of causes.—Would you attempt to remove diseases of the mind, by merely physical remedies? Would you, on the other hand, hope for the removal of merely corporeal diseases by the application of intellectual means? Would you sooth the mental anguish of remorse, without the consolations of religion, and assurences of divine forgivenness? Would you, in other words, attempt to destroy a poisonous variety of plants, without striking at the roots of their existence and vitality?

The mere pleasures of sense, as well as those of the intelleet, are susceptible of beirg rendered more intense, by the application of stimulants: in the varied and endless catalogue of stimulating powers, are to be found all the great *allurements* to dissipation and confirmed intemperance; but it will hardly be contended, that one grade of stimulants, possesses the same strength and adaptation of allurement, with all the varieties of mankind. Physically speaking, one man's system is excited to pleasureable sensations by snuff, the system of another by tobacco, of another by wine, of a fourth by spirits and opium, of a fifth by highly seasoned and stimulating food, &c. &c; and we are all perfectly aware, that a persistency in the use of any or all the above stimulants, will sometimes degenerate into a confirmed *habit of intemperance* in their use, too strong for the restraints of either the moral or intellectual energies of the self-devoted victims. You will frequently hear the devotees of any or all the above excesses, execrating the very agents they employ in wearing down their constitutions with incidental diseases and premature decay, and moralizing with the finest touches of elocution, on the heinousness and immorality of such dangerous and degrading excesses: and what does all this prove? Why, it demonstrates conclusively, that the *habits* of dissipation and intemperance, like all other derelictions from the standard of nature and philosophic moderation, are to be resisted in their *first formation*, and before they can acquire the resistless force of torrents, before which all human resolutions, and efforts of preservation, sink to rise no more! There are two periods of human life; there are two marked and distinct periods in the progressive excesses of dissipation and intemperance. In the rise of life, we act upon every thing around us, from a confidence in our own strength, and a consciousness of being able to master and shape our own destinies; in the decline of life, when the physical, moral, and mental energies begin to fail, we act upon less resolute and less confidential principles; in other words, we merely act on the *defensive*, and resort to expedients for warding off diseases, dangers and death. These two periods are strongly marked in the lives and characters of all men; from the general who achieves victories in his youth, and sustains defeats in his old age, to the man of intellectual powers and persuits, who, like the immortal Milton, writes a "paradise lost" in the meridian of life and intellectual resolution, and a "paradise regained," when the tremors of old age and irresolution have crept over him. This is a faithful picture, of a man of dissipation and intemperance. At first, he adventures on an excess, partly from the attractive force of the allurement, and partly from the consciousness of moral and intellectual resolution to withstand any temptation to dangerous indulgence. In the formation of intemperate habits, this is precarious and hostile ground: the Scripture says, "let him who stands, take heed lest he fall." The habit of intemperance is of slow or rapid growth, in proportion to the strength or weakness of our resolutions to withstand temptation. Where many and strong motives combine to retard our progress in excesses of intemperance, we advance slowly and almost imperceptibly to self-destruction. When the animation of youth, and the convivialities of conversation, are sufficient for the production of pleasureable sensations: when we are highly susceptible of impression from the varied charmes of nature; and while the brilliant prospects of a long and animated life, seem "to bid an eternal Eden smile around us," the temptations to degrading intemperance, are only those which enhance the intensity of other pleasures. But, in proportion as all these fairy prospects fade on the vision; in proportion as the repetition of these enjoyments causes us to lose the sentiment of novelty; and especially when satiety of such enjoyments produces lassitude and coldness, we invariably descend to more sensual and intense expedients for renewing sensations of pleasures: and unfortunately, for mankind, those expedients are too often connected with the dissipations and intemperance of the glutton, the epicure, the opium eater, and the drunkard. This descent to confirmed habits of intemperance, in all its varied stages of degradation need not be delineated; these graduated debasements are visible in every department of society; and are so common, as almost every where to have lost their novelty and impression.

I have not yet spoken of those dissipations, which seem to be connected with the energies and passions of the mind; and compared with which, the intemperate excesses of the mere animal appetites and passions of man, dwindle into a comparatively insignificant and ordinary character. Where the character of an individual is decidedly intellectual, there always will be discovered at an early period of life, a strong native propensity to an indulgence in intellectual pleasures, and in those passions which are more closely allied to the mental powers. I mean here those pleasures of the mind, which have their rise in the *memory,* the *understanding* the *imagination,* &c. and those which are the offspring of an indulgence in those passions of the mind, which we call *love, hope, ambition, &c.* With regard to the pleasures of *memory,* they are as various and unlimited as the objects by which we are surrounded in nature; they comprise every thing cognizable by all the senses of man, the impressions of which can be stamped upon the retentive faculty; and they embrace also, those recollections of our own conduct, which are fraught with the pleasures of a *good conscience.* It is absolutely impossible to define or limit the pleasures of memory, they embrace our parents, our earthly friends, and all the objects of our youthful attachments: the houses in which we were born and educated, the haunts of our youthful and innocent diversions, and all the objects of our early pursuits. The pleasures of memory also comprise, all we have learned of the heroism, the magnanimity, and the intelligence of the great warriors and sages of antiquity; they in fact embrace all the recollections of the mind, in its recognizance of all the objects and events which have ever been pleasing to us: and they particularly afford us happiness from a review of a *well-spent life.* But are there not pains as well as pleasures of memory! There are: and here commences the catalogue of dissipations, the first impulse to which is to be found in the mind. Was it an inherent baseness and brutality of native character, that rendered Robert Burns intemperate? Was it a bestial love of the liquid poison which finally destroyed him, that originated and confirmed those habits of intemperance which sent him to an early grave? No: his dissipations commenced in the convivialities and pleasures of a refined, delecate, and superior mind; and were confirmed into habits of intemperance too stubborn for the control of his moral energies, by the lowliness of his fortunes, the poignancy and vulgarity of his sufferings, and the *pains of his memory!* Why do we see a man like this, the prey of a morbid and confirmed melancholy? And why do we hear him warbling forth his distresses, when contemplating objects yet dear and painful to his memory, in the following inspired and tender straints: "ye mind me of departed hours—departed, never to return!" The fate of Robert Burns has been the fate of thousands whose names are lost to fame, and who have sunk into obscure and lonely graves, unpitied and unknown. Thomas Paine, once remarked, that one of the greatest miseries of human life, consisted in not being able to forget, what it was painful to remember: Mr. Paine's character was highly intellectual; his whole life had been devoted to conferring *political benefits* and *moral misèries* on mankind; and it is not merely possible, but highly probable, that the desertations of society on account of his theological writings, and the *pains of his memory*, led to those confirmed habits of dissipation and intemperance, which ultimately destroyed him. But, the instances just submitted to the reader, are but two out of thousands which might be adduced, to prove the influence of the *pains of memory*, in originating and confirming fatal habits of dissipation and intemperance. How many millions have sunk into the vortex of intemperance, from the influence of those pains of memory, called an *accusing conscience?* Physician:—"canst thou minister to a mind diseased," by medical prescriptions which can only affect the body?.

The pleasures and pains of the *understanding* come next under consideration; and present such a field for the investigations of philosophy, as can only be delineated in outline. Curiosity is the first passion, or rather emotion of the human understanding; it leads the mind to the investigation and scrutiny, of all the objects of nature and art which present themselves to man, betwixt the *cradle* and the *grave?* the emotion or passion of curiosity does more; it leads us to the investigation of objects beyond the boundaries of time, and impels us to attempt a revelation of the great enigmas of eternity itself! The mind of man is naturally attached to truth; and always experiences pleasure in the discovery of it, when the disclosure is found beneficial to comfort, health, fame, or enjoyments of any description; in all these cases, and innumerable others, we experience what may be called the *pleasures of the understanding*.

But has not the human understanding also its *pains?* I think so: we all know perfectly well, that the period of death must arrive: and does not this certain anticipation give pain to thousands? Is not the fear of death painful? I will admit that the uncertainty of the moment, wisely and benevolently hidden from us by Providence, in some measure blunts the painful anticipation of death: but what are the mental pangs of the convict, who is given to understand that he must be executed to-morrow! Both, the pleasures and pains of the understanding, have relation to the discovery of truth. Suppose a man be bitten by a serpent, of whose character he knows nothing; is he not alarmed? Suppose that he immediately discovers the reptile to be harmless: do not the mental pains of alarm cease; and does he not experience pleasure from the consciousness of security from danger? Here the pleasure of the understanding is derived from a beneficial discovery: but suppose he ascertain that the reptile by which he has been assailed, is of a venomous and fatal character, and that he clearly understands his immediate destiny to be death; are not his mental pangs identified with the pains of the understanding? I have not space, in a work like this, to go into a philosophical detail of the important truths connected with this subject; and regret to be compelled to differ from the authority of the great Dr. Rush, who alleges that the pleasures of the understanding have no antagonist in pain. A knowledge of facts, is the aggregate amount of the *truths* acquired by the operations of the understanding: where these acquisitions of knowledge develop consequences *beneficial* to human enjoyment and happiness, they are always productive of *pleasure* to the mind, through the medium of the understanding: but, where, by the operations of the understanding, the mind is brought into a full view of dangers and disasterous consequences, the results are always *painful* and *unhappy.* This I believe to be a full and fair statement of the case: and were it not, I would like to know, what influence in the religious reformation of mankind, could possibly be derived from *faith,* in the belief of future rewards and punishments! Ignorant of consequences, what to man would be the *happiness* or *misery* of either *prosperity* or *misfortune!* And how are either to be calculated without the operations of the understanding?—can a man even calculate the results of a plain question in arithmetic, without the operations of this mental power? It is alone by the pervading and subtile powers of the understanding, that we are enabled to feel the realitise, of either intellectual pain or pleasure, happiness or misery. The *memory* of man, acts upon nothing but facts and events which are past and gone: but the *understanding* operates also, on the present condition and circumstances of mankind, and even extends its views to futurity: and these are the reasons why the pleasures and pains of the understanding, are more intense than those of the memory. These are also the reasons, why we are led astray by the festivities of present dissipations and intemperance; and these are also the true reasons, why we resort to the banquit and the flowing bowl, to drown both past and present sorrows connected with the mind. Thus we see, that both joys and sorrows, are capable of producing habits of intemperance and dissipation: Physician: can your medical drugs restrain those Joys, or remove those sorrows which spring from the mind itself, when all the maxims of moral wisdom and philosophy have failed! No: you must resort to the restraining powers, and the consolations of religion and morality.

The pleasures and pains of the *imagination*, commence where those of the *memory* and the *understanding* terminate: and, there is this specific difference between them; the powers of the understanding and memory, operate on *facts* and *probabilities*, while those of the imagination, riot in the wild excesses of *fiction*, *romance*, and absolute improbabilities. The range of the human imagination seems to be unlimited; and what is very extraordinary, and something difficult to be accounted for, its vigour and creative powers, seem to be proportioned to the weakness and want of cultivation of the understanding. All the records which have descended to us from very ancient times, seem to favor the presumption that the empire of imagination, fiction and romance, in the dark periods of antiquity, gave a tone and character to the human mind; and that the early records of history, only teem with romantic fictions which defy belief, and with delineations of prodigies which never existed, because the philosophic *investigations* of the *understanding* had not yet corrected the *errors* of the *imagination.* It was probably for these reasons, that Homer in his "Illiad" admits and describes a plurality of Gods; and that Ossian's fancy saw the ghosts of departed heroe's. who had been slain in battle, half viewless among the clouds of night. Had the progress and improvement of Homer's understanding enabled him to arrive at the sublime conclusion which announces the existence of one *great first cause,* he never could have delineated in poetic numbers the distinctive characters of his fictitious deities: and, had Ossian not been ignorant enough to believe in ghosts, his imagination never could have deceived him into the belief, that those of his fore-fathers were witnessing from the clouds the sanguinary horrours of his battles? the fact seems to be, as I have said before, that the empire of imagination commences, where the matter of fact and philosophic operations of the *understanding* and *memory* cease; for I. think it will not be contested, even by men of ordinary intelligence, that it is impossible to imagine the *existence* of a thing which we are convinced has *no being:* or fancy a thing to be *true*, which we know to be a *falshood.* Can any man imagine that sugar is bitter, gall sweet, or that two and two make five? No: the truth is, that a knowledge of facts and. realities, destroys all the frost-works of fancy and fiction, and demonstrates clearly, that philosophy and science have nearly extinguished the fire of poetic genius. In other words, few men can be poets in this age of philosophic improvement, who will not borrow or steal from the old writers, or who cannot find subjects of poetic inspiration, on which little or nothing, is or can be certainly known. Newton or Locke, would have cut as contemptible a figure in poetry, as Homer and Ossian would have exhibited in astronomy and metaphysicks.

We all know that the fire of the imagination is weakened and destroyed by old age and experience; and that those who always deal in fictions, are always the victims of folly. The pleasures of imagination, are always the most brilliant and powerful in the youthful mind. and the reasons are obvious. This is the period when all impressions made on the mind, by disclosing to us the opening beauties of nature, and the imposing splendors of creation, are entirely novel and without alloy. This is the period when none of the cares and anxieties of life, overshadow and begloom the fiery prospect of fancied and endless felicities to come: and this too is the period, when our youthful *friendships* are untainted by a knowledge of the baseness and selfishness of mankind—and our loves of the supposed divinity of the female character, are unalloyed by those appalling discoveries of experience, wisdom and philosophy, which teach us, that every thing human is imperfect, and unworthy of our idolatrous devotions? These are the reasons why many modern philosophers have been of opinion, that the state of savage and uncultivated nature, as regards a more refined condition of the human mind, is much more conducive to human happiness than any other; for say these men, "where ignorance is bliss, it is surely folly to be wise." If these delusive fascinations of the imagination could continue through life, uncorrected by the bitter lessons of experience and wisdom; or if man could be so educated, as never to seek or experience happiness but in the *realities* of life and nature, the wild delusions of fancy, would never lead his judgment astray in the pursuit of happiness; nor would he ever be discontented with the moderate enjoyments which the *realities* of existence afford him. But, one of the most difficult lessons in wisdom and philosophy, is to be able to acquire and preserve through life, that balance of character which preserves to us, the innocent delusions of the fancy, without suffering them to interfere with, and ultimately to destroy our rational attachments to the colder realities of life: It is the want of this just equipoise, between phyilosophic moderation and strength of judgment, and the acute sensibilities allied to a cultivated imagination, that constitutes the real vortex in which so many men of enlightened and lofty genius have sunk to rise no more. Relying on the pleasures of imagination for happiness in early life; never dreaming that they are in a world of *sad realities*, which will involve them in misfortunes against which, nothing but the exercise of prudence and judgment can guard them; and continuing to enjoy the present moment, without looking forward to the probable and untoward contingencies of futurity—they are never aroused from their brilliant and illusory visions of fanciful and imaginary happiness, until they are overwhelmed with real miseries and misfortunes, and pressed upon by those imperious calls of want and necessity, which *cannot* be silenced by visionary or imaginary means. Here commence those *pains* of the imagination, those *lacerations* of sensibility, and those *horrible* anticipations of real and unmitigated suffering, which no human language can describe, and which are so often seen to goad the man of genius and superior endowments, to dissipation and intemperance, and precipitate him to all the desperations attendant on ruined fortunes and an early grave! This is the vortex that has swallowed thousands of the greatest men that ever existed; this is the bottomless ocean that has engulfed millions of the brightest and most useful men that ever had existence. It is useless to speak of the love of liquor being the cause of intemperance, as applied to men of lofty and powerful energies of mind; and it is worse than useless to attempt the reformation of such men, without *knowing* and *reaching* the real causes of their derelictions. Nearly all that has been written on the subject of intemperance, has been superficial and nugatory, and confined to the mere contemplations of its *effects*. Would you prescribe remedies for the mere effects of a disease, without knowing and striking at the real causes? Would you attempt to guard yourself against the pointed danger of an assassin, without paralyzing the *arm* that held it to your bosom? I will admit that you may remove the *diseases* and *habits* of intemperance, where they are merely connected with the corporeal system and physical sensations of men, and have nothing whatever to do with the mind, by the administration of medical drugs which will act on that corporeal system, and by the substitution of new bodily habits for old ones; but, beyond these points you cannot go by physical means, when you advance on the confines of the mind, and the intellect-al passions. Here you are in a new region, and must adapt your means to the origin and nature of the disease; you must employ the moral powers of dissuasive eloquence; the divine consolations of Religion, held out by Scripture, to erring and repentant man, and its denunciations against the conduct of the *self-destroyer;* you must employ the maxims of philosophy, and the admonitory precepts of true wisdom; you must sooth the victim of intemperate despair, with reasonable hopes of a better fate, instead of irritating him by abusive and degrading denunciations:—&c. &c. But, as this is a most important subject, I will endeavor to elucidate it a little further. When the causes of disease are connected with the mind and its passions, mere physical restraints, and even punishments, will amount to nothing in attempting a cure. There is a class of mankind, I will admit, who like children, whose *moral susceptibilities* cannot be acted upon, must be restrained from excesses, and even the commission of crimes, by ignominious corporeal terrors and punishments; this class of men always possesses more of the physical or corporeal, than of the moral and mental character, and must be acted on by pillories, whipping-posts, and sometimes gibbets. But, terrors and punishments which merely affect the bodies, have no influence with those men whose minds and passions are morbidly affected; or those who are under strong moral impressions of rectitude of conduct. The whole range of martyrs, who have suffered unspeakable tortures in the cause of religion and patriotism, demonstrate these facts.—Would you then attempt to restrain from intemperance, by mere corporeal and physical means, the man whose mind and its passions are affected? Certainly not; every man whose character is decidedly intellectual, feels that his native dignity is outraged, and degraded by corporeal and ignominious restraints or punishments, and will in nine instances out of ten, destroy himself to escape from his own sentiments of degradation. While the genius of conquest, in the person of Napoleon, was lowering by successive victories all the national banners of Europe, a French soldier of the line presented himself to the Emperor and desired to be shot.

When interrogated as to his reasons, he replied that he had been sentenced to receive ignominious corporeal punishment for some misdeed, rather than submit to which, he preferred *death;* the impression made on the mind of Napoleon was such, that ignominious corporeal punishments were immediately abolished throughout the French armies.

It is almost needless to remark, on those passions of the mind called *hope, love, ambition, &c.,*—that they are all productive of pleasures and pains, in proportion as their influence is bounded by moderation, or characterized by excess. The *pleasures of hope* have been finally celebrated by Campbell;. and are well known to have a powerful influence in blunting the miseries and misfortunes of mankind during life, and even in illuminating their anticipations of a happy immortality beyond the gravel But, the pleasures of hope have their counterpoise of evils and miseries: and when indulged in to excess, or founded on visionary and impossible principles, frequently terminate in disapointment and despair. Here wisdom, fortitude, religion and philosophy, are probably the only essential and efficient preventatives, against those intemperate palliatives of disappointed hope, which have led thousands to drown themselves, their fortunes, and their miseries in the *bowl.* The miseries of despair and disappointed hope, are seldom the portion of those whose *educations* have been moral and judicious, or who have been early taught to distinguish the *realities of life,* from those illusive and *visionary expectations* of it, which never can be realized, even by the greatest prosperity. The visionary gildings with which youthful feeling and animating anticipation invest the untried scenes of life, always dissolve before the lessons of wisdom and experience; and where these privations are followed by positive misfortunes from which there exists no hope of redemption, intemperance almost invariably succeeds, as the only remedy by which temporary alleviation can be obtained. But this conduct is founded in short-sighted and desperate policy; because to the mental pangs of misfortune, are always added the miseries of corporeal disease.

Love is likewise an intellectual passion, and like hope,

is productive of pleasure and pain, happiness and misery. I have before spoken of this passion, as connected with the enjoyments and happiness of man; it now becomes my duty to take a brief view of the sombre colorings of the picture, and to develop some of the causes with which its miseries are connected. Love is always founded on perceptions of *real* or *imaginary* perfections; when this elevated and ennobling sentiment is based on the perception of qualities which really exist, it invariably leads to happiness, and is an unerring indication of superior wisdom; but when it is founded in errors of the imagination, and in the false perception of merely visionary qualities which have no existence, it generally eventuates in misery, and is a decided mark of over-weening stupidity and folly. The first step to misery in wedded love, where the qualities of either of the parties are not sufficiently noble to *sustain the passion*, is the discovery of blemishes of person, disposition, mind or character which were not known previously to marriage. This discovery produces a chill of the affections, which leads to a more narrow and scrutinizing investigation of the causes of our having been decided. If they are found to have originated with ourselves, we invariably undervalue and detest our own judgment which could suffer us thus to be deceived, and immediately become dissatisfied with ourselves: and it requires no great exercise of wisdom to know, that those who are dissatisfied with themselves are displeased with all those around them. On the contrary, if it is found on investigation that we have been deceived by the *hypocrisy* of the individual to whom we are tied by bonds which death alone can dissolve, contempt and detestation are the inevitable consequences; for it is no more possible, for a man or woman of moral discernment to *love* an unworthy object, knowing it to be such, than it is for a human being to *hate* the presence of virtue combined with peerless beauty. Here then commences that series of domestic and conjugal miseries, which defies and bafles the power of mere language to describe: and the parties soon become estranged from and perfectly hateful to each other. Home becomes a hell; the tavern and gaming table are resorted to; to bad company; habits of intemperance succeed; and the event is *death*, by confirmed habits of intoxication, or *life* embittered by negligence, disease, poverty, and want! I am the more particular in mentioning the effects of *love to hatred* turned," and in tracing those effects to their causes, not only because the picture which is true to life may be instrumental in preventing deceptions and *hypocrisy in courtship*, but because it may have a tendency to illustrate the eternal truth, that no miseries can ever be drowned in the midnight howl, unless the chalice contain the poison of death itself?—I said that love was always founded on the perception of real or visionary perfections, with that founded on amiable and noble qualities, I have here, nothing to do, because it is always. permanent, and always unshaken by misfortunes. This position requires no further proof, than can be found in every country, and in the sphere of every man's observations on life. Where, however, the attachment is founded on illusory perceptions, it is not only shortlived in itself, but eternally liable to destruction by variations of fortune. Some persons, indeed all individuals of the human species, are formed by nature, for enjoying the felicities of attachment and love. With these elementary principles, and with a heart alive to the tenderest sensibilities, the devourer of novels and romances, in which the human character is invested with perfections that never pertained to it, is peculiarly liable to miseries and misfortunes in love. I say once for all, and wish it to be borne in mind by the reader: that no inordinate and excessive passion, not even that of love itself, was ever the offspring of correct perceptions of human nature, *such as it really is.* Where is the man or woman of reflection, who does not know that human nature is not perfection; and who is not perfectly convinced, that it is a compound of personal and moral beauties and imperfections. Those who are in time trade acquainted with these philosophic truths; and have early learned to know that man is a compound, to say the best we can of him of virtue and vice—strength and weakness—wisdom and folly, will never experience any of the passions in their extremes.

Their loves and hatreds, their friendships and enmities, and indeed all their other passions, are *true to nature*, and therefore, always characterized by moderation. Loves and hatreds are only felt in the extreme, because in the former case, we are blind to imperfections which really exist; and because in the latter instances, we shut our eyes against many noble traits of character, which would mitigate our unqualified hatreds. The same may be said of our friendships and enmities; and indeed of all our other passions: even the sneaking scoundrel *avarice*, if he did not overrate the objects of his desires, would abandon his swindling propensities, and relax his gripe on the miseries and misfortunes of mankind. It is the immoderate overrating of the objects of our passions, that produces all their excesses; against which no human being can be guarded, unless through the medium of wisdom and intelligence, which alone can stamp the *genuine value* on every object of human desire or pursuit. Few instances are to be found on record, where the miseries of disappointed love have been experienced in the extreme, by persons whose errors of imagination had been corrected by experience, and the acquisitions of true wisdom; and even where all the agonies of disappointed love have been felt in their excesses, they produce different effects upon the different sexes. On woman, they induce a disposition for retirement and a solitary life; which sometimes end in confirmed melancholy; sometimes in insanity, and not unfrequently in a *broken heart*. With man, on the other hand, the excesses of unfortunate love produce very different effects, they urge him to mix in crowded assemblies, in the hum of business, and in the haunts of men: they dispose him to attempt a forgetfulness of his miseries, by exploring new scenes of life, in countries to which he is a stranger; by encountering the dangers of the field and flood; and by drowning the memory of his misfortunes in the oblivion of the bowl!

Of the miseries of *ambition*, and the excesses to which they lead, the space allotted will not allow much to be said. Like love, the passion of ambition, both in moderation and excess, depends for strength on the value we set on objects of ambitious desire. To those whose wisdom teaches them the true value of earthly objects, the passion of ambition is always productive of enjoments; but, when an over-estimate of the objects of ambitious pursuit, arises from false, though dazzling perceptions of those objects, the passion always acquire an uncontrolled dominion in the human breast, producing misery to the individual, and frequently the most dreadful desolations to society and mankind. When ambition is confined to moral bounds; in other words, where it is restricted to *doing good*, it becomes a powerful auxiliary to religion and morality, and to the peace and happiness of mankind.

"But, talents angel bright, if wanting worth,
Are shining instruments in false ambition's hand,
To finish faults illustrious, and give infamy renown!"

Where ambition is laudable, and restricted to beneficent and moral objects, it serves to dignify and adorn the human character: and even, where thus characterized, it meets with failures and disappointments, it produces no serious and lasting miseries to its votaries.. The real passion of ambition is of a heaven-born character; it is founded in a strong desire to be remembered with gratitude and admiration by posterity and future ages—and is the legitimate offspring of a vital and deep-seated sentiment of *immortality?* We see its indications in every department of life, and in every age of the world. The monumental inscriptions of ancient times; the mummied catacombs, and the great pyramids of Egypt themselves, bear witness of the universal prevalence of this all-absorbing sentiment of immortality, and of the dreadful contemplations which accompany the anticipations of being swept from human memory by the hand of time! The desire to be remembered, is as obvious in the schoolboy who inscribes his name on a tree or a rock, as in the lofty and headlong careers of Charlemagne, Alexander and Napoleon:—who desolated nations and overturned empires, to give their achievements to posterity and future ages.—When the passion of ambition, of whatever grade, or to whatever objects directed, is disappointed in its expectatations, it invariably leads to dissatisfaction with life and mankind, and frequently plunges its votaries into the vortex of intemperance and debauchery. These effects are not only confined to the ambition of men possessing lofty and powerful energies of mind, whose objects of ambition are correspondent in elevation, but they are discoverable in all the inferior orders of society, and in all the subordinate ranks of intellectual power; they are in fact, as observable in the *Cæsar* who is disappointed in the possession of an imperial crown, as in the humble votary of literature and science, or the hook-fingered and swindling devotee of avarice, with whom wealth is the idol of adoration! Let any of these men, be finally and permanently disappointed in the first and great objects of their ambition, and if they are destitute of resolution, fortitude, wisdom, and philosophic energy of intellect, they invariably sink in the whirlpool of intemperance, debauchery and sottishness:—Alexander the great, died from the influence of a fit of intemperance, because probably he had no more worlds to conquer: and it is needless to advert to the thousands of instances which every where present themselves, of men of all ranks and grades of life, who sink into insignificance and obscurity, from the effects of intemperance brought on them by disappointed ambition.

I have now, I think, shown some of the various causes of intemperance, and probably to the satisfaction of reflecting men, traced some of them to the physical and mental constitutions of men, as far as it is practicable to be done by observations of mere *effects.* In this brief essay, by no means correspondent with the importance of the subjuct, I have neither followed nor profited by the hacknied theories which have heretofore been published; I have endeavored to view human nature as it is, and to remark the developments of the causes of intemperance, such as they have appeared to me in my medical pursuits; and if I have not been as successful as might be desired by medical men who are the real friends of humanity, I may at least have furnished some materials which may be useful to such fathers of the profession, as Mitchill, Physic, Hossack, and many others, who are engaged in developing the mysticisms of medical science, and rendering them intelligible to mankind.

REMARKS,

PRELIMINARY TO THE

MEDICAL PORTION OF THIS WORK.

I have now done with the passions most material to be thought of in a work like this. I think I have spoken of them as they deserve; and as being the real causes of very many and obstinate diseases; and I also think, without any sort of vanity on the subject, that I have taken views of them which are not only new, but such as will be satisfactory to men who are pleased with *common sense*, and *matter-of-fact* disclosures, instead of visionary theories, and old doctrines that have been worn thread-bare by repetition. Where I have found the *essences* of the passions beyond the reach of investigation, I have freely confessed the truth; being determined not to veil my ignorance of what is most likely hidden from us by divine wisdom, by long sounding words, which, when explained would make men of common sense laugh at medical quackery, and by technical language which means next to nothing. I have spoken of the passions as I have seen and witnessed their effects on the human system, and on the peace and happiness of society generally; and particularly as regards intemperance, or rather excess in fear—joy—anger—jealousy—love—grief—religion—gluttony and drunkenness, I have ventured to go as far into some of the remote and constitutional causes of them, as I possible could without running into mere theories, not supported by the experience of mankind. In treating of them, I have been limited much by want of space; and have therefore in some instances, been compelled to comprise as much information as possible in a few words; and I must also observe here, that on intemperance, religion, love, jealousy and anger, I have extended my remarks further than on the rest of the pasions; because I consider them of vastly more importance to the *health* and *happiness*, and to the *diseases* and *miseries* of mankind, than all the rest of the passions put together. I have classed Religion and Intemperance under the head of the passions, because all our desires and aversions become passions, when they become too strong to be controlled and moderated by moral sense and reason; and if even these were not the facts, *mere names* are nothing but blinds, frequently placed by the learned between the reader and the *realities of things*, to conceal the naked poverty and barrenness of the sciences, as professed by literary men. If our education consisted more in a knowledge of *things*, and less in a knowledge of mere *words* than it does, and if the great mass of the people knew how much pains were taken by scientific men, to throw dust in their eyes by the use of ridiculous and high-sounding terms, which mean very little if any thing, the learned professors of science would soon lose much of their mock dignity, and mankind would soon be undeceived, as to the little difference that really exists between themselves and the *very learned* portion of the community. I am the more particular on this subject, not because I wish to lower the public opinion respecting the real value of medical knowledge, but because the time has arrived when the *hypocrisy* which has attached itself to *religion*, the pettifogging *dissimulation* which has crept into the practice and science of law, and the *quackeries* which have so long disgraced the practice and science of *medicine* are about to be scattered to the four winds of heaven, by the progress of real knowledge, and the general diffusion of useful intelligence. The great body of the people are beginning to find out as I before remarked in substance—that when we take from the learned sciences all their technical and bombastic language, they immediately become plain common sense, very easily to be understood by all ranks of men. I have also said, and I again repeat it, that the really valuable materials in medicine, and those which are the most powerful in the cure of diseases, are few and simple, and very easily to be procured in all countries; and on this subject, I will say something more which may probably, be considered new. I not only believe, that every country produces, or can be made to produce, whatever is necessary to the wants of its inhabitants—but also whatever is essential to the cure of diseases incidental to each country; it is by no means probable, that an all-wise Creator would create man with wants he could not supply, and subject him to diseases for which there were no remedies to be found in nature, and in all the different countries and climates of which he is an inhabitant. If such were not the facts, how miserable would be the condition of the human species; eternally harrassed by the calls of wants which could not be satisfied, and afflicted with diseases for which they could find neither the means of alleviation nor cure? How did the Indian Nations of this country become so populous and powerful, unless from finding the means of supplying their wants, and of mitigating and curing their diseases, on the soil and in the countries which gave them birth? The fact is, that this country, like all other countries, produces spontaneously, or can be made to produce, by the genius and industry of its inhabitants, all that is required by the wants of the people, and all that is essential in medical science; and the sooner we set about finding out, and fully exploring the resources of our own country, the sooner will we be clear of the abuses and countless impositions in the adulteration of medical drugs; and the sooner will we be exempted from individual and national *dependence* on other nations. There are many drugs that come from a broad that are made good for nothing, by adulterations or mixtures before they reach us, or lose their virtues by long standing and exposure; and any professed druggist if he will tell you the truth, will tell you the same; and these among many others, are the reasons why, I mean to be very particular in showing you, as respects the plants, and roots, &c., of this country, not only how great are our resources, but how easily we can evade roguery and imposition, and obtain pure and unadulterated materials in medicine, if we will be industrious in developing the real resources of this country. The science of botany, like many others I could name, has dwindled into mere mumery and hard sounding names of plants, &c. I can find you, indeed you can easily find them yourselves, very many individuals profoundly learned in botany, who can tell you all about the *genus* and *species* of plants and herbs, and can call them individually by their long Latin names, who can tell you nothing whatever about their use to mankind, or whether they are poisonous or otherwise; and I want to know whether such information, or rather such want of information, is not mere learning without wisdom, and science without knowledge. But why need I speak of the science of botany alone, as having sunk into frivolity and superficial nonsense; the same may be said of many other of the sciences, which were in their origin and early progress useful to mankind. Real knowledge consists in understanding both what is *useful* and what is *injurious* to mankind; and true wisdom amounts to nothing more than appropriating to our use whatever is beneficial, and avoiding whatever is injurious to our enjoyments and happiness: this is the true distinction between *common sense* and *nonsense*: if you will have the same idea in finer language, between *wisdom* and *folly*. For the common and useful purposes of mankind, the refined fripperies and hair-drawn theories of mere science, are of no use whatever; indeed they never have had much other effect, than to excite a stupid admiration for men who pretended to know more than the mass of mankind: and it is this stupid admiration, this willingness to be duped by the impudent pretensions of science and quackery combined, that has led to impositions and bare-laced frauds upon society, without number. Wherever *artifice* is used, it is either to cover defects, or to perpetrate impositions and frands; and if you wish to know how much of this artifice is in vouge in the science and practice of medicine, ask some physician of eminence to give you in plain English, the meaning of those mysterious and high-sounding names you see plastered on bottles, glass jars, gallipots and drawers in a drug-store, or doctor's shop. There you may see in large and imposing capitals—*Datura Stramonium*, which simply means stink-weed, or vulgarly Jamestown weed: *Tanacetum Vulgare*, which in english means Common Tansy:

Chenopodium Anthelmenticum, good heaven, what a name for Jerusalem Oak: *Spigelia Marilandica*, which means nothing more nor less than Pink Root: *Alium Sativum*, which means Cloves of Garlic: and who would ever suppose, unless he were previously iniciated into the sublime mysteries of the "Physicians' Materia Medica," that *Cantharis Vittata*, was the Potatoe Fly—that *Hedeoma Pulegioides*, was merely the common plant Pennyroyal: that *Phytolacca Decandra*, was nothing but Poke-weed: that *Panax Quinquefolium*, was nothing but Ginseng: that *Rubus Villosus*, meant in plain English, the Black-berry: that *Upatorium Perfoliatum*, was nothing but Bone-set: that *Polygala Seneka*, was Snake Root: that *Laurus Benzoin*, was no more than Spice-wood: that *Asarium Canadense*, was Wild Ginger: that *Babtisca Tinctoria*, was only another name for Wild Indigo: that *Hydrastis Canadensis* was nothing but Yellow Root: that *Podophyllium Peltatum*, was merely the May Apple, or common Jalap of the shops: that *Sanguinaria Canadensis*, was no more than the Puccoon, or Blood Root, well known to every old woman in the state: that *Cornus Florida*, was nothing but Dogwood: that *Gillenia Frifoliata*, was merely Indian Physic: that *Symplocarpus Fœtida*, was nothing but Skunk Cabbage: *Anthemus Cotula*, was the Wild Chamomile. that *Lobelia Inflata*, was nothing but Wild Tobacco: that *Comptonia Asplenifolia*, was only the Sweet Fern:—and so on to the end of the chapter. But on consideration of the importance of this information, I will add a few more instances of the shameful impositions practiced on the mass of the people, by the quackeries connected, with medical science. They are as follows: *Oleum Ricini*, meaning Castor Oil: *Unguentum Picis Liquidæ*, meaning Tar Ointment: *Oleum Terebinthinæ* meaning the Oil of Turpentine: *Zanthoxylum Clava Herculis*, meaning the common Prickly Ash of our country: *Sal. Nitre*, meaning Salt Petre: *Tartarized Antimony*, meaning emetic Tartar; *Sulphat Soda*, meaning nothing but Epsom Salts: *Ruta Graveslens*, meaning our common Garden Rue: *Salva Oficinalis*, the common Sage, *Sambucus Nigra*, common Elder: *Serpentaria Virginiana*, Virginia Snake-root. *Myrtis Pim-*

ento, common Pepper: *Elmus Americana*, meaning Red Elm: *Aqua Calcis*, meaning Lime-Water: and *Carbo Ligni*, *Charcoal* of *Wood!!* These I think, are fair specimens of the useless technical terms and phrases, with which the science of medicine has been encumbered, by a policy hostile to the interests of every community; in which the reader will easily distinguish, if he will look one foot beyond his nose, not only that big words and high sounding phrases are not superior wisdom, but that three-fourths of the whole science of physic, as now practiced and imposed upon the common people, amounts to nothing but fudge and mummery. In fact, it has always seemed to me, whenever I have reflected seriously on this subject, that all these hard names of common and daily objects of contemplation, were originally made use of to *astonish the people;* and to aid what the world calls learned men, in deceptions and fraud. The more nearly we can place them on a level in point of *knowledge*, the happier we would become in society with each other, and the less danger there would be of *tyranny* on the one hand, and submission to the degradations of personal slavery on the other: nor are these all the benefits that would certainly arise from a more equal distribution of useful information among the people. We all know perfectly well, and if we do not we ought to do so, that there are two ways of acquiring a greater name than common among men. One is by putting on affected airs of superior wisdom, and the concealment of weakness and ignorance to which all men are subject: and the other is, by exhibiting to the world, grate and useful energies of mind and character, of which nothing can be more decisive proof, than success in our undertakings. But this is not all; the less we know of the weaknesses and imperfections of what the world calls *great men*, the more we are disposed to overrate their merits and wisdom, and to become their humble followers, admirers, and slaves. This is the reason why I wish to impress upon your minds, the simple and important truth, that there is not so great a difference between men as there appears to be; and that you are always to find out in the characters of men, the difference between *impudent presumption*, which seeks to blind you to defects, and modest and *unassuming merit*, which is above hypocrisy and deception. On the other hand, I wish you to remember, that the *more* we know of the ignorance and weaknesses of *great men*, ignorance and weaknesses which they all have, however they may try to hide them, the more easily we will feel ourselves on a level with them, the less we will be compelled to think of their assumed superiority, and consequently the less danger their will be of our becoming their most humble followers, their tools of dirty purposes, and in fact their slaves. The fact is, if we could always strip the fine coat, the ruffled shirt, the well blacked boots, and what would be better than all, the hypocrisy and presumption, from about those who pretend to lord it over us: and if we could always hit the true medium of truth and justice, in forming our opinions of each other, there would be much less fraud in this world than there is: for you may rest assured, and I desire you most particularly to fix it in your memory, that no man or junto of men, ever yet attempted to cheat or impose on your credulity, without first forming a contemptuous opinion of your discernment; in other words, all attempts to cheat and deceive you, are direct insults to your understandings.———With these remarks, in which I have been as plain as possible in point of language; in order that you might the better understand my meaning, I will now go on to describe to you, in as plain language as can be made use of, all the diseases we are mostly liable to in this country, and all the best remedies for those which are brought to us from other countries. I intend also to describe particularly all the roots, and plants, and so on, which we have about us, in our gardens, barnyards, fields and woods, which are useful in the cure of diseases. These will be important considerations, because I am convinced we have many things the most common about us, that as medicines, are as good as any in the world, and the knowledge of which, by the people themselves, will enable them to cure their own diseases in many instances; and avoid many and great expences. The language I will make use of, as I said before, will be extremely plain, the object of the work being, not so much to instruct the learned as the unlearned; nor will I regard in the slightest degree, any of those petty critical remarks, which may be made on such language, provided I succeed in adopting language which can be understood by those for whom this work is intended. And here I cannot avoid remarking, that since this work of mine was commenced, and measureably finished, I have received from New York, the first number of a periodical work on the same plan that this is, to be written by some of the greatest medical men in the United States, some of whom are Mitchell, Hossack, Mott M'Neven, &c. These gentlemen as well as myself, are convinced that the time has come, when all the mysteries and technical language of the science of medicine, must be made plain to the people of this country, and when the old frauds, and quackeries of the profession must be laid down, and discontinued in practice. I am gratified that men whose names have so much weight, have undertaken to make the science of medicine plain; because otherwise, I should have stood alone in the great attempt, and had to contend with all the petty critical remarks, of all the petty professors of the science, and all those who wish to make a mystery, of what every man in the community is fully able to understand if well explained.

Before concluding these observations, it may not be improper to make some remarks, intended for the more youthful portion of those into whose hands this work may fall. Some of the diseases I am compelled to mention and explain, necessarily relate to a sex whose weaknesses and delicacies of constitution, entitle them to the highest respect, and the most tender consideration; nor can any youth be guilty of a more flagrant breach of humanity, nor more completely disclose a brutal and unfeeling disposition, than by manifesting a wish to turn into unfeeling ridicule, the diseases and calamities of women: I would at once pronounce such a young man a brute, a poltroon and a coward. But I am confident there are few if any such in this country, because there are few or none who will not recollect, that their venerable mothers were of the female sex, and that they have probably sisters and other relatives of the same sex. I wish the younger portion of my readers also to recollect, and I most respectfully request them to do so—that when perusing my book, on the various diseases to which the human body is liable, as to their uncertainty of life, and the slender thread on which it hangs. I wish them to remember, how unknown to them are the vicissitudes ofthe world; how easily they may be thrown into strange lands, destitute, friendless, and afflicted: I wish them to engrave on their minds, that sacred rule of doing all things to others, which they would wish others should do unto them: that they would always let the tear of sympathy drop for their fellow-creatures in affliction and distress, and always let their hearts melt at the tale of human woe, for which God will bless them in all their works.

ON SLEEP.

"What better name may slumber's bed become.
Night's sepulchre, the universal home,
When weakness, strength, vice, virtue sunk supine,
Alike in naked helplessness recline;
Glad for a while to heave *unconscious* breath,
And wake to wrestle with the *dread of death.*"—

To exist as it were between death and life; to rove in imagination, unfettered by the cold and strong realities of waking existence, through a boundless realm of visions which seem real; this is what we call sleep, without knowing much of any thing about its causes. The real cause of sleep has been a matter of much guessing and speculation with medical men; even very *learned philosophers* have disagreed in opinion respecting the cause of sleep, and nearly all the little we know on the subject is, that when the sable curtain of night is drawn around us, the mind and body worn out and exhausted by the fatigues of the day, sink into soft repose.

Napoleon, whose genius seemed capable of seizing every subject of contemplation with a giant grasp, remarked while distinguishing between *sleep* and *death*, that sleep was the suspension of the *voluntary* powers of man:—and that *death* was a suspension of those that were *involuntary.* This was probably the most correct distinction between sleep and death, that has ever to my knowledge been drawn by any man; and I will endeavor to explain as clearly as possible, what I think he intended by it. When we lie down to sleep, we voluntarily exclude the operation of the senses; in other words, we see nothing, hear nothing, feel nothing, smell nothing, taste nothing: and endeavor to *think* of nothing—this is as far as we can go in the matter, for no man can possibly tell when he falls asleep, or in other words, when an entire suspension of the voluntary powers of the body and mind ţkes place. While in this situation, however, we know ,ıat the sleeper breathes, his heart beats, the blood cir- ,ulates, that the stomach digests its food, and that perspiration takes place: now, as the will of the sleeper has nothing to do with these matters, they depend upon the involuntary powers of the human system, and when these powers cease, *death* takes place. This is as far as we can go as regards sleep and death, for as to dreams and their causes, a'l we :an tell about them is, that during sleep the mind and im- ·gination act with such brightness and power, as to leave trong impressions on the waking memory; I say the mind ınd imagination, because we not only distinguish objects as f they were present, but because we can and sometimes actually do reason about them and that too very correctly.

It is impossible for us to enjoy good health, unless blessed with sound and refreshing sleep: without sleep the whole frame is thrown into disorder, and a strong disposition to disease; and the mind is much confused and weakened. Without the due repose of sleep, the appetite for food is depraved and sometimes lost; the health and strength fail; and the spirits become distressed and melancholy in the extreme. The acrid matter is thrown off during sleep, insensible perspiration is increased, and the body increases in growth in ı greater degree than when awake and actively employed. You are much taller in the morning when rising from a re- 'reshing sleep, than during or after a day of severe fatigue. Sleep assists much in the cure of diseases, and may be considered, if sound and refreshing, a favorable symptom of recovery in sickness. It is a welcome visitor in fevers, because it diminishes the rapid motion of the blood, and consequently cools and refreshes the system. It is of infinite benefit in dysentary or flux, because it restrains the frequency of the stools; also in female diseases—in consumptions, rheumatisms, pleurisies, and in flooding; in fact, the cure of almost all diseases require sound and refreshing sleep, and so well known was this fact to a physician of great eminence, that he seldom or never gave his patients operative medcines, before he had produced sound sleep by the admin- ·stration of an opiate. The body receives nourishment during sleep; and this is the reason why the growth is greatly promoted by sleep; all men who are inclined to obesity or fatness sleep much. All young plants grow in the night time; indeed all young aimals grow in the night while sleeping; and this is the reason why children require more sleep than grown persons.

I have already told you in my Introduction, that man is a creature of *habit*, and may therefore accustom himself to almost any thing by practice. Napoleon had an alarum watch, for the purpose of awaking him at any hour he chose. During a campaign, one of his field officers entered his tent at 2 o'clock in the morning, having some important business with him. Contrary to his expectation, he found the emperor up and dressed, and employed in laying off the plan for the battle of the next day, and addressed him thus: "you are up late emperor." O no, said Napoleon, "I have just risen; my sleep is over." After calling for his coffee, his usual practice immediately on rising, he communicated to his officer the method he had followed, to ascertain the time of sleep required by his constitution. "I had," said he, "been accustomed to awake every night after sleeping five or six hours, and to continue awake during the remainder of the night. This led me to believe that I remained longer in bed, than nature and my constitution required; and determined me by this alarum watch, to abridge my hours of sleep *ten minutes* each night, by rising ten minutes earlier. I soon discovered how much sleep nature required, by the length of time I slept soundly, which was only five hours. I have since continned this practice, and find my health good, and nature sufficiently restored and refreshed by it. When in actual service, and my mind much employed, my usual time of sleep is but four hours, from eleven till three inclusive, &c." As in all other cases, too much or too little sleep, produces injury to health and strength of body and vivacity of mind and feelings. The bed in which we sleep for comfort and health is very important: the use of feather-beds, particularly in the summer season, is extremely unhealthy; and how persons can lie snoaring, soaking and sweating, in a huge feather-bed for eight or nine hours at a time, which is usual with many of the wealthy people of the western country is to me perfectly astonishing; and I wish them to understand distinctly, that by so doing the following consequences inevitably follow. Their flesh becomes soft, flabby, pale, and weak; the digestive organs of the stomach become relaxed, feeble, and of no account, as is proved by the want of appetite; in fact, the whole muscular and nervous systems, become so impaired and lost in tone and vigor, as to be incapable of performing the duties assigned to them by nature. A mattress made of shucks, nicely cleaned and hackled, forms a delightful bed for summer; and if you would enjoy sleep to the extent which is essential to health and strength, avoid a feather bed as you would the plague, and sleep on mattresses of some kind, or on a straw bed, or even pick out the softest plank in the floor and stretch yourself on it. It is worthy of observation that most persons who sleep hard, are more healthy and lively than others: look at the Indians who sleep on deer and bear skins; look at soldiers who sleep on blankets; and at wagoners, who always on journies, sleep on hard mattresses on the floors of houses, or on the hard ground in tents. And it is worthy of particular remark, that a hard bed promotes digestion, and prevents incubus or night-mare, that demon of digestion which is a scourge of thousands. All asthmatic persons, or in other words, those who have the phthisic, should sleep hard, and in refreshing and pure air; feather beds in close rooms are murdering thousands of these people by inches. Many people are subject at night to palpitations of the heart, shortness of breath, which seems to threaten suffocation, great anxiety and depression of spirits, uneasiness for which they cannot account, tremors, and so on, usually called nervous. These people ought always to sleep on hard beds and in pure air: and they ought always, in warm weather, to wash or sponge their bodies with cold water, taking care immediately after, to wipe themselves dry with a coarse towel, and then to use the flesh-brush; this course of proceeding, will just before going to bed, produce sound and refreshing sleep. Warm bathing of the feet before going to bed, is of infinite service in causing sound sleep; the bath ought to have a little salt in it, and to be continued fifteen or twenty minutes; after which the feet ought to be wiped dry, and well brushed with a flesh-brush: persons subject to cold feet, and those much advanced in age, will find much benefit from the flesh-brush, and from wrapping their feet in well dried flannel before going to bed. When we lie down to sleep, every painful thought and unpleasant circumstance, should if possible, be banished from the mind; and we should always endeavor to turn our meditations into channels, which will leave tranquil and soothing impressions behind them when we fall asleep. Dr. Franklin's rules for sleeping well, and having pleasant dreams, are very plain: he says—"eat moderately during the day, and avoid heavy suppers; sleep on a hard bed with your feet to the fire, especially in very cold weather; and above all, during the day, take sufficient exercise. If you awake from a sense of uneasiness or accident, and cannot again compose yourself to sleep, get out of the bed and throw open the bed-clothes, and expose your naked body to the action of the cold air, there is no danger of taking cold. When the cold air becomes unpleasant, return to bed; your skin has by this time discharged its perspirable matter, and you will soon fall asleep, and your sleep will be sound and refreshing. I have frequently tried this method with success, and find after exposing my body to the cold air, a quick desire to sleep. I therefore recommended it as free from any danger of taking cold. Persons unaccustomed to this method, should gradually accustom themselves to a free circulation of air. The higher and more airy the bed-chamber, the better for health." As man is the creature of habit, he may bring himself gradually to bear almost any exposure; but great and sudden changes in our habits should always be avoided. Small close bed-rooms, and particularly bed curtains, should always be avoided, and for this reason; in close rooms and curtained beds, you breathe unchanged air, which has become impure from previous breathing. As boiling water does not grow hotter by longer boiling, if the particles that receive greater heat can escape, so living bodies do not putrify and become corrupt, if the particles as fast as they become corrupted, can be thrown off. Nature always expels much bad and corrupted matter, by the pores of the skin and lungs: you may easily prove this to yourself, if your nose is sufficiently sharp, by catching a scent of the breath and sweat of many persons. In a free and pure air, the corrupted perspirable matter from the skin is immediately carried off; but in a close room or bed, or in a dirty bed even in pure air, these particles of bad matter are not carried off, and sickness is nearly always the consequence. Dirty rooms and beds, cause a great deal of disease, and persons cannot easily be too cleanly, in their habits, if they wish to be healthy; but I will say more on this subject when I come to speak of *baths.* In close rooms or dirty beds, we breathe the same had and corrupted air, over and over again, so that at every moment it becomes more injurious. *Confined air*, when saturated or filled with perspirable matter, must remain with us, and produces many of our diseases. Persons who are inclined to bc fat, or who are in reality so, should sleep on hard beds—take a great deal of exercise—never sleep more than five or six hours—and use well the flesh-brush, particularly over the *joints.* By these means, together with preper regimen, which means food and drink the bulk of the body may be reduced, and the flesh made firm and strong.

Nothing undermines and destroys the health and constitution, with so much rapidity as want of sleep; gamesters, courtezans, debauchees, and infact of all those who lose much sleep, prove by their pale and sallow complexions, the want of "nature's sweet restorer." Many instances have been known in London and other large cities, where the waiters and servants in gaming houses, have become absolutely insane or crazy for want of sleep. A person by long sitting up and losing sleep, may at length become unable to sleep, from extreme irritability of the nervous system; therefore persons of an irritable habit, should always be cautious of such circumstances. I have known many instances of apoplexy being produced by want of sleep: persons should therefore, when such cases are apprehended, to bathe their feet in warm water when they lie down, and take a dose of cooling medicine, such as Epsom Salts; or in case of fever to lose a little blood, and take a slight opiate. More, however, will be said on the subject of sleep, and its diminution and excess, under the head of *exercise.*

EXERCISE.

If you would enjoy health, take *exercise* and be temperate; and if you attend to these things properly, you will have but little use for either physicians or medicines.—Temperance, exercise and rest, are the sure guarantees of sound health and vigour, if you have naturally a good constitution, and almost the only *sure means* of amending and preserving a weak and deficient one. Persons who take proper exercise, and combine that exercise with temperance, are seldom sick; and those who fly to medicines on every trifling cause of complaint, in nine cases in ten, might relieve themselves, by abstaining from food for a short time, living on light diet, and taking as much exercise as will cause perspiration, without impairing their strength by excessive fatigue. Exercise, for the purpose of producing perspiration, and throwing off the excrementitious or bad matter from the system, is much better than any merely medical means; not only because it is the means which nature herself prescribes, but because, unlike medical drugs generally, it strengthens instead of weakening the system. We are always to suppose, from the fact of the horrible fetor or stench which arises from the bodies of those on whom fever has just been broken, that the retention of that bad matter in their systems contrary to nature, was the real cause of their febrile or feverish disorders; and does it not follow, that by getting clear of that matter by natural means, before it has time to accumulate and produce malignant and obstinate diseases, is much better than to *force the vital organs* into a destructive action for producing the same effect? In other words—do you not know, that when you force the stomach into laborious action, or indeed any other vital organ of the system, that you always weaken and impair its energies, and lay the foundation of many diseases, to which the system under other circumstances, would be a stranger? A person of common size, and in good health, will perspire or sweat, from three to four pounds weight in twenty-four hours, if proper exercise be taken, and the fact is, that there is more in proportion of all the fetid matter of the system, discharged from the skin in perspiration or sweat, than there is by the stool and urine combined: and can you not as easily see as I can tell you, that unless this bad matter is thrown off from the body by *exercise* and *perspiration*, that the fluids of the body will become greatly corrupted, and all its vessels oppressed and morbidly irritated, and that disease must and will follow? There is no *witchcraft* about the disease to which we are all liable; they are all matters of plain reasoning between causes and effects, to the full understanding, of which, every man is as competent as any other man. Are we not witnesses daily and hourly, of the beneficial effects of exercise, in the cure of diseases in which both medicines and medical men have failed? Half the diseases of delicate women, and in fact nearly all the diseases connected with hysterics and hypochondria, arise from want of due exercise in the open, mild, and pure air. Instead of stewing in a close room, and indulging in moody and gloom anticipations: and instead of lying in a huge feather-bed until nine or ten o'clock in the morning, dosing through morbid dreams and vainly courting sleep, the woman of delecate nerves and infirm health, and the gloomy hypochondriac who has probably not sweated for months together, ought to spring from the feathered couch at day-light; view the opening and brilliant landscapes of nature, just kindling into life and beauty under the beams of the rising sun—and breast the pure mountain breeze!

I have just told you, that exercise will not only preserve your health if you have a good constitution, but that it will frequently give healthy action and strength to a weak and deficient one. Cicero is described by Plutarch, as being at one period of his, life, thin and weakly; so much so indeed, from the debility of his stomach, as to be able to eat but once a day, and that a very small quantity. In this debilitated and weakly condition, he traveled to Athens for the recovery of his health, and so great were the effects of his exercise, that together with the gymnastic exercise of the place, he became firm and robust—and his voice, which had before been squeaking and harsh, was changed for melodious, deep and sonorous tones. The same writer, Plutarch, describes the great Roman warrior Julius Cæsar, as being originally of very delecate health, pale and soft skin, and of very feeble constitution by nature, and subject to fits; but that by a military life, using coarse diet and great exercise, he not only became inured to the hardships and exposures of war, but healthy, active, vigorous and strong. It is not worth while to give any more instances, of the powerful influence which exercise has on the human system; if you wish to know more about it, look at the brawny arms and strong chests of sailors, who are always pulling ropes, and contending with the winds and storms of the ocean; look at the strong figure of the sturdy woodman, who makes the forests bow to the sound of the axe; and indeed at all persons who are engaged in active and laborious callings: and then, by comparing these people with those who are always confined to their houses, to books and sitting postures, and to trades which prevent them from moving about, you will be able very easily to see the effects of exercise much better than I can describe or tell you of them. I feel confident in saying, that by exercise on horse-back for women, and exercise on foot for men, together with some attention to food and drink, this dreadful disease called *dyspepsia* or *indigestion*, which paralyzes both body and mind, and makes existence itself a burthen, together with the whole train of nervous diseases to which we are subject, may be cured completely without the aid of medicine, by laying down and following systematic rules for exercise, rest, and diet.

All the quack medicines of cleansing the blood, which you perceive in the news-papers, are mere impositions on the public. Such medicines have their day, and then die off to make room for new catalogues, without any benefit except enriching the imposters who invent them. The sure remedies for impure blood, and consequent eruptions of the skin, are those which nature prescribes, and which simply are *exercise, temperance*, and *cleanliness* of person, if you will mind these things, you need care nothing about *cosmetics* and *lotions*, and such nonsense, which always sooner or later do immense injury. We see daily and almost hourly, persons who have been accustomed to exercise and labor in their youth, changing their former modes of life for those of ease, wealth, refinement, and idleness, &c.,—and we very soon also see, that these persons immediately begin to sink into all the diseases which arise from the corrupted habits of body, merely for want of their accustomed exercise and active habits; diseases to which they would probably not have been liable, had they continued in their original habits of exercise and useful industry. We see them immediately laboring under morbid eruptions of the skin, jaundice, nervous irritability, palsy, indigestion, consumptions, and heaven above knows what more diseases too tedious to name. In all these cases, let me urge upon you the vast and unspeakable importance of exercise, and regular diet, by which last I mean, never touching spiritous liquors of any kind. Follow the French rulese in these respects, and you will enjoy all that sprightly vigor of mind, and buoyant elasticity of health and feelings for which that people, are celebrated in all parts of the world. The French people, from their habitual taking exercise, and nearly always being temperate in eating and drinking, are exempted in a great degree from those diseases which arise from want of exercise, gormandizing on strong food, drinking spirituous liquors, and sleeping immoderately and in close chambers. In these respects, nearly all the rest of the world ought to take lessons from them. We all know very well, that due exercise and rest, combined with light and temperate eating and drinking, always produce cheerfulness and serenity; and how do they do so? Why, simply by preventing obstructions in the system; and by removing them whenever they present themselves. You seldom find a

Frenchman gloomy, oppressed in his feelings, despondent—No: and for these good reasons, he seldom omits to be active in his movements; to take exercise and proper rest; and above all, he seldom eats heavily, and immediately lies down to snore away ten or twelve hours, to the exclusion of exercise beneficial to health. We all know very well, that sluggardism or sedentary habits, and want of exercise in proportion to our strength, produces uneasy and bad sleep, costiveness of the bowels, a dry and feverish skin, and a thousand other things connected with obstructions; and we all know just as well, that exercise duly taken, will always produce sound and easy sleep, that it has a tendency to open the bowels and to keep them open and regular, and to remove all obstructions of the skin, of the lungs, of the liver, &c. &c. to the end of the chapter: and yet we will lie in bed, or sit about in a close warm room, breathing an atmosphere sufficient to poison us, and gorge our systems with medical drugs, enough to destroy the whole tone and energies of the stomach and bowels! I say again; instead of the medicines always used to remove obstructions, to make sweat flow, to make the blood circulate freely, and to excite all the healthy sensations and excretions, take *exercise* in the pure air, live temperately on light diet and drink, never provoke sleep by any other means than natural ones, and sleep no more than is necessary to renovate the system. Under such circumstances as these, you will have no use for mercurial purges, nor any medicines save those of a simple and harmless character. Morning and evening are the proper times for taking exercise; rise early and walk from one to two miles; in the evening also devote an hour to exercise in the open air. You may also use weights of from five to six pounds, which, when taken into the hands, are to be thrown backward and forward so as to produce an action in the chest; this exercise is properly adapted to persons of weak breasts, and particularly to females. I have frequently seen persons so extremely weak in the chest, and so what we call *short-winded*, as to be unable to ascend the smallest hill without getting out of breath; and who, by the use of these weights a short time, have become so much improved as to be enabled to ascend the highest hills without inconvenience or oppression of the chest. The great object of exercise: and it will always have those effects when judiciously taken, are to increase and regulate the secretions and excretions, by the skin of the kidneys, &c. &c.—to give power to the muscles; to impart tone and strength to the nerves; and where a person is fat and unwieldly in size, to reduce the superfluities of flesh and fat; to reduce the quantity of blood, and to make it thinner and lighter. The other benefits resulting from exercise are, good appetite, good and easy digestion, tranquility and serenity of mind and feelings, pleasant and refreshing sleep, astonishing increase of strength and wind in breathing, &c.—I have seen a boy on the Mediterranean, his carriage being filled with passengers, run by the side of his horses at considerable speed for ten and fifteen miles together, without being fatigued at the end of the journey, or being the least oppressed for the want of breath. These boys subsisted on a few bunches of grapes, and a small flask of wine, daily, both of which they carry suspended from their necks. The cheerful dispositions of these poor boys, and their great breath and strength, convinced me fully of the great benefits arising from diet and exercise. The advantages of the training system, are not confined to pedestrians or walkers—or to pugilists or boxers alone: or to horses which are trained for the chase and the race track: they extend to man in all conditions; and were training introduced into the United States, and made use of by physicians in many cases instead of medical drugs, the beneficial consequences in the cure of many diseases, would be very great indeed.

WARM OR TEPID BATH.

It is impossible to find language to express in adequate terms, the importance of this powerful preserver and restorative of health—the great and almost indescribable luxury, the *bath*.

Considering its importance to the preservation of health, and the cure of very many of our most afflicting diseases I am truly astonished that the warm or tepid bath should be so little used in the western country.

Warm baths are such as have a temperature between the 76th and 98th degrees of the thermometer; but, persons having no thermometer, indeed there is no need of one for regulating the temperature of the water, have only to consult their own sensations in entering the bathing tub: because their own temperament in contact with the water, will immediately advise them of the temperature required: the only inconvenience that can ever be experienced in using the warm bath, will be in being compelled to leave its comforts. The usual time of bathing is from twenty minutes to half an hour; but with regard to the time, it is not material: the feelings and sensations of the bather will better determine this point than I can tell him. The warm bath, contrary to the general opinion, does not heat the body; it has on the contrary an opposite effect, inasmuch as it obviously abates the quickness of the pulse, and reduces the pulsations in proportion to the time we remain in the warm water.

When persons have travelled a long journey, and feel much fatigued, or over heated by exposure to the sun, or their minds are much disturbed, the bath will be found an excellent remedy for invigorating the whole system, and at the same time reducing the irregular and quick action of the blood. Indeed I feel confident, that in thousands of instances, if the bath were used in the first symptoms of those irregular and feverish feelings which prey upon the mind and body, very many persons would escape sick beds. During my practice in Virginia, I escaped the fever prevalent in Botetourt county, called the *lick fever*, in several instances after having felt distinctly all the symptoms of that disease, by the speedy use of the warm bath, and gentle purgatives of epsom salts. Had I not used the bath, I feel confident I could not have escaped this dreadful and malignant disease, being exposed during its prevalence, in attendance on a great many patients. The warm bath is of very great utility, to persons troubled with eruptions or breakings out of the skin, such as itch, and indeed venereal sores. In hyochondriacal, hysteric, and insane cases—and infact on persons laboring under madness, the beneficial effects of warm baths are always visible: in scorbutic and old ulcers or sores, when attention has been paid to regimen, the utilities of the bath are equally great. In palsy and all nervous diseases, I recommend warm bathing as one of the most effectual remedies.—Doctor Charleton of Bath in England, states, that out of 996 paralytics most of whom had resisted the powers of medicine, 813 were benefited by the application of the warm bath at the hospital of that city. In a great variety of chronic or inveterate complaints, such as billious diseases, derangements of the liver, and of the stomach and digestive functions, it is impossible to describe to you its useful effects; and I solicit you with every sincerity of heart, to use the warm bath individually, and in your families, as one of the efficient preventives and cures of disease which is in every man's reach. In using the bath with some system and regularity, you will ward off many hours confinement by ill health; save the expense of many a Doctor's bill; and prevent you from having a ruined constitution, and a stomach worn out by swallowing medicines: for I do assert, without fear of contradiction, but by the *ninnehammers* of the profession, that if the warm bath were more frequently used, with proper abstainance from food, on the approach of fever, and many other diseases which I shall enumerate under their proper heads, in five cases in ten, medical assistance would not *be required.* In all cases of debility from spasms—in pain—in cholic—in cramp—and in anxiety and restlessness, the bath will relieve and tranquilize the system. In hectic or consumptive fever, I have found it of great benefit from the fact of its lessening the heat; and most particularly beneficial, when the liver was connected with this dreadful disease. In dyspepsia or indigestion, this terrible disease which makes life itself a burthen, the bath is a valuable assistant and comforter in the cure.—All young persons who manifest a disposition to stop at a premature point of growth, in other words, to remain pigmies for life, should use the bath; because it always promotes the growth of the body, increases the proportions of the limbs, and adds much to the muscular powers. On the subject of *barrenness* I have reflected much; and as it seems to be the anxious wish of many of the wealthy to have offspring, the remark or seasonable hint, that the bath is admirably adapted to the want of increase of family, may be quite sufficient without descending to particulars.

The ancient Greeks, Romans, and Germans, as well as the Persians, Turks, and modern Egyptians, enjoyed the comforts and benefits procured by bathing, in a degree of which we can scarcely form an idea. The Freuch owe much of their cheerfulness and vivacity of disposition to the warm bath; and you could not inflict on Frenchmen or French females, a greater punishment than to deprive either, of the warm bath which they always prize as a component part of their existence. The soft, delicate and beautiful skins, for which the French females are so much celebrated, are very much owing to tepid bathing, being far preferable to all the cosmetics and other preparations sold for the purpose of whitening and beautifying the skin. The habits of persons are very different as to perspiration or sweating: some perspire very much, and others very little: from some, no offensive affluvia arises in perspiring, whilst from the bodies of others, there arises a perfect fetor—and I must here say, that of all possible putrid smells; that arising from the perspiration of the human body, is the most dreadful; and to such persons as have a fetid perspiration, I do most certainly know, that the frequent use of the warm bath would be of immense service. It would not only prevent strangers from becoming disgusted with their society, but be a great auxiliary in promoting their health, and removing that most unpleasant smell which salutes the nasal organs with a perfectly sepulchral stench! This uncleanliness, or want of cleanliness, exhibits itself as frequently in the drawing-rooms and festooned halls of the great and wealthy, as in the humble cottages of the obscure and needy; and sometimes produces disgust which neither time nor circumstances can remove.

Let me then, *again*, and with every desire for your happiness, and every delicacy of sentiment I am master of, urge upon you the simple fact, that *cleanliness* is the very best of perfumes—and that all those which are imported from the east, are inferior to the pleasant and native smell of the skin, when perfumed by the use of *soap* and *water*. I ought here perhaps to close my remarks; but I feel it a solemn duty I owe to my fellow beings to be candid, and as I have pledged myself to do, to inform them plainly of whatever I know to their advantage. I have absolutely known many matches in wedlock, completely destroyed by the discovery of a want of cleanliness—and many married persons rendered miserable and highly obnoxious to each other, by this lazy, indolent, and I will add, this dirty trait of character: for it is well known to all keen observers of mankind, that *moral purity* and *cleanliness of person*, are nearly always found combined.

Every family, rich and poor, ought to have a bathing machine, improperly called a tub. It is easy of construction and very simple, being in shape like a child's cradle without rockers, about six feet in length, and of width sufficient easily to admit the body, with a hole in the bottom near the foot, to let the water pass off after being used, it may be constructed of wood or tin, and if of the latter, ought to be painted to prevent rust. Where it is made of wood plank, the seams or cracks ought to be filled with boiling tar or pitch to prevent leakage. Rocks properly cleansed previously to being heated in the fire, afford very easy means of heating the water to any temperature, and will always enable the bather to take the bath with very little trouble.

Most wealthy persons imagine, when they have furnished their mansions with splendid mirrors, Turkey carpets, sophas, and various other decorations which soon tire after the novelty of seeing them ceases, that all things are complete; but, I say, that unless they have a small room appropriated to bathing, in which the necessary apparatus can be found fitted up for use, their houses want one of the most necessary appendages of comfort and health: and that they ought to be charged with the responsibility, of many diseases which afflict their families, for want of this *fountain of health.* The construction of public baths, has from the remotest ages been considered an object of national attention; and most sincerely and ardently do I desire, that NASHVILLE, a city of public spirit, and cordial support of every thing useful; a city whose kind hospitality endears it to the warm recollections of every stranger who visits that metropolis, may shortly construct a public Bath, whose beautiful structure will be admired as a public ornament, and its utility fully established as the harbinger of health to its citizens, which may operate as an example in the introduction of this luxury into the western country.

The warm or tepid bath, should be used about twice or three times a week in summer; in winter once a week is sufficient. It ought to be used in the morning, at noon, or when going to bed.

Having now given a concise account, of some of the benefits of this hath, I shall next show by a brief statement of facts, the method of bathing practised by the hardy Russians. They have sweating or vapour baths which are resorted to by persons of all classes, rich and poor, free of expense, because these baths are supported and kept up by the government. Here mingle together the beggar, the artizan, the peasant, and the nobleman; to enjoy the luxuries of the steam or sweating bath, in both sickness and health. The method pursued to produce the vapour bath, is simply by throwing water on red hot stones in a close room, which raises the heat from 150 to 168 degrees, making when at 168—above a heat capable of melting wax, and only 12 degrees below that for boiling spirit of wine. In this tremenduous and excessive heat, which on an American would produce suffocation, the Russian enjoys what to him is a comfortable luxury of the vapour bath; which shows clearly as I have before observed, the wonderful force of habit among mankind. In these bath houses are constructed benches, on which they lie naked, and continue in a profuse sweat for the lapse of one and sometimes two hours, occasionally washing or pouring over their bodies warm or cold water. During the sweating stage, the body is well rubbed or gently whipped with leafy branches of the birch tree, to promote perspiration by opening the pores of the skin. A Russian thinks nothing of rushing from the bath room dissolved in sweat, and jumping into the cold and chilling waters of an adjacent river: or during the most piercing cold to which his country is liable in winter. to roll himself in the snow; and this without the slightest injury. On the contrary, he derives many advantages from these sudden changes and abrupt exposures; because, he always by them hardens his constitution to all the severities of a climate, whose colds and snows seem to paralyze the very face of nature. Rheumatisms are seldom known in Russia, which is certainly owing to the habit of thus taking the vapour bath. The great and sudden transition from heat to cold, seems to us very dangerous and unnatural; but I have no doubt the Russians owe their longevity, their healthy and robust constitutions, their exemption from certain moral diseases, and their cheerful and vivacious tempers, to these baths and their generally temperate mode of living. A learned writer has justly remarked, and not without cause, that it is much to be lamented, "this practice of bathing should have fallen into such disuse among the modern nations of Europe; and that he most sincerely wishes it might again be revived in our towns and villages." When we look back and see the benefits that the old physicians derived from this remedy of nature's own invention, and the many cures formerly affected by the use of the bath; and that Rome for five hundred years together had few physicians but baths, we cannot avoid being astonished that they should ever have fallen into disuse, from the prejudices and negligence of mankind.

COLD BATH.

The cold bath is one of the most important medical remedies, presented from the friendly bosom of nature. The cold bath means cleansing or washing the body with cold water, of a temperature varying from the 33d to the 56th degree of Fahrenheit's thermometer or the usual warmth of our river water during the summer months; but the entrance of spring-branches into the river should be avoided by persons bathing, because it produces a sudden change of temperature, from an agreeable warmth a to cold and chilling sensation.

Bathing in cold water during the warm season, is a preventive against disease; particularly fevers, by lessening the heat of the body; it cleanses the skin from its impure and acrid contents, thereby removing a primary source of disease: the bath braces the solids which were before relaxed by heat, restoring and tranquilizing the irritability of the nervous system, and greatly exhilarating and cheering the spirits with an increase of strength and bodily power. If the bath has been serviceable, you will quickly feel after leaving the water and rubbing well with a coarse towel, the most pleasant glow or increase of heat, with a delightful serenity and cheerfulness; but if the bath has been injurious, you will feel the contrary effect to that which I have described: and you must of course discontinue its use, and apply the tepid or warm bath in its stead; the effects produced by the cold bath when they prove injurious to the bather, are directly the contrary to those which I have before described —such as heaviness and depression of spirits—respiration or breathing becomes impeded—livid or dark appearance of the skin–nails purple–the lips change their florid appearance to a pale or purple color: and the countenance assumes a cadaverous or ghastly color, accompanied with head-ache. In such a case, the bather should immediately take plentifully of warm toddy, made of spirits of any kind, or if a cramp in the stomach. which sometimes takes place from the cold bath, thirty or forty drops of laudanum for a grown person, with warm toddy, together with the application of warm salt to the stomach, will give immediate relief. Moderate exercise should always be taken after bathing so as to restore the equilibrium of the circulation, and produce a reaction in the vessels and muscles. The morning is the best time for bathing; or two hours before sunset, if in a river;

as the water has then from the rays of a summer sun, acquired an agreeable warmth. When the sun has disappeared, or evening begins to throw her mists over the waters, it is imprudent to bathe, owing to the dampness of the atmosphere, which is apt to produce a chill followed by fever.

The rules for bathing are, to enter the bath on an empty stomach; or in other words, sometime after eating; wet the head first, and if the bathing place is free from impediments, dive in head foremost, so as to make the impression uniform; for you will feel the shock less by boldly entering it, than by reflecting and acting slowly and timidly, by which you might produce dangerous consequencas by propelling the blood from the extremities to the head, inducing apoplexy.

The time of remaining in the bath should always be short, and must be determined by the constitution, and the feelings of the persons themselves, as healthy persons may continue in the bath longer than those who are weakly and in bad health. It is improper and unsafe, to remain in the cold water longer than a quarter of an hour at most, during the hottest day in summer as the principle object in cold bathing in the influence and effect produced by the first impression made on the system.—and should the cold bath be advisable in spring or autumn, which is sometimes the case, one or two minutes at most will be sufficient; when the bath is necessary at these seasons, it will be advisable to use the shower bath as hereafter described.

On the use of the cold bath, considerable judgment is required, as many serious and lingering complaints have been produced by the injudicious use of this remedy, and many diseases brought to a fatal termination by its improper application, I shall therefore described as plainly as possible, the different effects produced in the different constitutions, and the diseases for which it is beneficial.

On aged and thin persons, it acts more powerfully than on corpulent and fat persons; therefore a fat and young person can remain double the time in the bath to one that is old or of delicate constitution. The remark which I have before made, should be attended to by person of stout or corpulent habits, particularaly those of short necks should always wet the head and enter the bath courageously, so as to prevent the determination of blood to the head: persons of sanguine temperament should be particular as to these instructions.

Persons whose lungs are affected, or those laboring under breast complaints, should by all means avoid cold bathing; because by using it, they always advance the disease, and cut short the thread of life. In oppressions of the breast, or difficulty of breathing, short or dry coughs, &c., the bathing in cold water is highly detrimental and improper—obstructions also in women, or stoppage of the menses or courses—also persons of a scorbutic habit, or those afflicted with old sores or ulcers, or vitiated state of the system, gout or rheumatisms, pregnant women; in hemorrhages or discharges of blood from the lungs, in all kinds of inflammations internal or external, the cold bath is dangerous, and frequently confirms disease which ultimately results in dissolution or death. Its benefits are always found in a debilitated state of the system, when unconnected with the diseases I have mentioned; particularly those whose systems have been relaxed by sedentary habits, requiring tonic or strengthening remedies. I have frequently in one or two dangerous cases, used the cold bath with females, in an advanced stage of life; when nature was about to leave them, or in other words, when a heavy flooding from the womb was about taking place.

The application of cold water, (and frequently ice,) has been resorted to in profuse discharges of blood from the womb; with considerable advantage; cold water being a powerful astringent. When infirm or aged persons take the cold bath, they ought to take moderate exercise before using it, so as to increase or produce the action of the vascular system, for by this moderate heat, you produce re-action under the shock, which might not otherwise take place. Understand me, I meau gentle exercise: not such as to produce sweating, although it is perfectly safe to enter the cold bath after a moderate walk or ride. It would be highly dangerous to go into the water when sweating, or laboring under fatigue; because your body, from fatigue, is losing heat rapidly by sweat; but it would by this, lose suddenly what remains of heat; and therefore you would *counteract* the benefits which would otherwise, result from a *judicious* use of this valuable remedy if properly applied; therefore, neither previous entire rest, nor exercise to overheat, can possibly be proper. But, go between these points moderately, and you will receive all the advantages the *cold bath* of this description is capable of bestowing on the human species.

The *cold bath*, is somestimes used as a *shower bath* with great success; it means the falling of the water from a height of seven or eight feet, in a shower similar to rain. The construction of this bath is very simple. Fix a box that will hold water, or a large tub will answer: bore the bottom full of holes made with a large gimblet—let the box or tub be placed above your head, the distance above mentioned, and let the water be thrown in—you being under it stripped of your clothing—or from delicacy to exposure of your person, have a box made with a trap-door underneath, so that by pulling the string, the trap-door will fall by a hinge, and permit the water to fall on your body. In the northern cities, the shower bath is constructed in this way, so that the water is always ready in the box, while you are preparing by stripping yourself, when, by pulling the string when you are ready, you will receive the bath on your body. The shower bath produces the best effects when used early in the morning, after which, you should take a moderate walk, or exercise on horse-back. By making the water salt, that is with common salt, well mixed, it will be doubly beneficial, answering the fine effects produced by sea bathing. In such a case, the salt should be boiled the night before with water, to give it the strength and qualities of sea water. After leaving the bath, rub well with a coarse towel. The advantages of this method are greatly superior to the other methods of bathing, where the effects required to be produced are powerful; for although the bothing in a river covers the surface of the body more uniformly, yet, this circumstance by no means detracts from the excellence of the former, because those intermediate parts which the water has not touched, receive an electric and sypathetic impression, in a degree similar to those brought into actual contact, and as every drop of water from the shower bath operates as a partial cold bath, its vivifying shock to robust individuals is more extensive, and better adapted than any other method of bathing. I will now describe why this bath is better than the common method of bothing, together with its safety and advantages. In the first place, the sudden falling of the water may be used as often as you like—prolonged or shortened at pleasure according to your feelings, your constitution, your disease, or your gratification. Second: your head and breast are much secured; as it descends to your hands and feet, the circulation is not impeded, breathing is less difficult, and a determination of blood to the head and breast is prevented. Third: when the water falls in this way by single drops, gliding in succession over the body, it produces the most thrilling and delightful sensations, stimulating the whole system. Its being always easily obtained and near at hand, gives it additional advantages. Lastly: the degree of pressure from the weight of water is prevented; nor is the bath dangerous—the fluids and circulation never being interrupted by it. Besides—it is free from injuries to which bathing in rivers and creeks exposes us. In closing my directions and advantages from the shower bath, I recommend the salt bath particularly, as one of the finest remedies in fits. in deafness, and for rickety children, or those afflicted with a disease called St. Vitus' dance, a nervous affection. The great benefits resulting from the judicious use of the shower bath, have been fully felt and acknowledged in the city of New York, by the first and ablest physicians of that city, of improvements and great discoveries in medical science.

FOOD.

Food means any thing, which, when taken into the stomach, goes to the support and nourishment of the human body; and we all know perfectly well, that all other animals, as well as man, require food to give them support—health—and strength. All animals below man, seem to be confined to particular kinds of food to support them; and this appears to be the reason, why naturally wild animals are confined to particular climates, unless under the care of man: and, the simple truth, that man makes use of so many different kinds of food, shows that his Maker intended him to live every where, and to have dominion over all the beasts of the field, the fowls of the air, &c. as the Scripture expressly says. But I will endeavor to explain this matter a little further, so as to be more easily understood. Fish cannot live out of the water; birds cannot live out of the air; nor can any mere land animal, such as the elephant—the lion—the horse or the cow, live in either the air or the water: and further still, on this same subject, we see very plainly; that a sheep cannot eat meat, a wolf or a lion cannot eat grass' &c. In fact you may look at all the animals in nature, and you will see as I said before, that all below man, are confined to the particular countries and places where they can find food, and shelter from their enemies; and that to *man* alone is given the whole surface of the globe, because he can live every where on it, and easily find subsistence or food to support him. He can eat fish from the waters—he can eat birds from the air—he can eat the animals of the land—the herbs, and vegetables, and roots, and grains, of the fields and woods, &c. &c.

I shall now endeavor to explain as plainly as possible, because every person is interested in knowing it, what physicians call the "*process of digestion*," which means in other words, the changes which our food goes through when taken into the stomach. First, the food being masticated or chewed, and mixed in the mouth with the spittle called the saliva and air, is next received into the stomach, where it is exposed to the action of a kind of liquid, called by physicians, *gastric fluid*, which is a powerful solvent of anamal and vegetable matters. After remaining in the stomach a short time, it becomes a soft gluey mass, having undergone a change or decomposition in the stomach—which may be termed fermentation. From the stomach it passes in to the intestines, where it is subjected to the power or action of the bile: here it undergoes still further changes, by forming a white milky fluid, called by medical men, chyle. This milky fluid is sucked up by a numerous quantity of little vessels, called medically, absorbent lacteals. These little vessels, are in the intestinal canal, and all the food as it passes is subject to the influence of the mouths of these little vessels, which suck up this milky fluid called chyle. These little vessels have many communications; so many that it is impossible to trace them—being formed with such delicacy of structure, and so very small: after many communications with each other, they at last end in one common *trunk*—from which the chyle is conveyed into the *blood* near the *heart*. It is here mixed with the blood, and becomes subject to the power of the heart and arteries, or in other words, large blood vessels. It is then circulated through the lungs: here many changes take place by breathing the air or common atmosphere. After this, it joins with the great circulating mass, and becomes itself blood, this being the great fountain from which the body is formed and strengthened.

Food, then, we see very plainly, is intended to suppert nature—promote the growth—and to give strength—and to renew the waste of the system. The structure of man's body; his inclinations; his instincts; and the gastric fluid, intended to digest both animal and vegetable food—show that the Creator has intended man to receive his food from the animal and vegetable kingdoms. But of vegetable and animal food, animal is the most nourishing. It is putrescent and stimulating, and highly injurious to live on any length of time, without a due proportion of vegetables; for it overheats and stimulates so much, as at length to exhaust and weaken the whole system, which in the first instance, it gave vigour and support to. Persons who have lived for any length of time on meats, become oppressed, heavy and lazy; the tone of their systems are impaired, the breathing is hurried on the least exertion, the digestion is destroyed, the breath smells bad, the gums sweil, the limbs lose their action and become swelled, and soon break out in sores, (this disease is called *scurvy*) and sailors are much subject to it on long voyages when deprived of vegetables. A German received a premium of twenty thousand pounds sterling, for introducing *sour crout* or pickled cabbage into the British navy. This vegetable is an antidote or preventive against this dreadful disease calld *scurvy*, which, for a length of time destroyed thousands of sea-men on long voyages, who were compelled to subsist on salt provisions. All acids are considered good in scurvy. A diet of vegetables entirely is not sufficient to raise the human system to all the strength and vigour of which it is susceptible: and when used alone without any meat, produces flatulence and acidity of the stomach, muscular and nervous debility, and a long train of hysterical and hypochondriacal disorders. This shows the importance of a proportion of each being intended for man. We find some Eastern nations, who live entirely on vegetables, seldom robust but very active. This accounts in part, for the cheerful disposition of the French, whose vegetable and animal food are generally mixed, and boiled to the softest consistency. A mixed diet of vegetable and animal food is therefore best suited to the nature of man. The proportion of these, must be regulated according to the manner in which they agree. Persons who are fat, plethoric, or sanguine, should use but little animal food: those on the other hand, who are weak and nervous, may use more animal food. In all inflammatory and acute diseases, where inflammatory action exists, meat is hurtful. Meats which I shall hereafter describe are beneficial, more so than vegetables, for persons who are subject to indigestion; particularly wild meats, such as venison, or any wild game, such as birds whose flesh are white—the partridge, quail, pheasant, wild turkey, &c: the flesh of these is of a most agreeable and delicate flavour, little heating, and when young, very nourishing and easily digested. In fact, all wild animals are more easily digested than tame ones, with the exception of water fowls, and such as live on fish &c. whose flesh is oily, strong flavoured, but heavy and difficult to digest, &c. By the abuses of cookery, by which I mean the uses of high seasoning and sauces, the simplest food may be rendered heavy and indigestible. The frog is not used in this country, but looked upon with disgust, and to name it as an article of food, would almost turn the stomachs of many. In France, on the contrary, it is considered as one of the greatest delicacies, and frequently sell at a guinea a dish. The hinder legs alone are made use of in France, and other countries where it is made use of as an article of food. The flesh has a white and delicate appearance, and there are men in France who obtain a livelihood by catching them. I have frequently seen them engaged in this employment, which is very simple: they bait a hook with a piece of red flannel or silk, at which the frogs will bite like fish, and are thus as easily caught. I have merely mentioned this not by way of recommending them as a diet, but to show the variety of tastes and habits of different countries.——The flesh of the soft-shell turtle, which is caught in our own waters, is tender and nourishing, and more to be considered as one of the delicacies of Tennessee, than any thing else we have; and if properly dressed, affords a most excellent dish, and one very easy of digestion. The flesh of all young animalsis the hest and most easily digested: mutton or lamb, next to the flesh of the kid, is superior to any known. Veal is delicate, and better than beef as to digestion; but neither can be good for persons of weak digestion. I have mentioned venison as being very easy on the stomach; indeed it is so very easy of digestion, that I think *dyspepsia* itself might be cured by it, when accompanied by the exercise of hunting the animal which affords it. Pork is a food which is too much used in Tennessee, by persons of delicate and feeble constitutions. There is more pork meat used in East Tennesse than in any part of the United States of the same population; and it is to this vocarious habit of gormandizing pork at every meal, we are to attribute the many serious forms of congestive fever which prevail here, to say nothing about scrofula, palsy, apoplexy, indigestion, and so on. Pork is a food highly nutritious, but from the fat with which it abounds, by no means easily digested. It is in fact the strongest of all animal food, producing to weak and delicate stomachs, acidity and unpleasant belching or eructations; and therefore should be cautiously used by persons laboring under dyspeptic symptoms or indigestion, and those whose bowels are weak. Pork can be alone adapted to men who labor hard, because it requires activity and great exercise to digest it. Bacon is a coarse heavy food, and also difficult of digestion; and like pork, only fitting food for persons who have to labor hard. Ham is also a heavy and strong food, and should be carefully avoided by all persons of weak stomachs, even when it is cured in the very best manner. The young pig is more wholesome, and affords a much more delicate and light food than the old animal. The rabbit and squirrel, afford an excellent dish, easily digested, and admirably suited to the stomachs of those who are delicate and yet require animal food. But the fact is, all persons who have an impure state of the blood, those who have sores, or wounds, or breakings out on the skin, should by all means refrain from the use of all animal food, and particularly from *pork*. Fish, as a diet, is difficult of digestion; it is of all animal substances, the most putrescible, and ought not to be allowed to weak patients, or persons recovering from acute diseases—and the reason why dyspeptic persons should avoid it is, that the fat of fish is harder to digest than the fat of any other animal, and quickly becomes rancid. It frequently disagrees with many constitutions—producing flatulence or wind—sickness and weight at the stomach—and sometimes vomiting: and I have frequently known it to produce a general disorder of the whole system, accompanied with short but regular paroxisms of fever, and sometimes a breaking out on the body resembling the nettle rash.—It is a very common saying, in allusion to the use of spirits, after eating plentifully of fish, that it requires something to swim in; this shows that it is a dangerous diet to more than sickly, delicate, and dyspeptic persons.—Fish which abound in oil, called the red-blooded fish, are more stimulant and nutritive than any other; but much heavier and more apt to disagree with the stomachs of weakly persons than any other: the fact is, that dyspeptic persons ought to avoid fish altogether, and under any possible forms of cookery. Diet depends very much upon the manner in which it is cooked. The most simple food may be convirted into a poison, by the pampering and studied artifices of epicures and cooks. This is the reason why the French cookery is superior to that of the English, or even to our own. The French use all the innocent herbs and plants of the garden, while the English and Americans, season their food with highly stimulating spices, calculated to destroy the coats of the stomach.—During my residence in Franch, I recollect but two cases of dyspepsia or indigestion. This is certainly owing to the manner in which the French live. The qualities and quantities of our food, with the manner of cooking it, should be strictly attended to; and by so doing we would escape some of the most dreadful diseases incidental to human life. The more simply we cook and dress our food, the less of it the stomach requires to be satisfied; for by stimulating the stomach with high seasonings, we produce an *artificial appetite*, and rouse it to the requisition of more food than the system requires; and by overloading and oppressing its powers, weaken and finally destroy them. To enjoy good health, we ought always to leave the table with some appetite; nor ought we ever to partake of any dish, however palatable, which we know from experience to disagree with us. The more plain the food we use, the more easily will it be digested, and the less we will desire. The various dishes given at parties, consisting of pies, puddings, tarts, ice creams, floating islands, sometimes called, and very properly, *trifles, &c. &c. &c.* are just so many poisons calculated to destroy the stomach, and entail upon the dyspeptic a life of misery and disease. In the western country I have witnessed, especialy among females, that the disease called dyspepsia or indigestion, prevails very much. I would therefore particularly urge upon them, as they value their health and lives, to avoid all this *farrago* of fashionable deserts; for by so doing, and living temperately and abstemiously, they will establish firm constitutions, which will be entailed upon their offspring, extend to themselves the inestimable blessing of health, and enable them to reach the winter of a good old age.

FEVER:

AND GENERAL REMARKS.

It is almost impossible to describe *fever* correctly; because it shows itself in so many various ways and forms. To judge of its presence, we are to notice particularly the following appearances and indications: the state of the pulse—the skin—the color of the face—the change of feature—the eyes—the tongue—the breathing—the appetite—the state of the stomach and bowels. There is generally great thirst, and pain in the head—soreness all over the body, as if beat with a stick, or as if a person were fatigued after a hard day's work—a desire to sleep constantly—and sometimes a great increase of strength accompanying fever. By these symptoms you are to judge of this disease.

The most distinguished medical men have differed in opinion as to the *cause* of fever: and to this day, I must honestly confess, that physicians are much in the *dark* as to this subject. Doctor Brown a distinguished physician of Europe, thought it arose from a want of stimulant in the blood vessels—or an excess of it. Doctor Rush, our distinguished countryman, thought there was in fever but one disease morbid or convulsive action in the blood vessels. Doctor Chapman, professor in the University of Philadelphia, thinks that most diseases originate from the stomach. My experience in medicine convinces me, that this eminent practitioner of medicine is correct. The first impression is made on the stomach by medicine, which acts instantly by sympathy: It is the general reservoir which receives those medical remedies by which the disease is to be subdued; consequently, there is great sympathy between the stomach and the the whole system—and many cases, supposed to be liver diseases; on a minute examination, you will find to originate in the stomach. It is impossible to describe the close connexion between the liver and the stomach. On this subject particularly, pay attention to the stomach first, and you will discover the primary cause of the disease: I will therefore describe, plainly and faithfully, the symptoms of such fevers as are common amongst us, so that with a little care and common judgment, the reader will be enabled to discover by the symptoms, the causes of such fevers as prevail amongst us: nor do I consider that those fine and hair-drawn opinions of fever given by physicians generally, are of any benefit to mankind, but on the contrary, serve to bewilder and lead astray. The great secret of medicine is to discover the first cause of disease and in the next place to apply the remedies properly: and to do these things as they ought to be done, let your judgment be exercised with clearness, caution, and firmness; and to give you firmness, be conscious that you are endeavoring to act for the best—as there is not so much difficulty in medicine as many imagine; if you will but attend to the causes of the diseases, and watch the effects of the remedies. The fact is, that a man of good common sense and judgment. who will take his station at the bed-side of the patient —be minute in his inquiries as to the habits of that patient—know when and how he was taken sick—ascertain all the apparently small particulars as to the pains first complained of—and without what is called a learned college education, you will, in nine cases out of ten succeed, when mere theorists who prescribe for the *names* of diseases, without understanding them, will absolutely fail. On conversing with a sick persou, ask the following questions, if the situation of the patient enables him or her to answer; and after awaiting the subsiding of any strong excitement your presence may create. How were you taken? When were you taken? Where did you feel the first pains? What were your feelings for several days, previously to being taken sick? Is your mind disturbed in any way? What are your general habits? Are you temperate in eating and drinking? What have you eaten for several days before being taken sick? How and when have you been exposed? Do you recollect how you felt when you were first taken sick? What has been your general health? Or if the patient be a female; have you been regular in your monthly periods? Is there any suppression of urine? This is a delicate matter with females; because from delicacy of feeling, they frequently conceal it. How is the state of your bowels? These are important matters, and require candid statements from the sick. By thus minutely inquiring into the state of the system, you strike at the root of the disease, and get on the right track; for thousands have been killed by physicians, for want of this accurate knowledge, or mistaking the disease.—There are many other circumstances which should be known; and, which your good judgment will not fail to point out to you: and I need not add, that the necessary information should be obtained from some experienced person of the family, if the patient should be in a deliririum, or too young, or too sensatively delecate to give it. From what I have before observed, that *fever* shows itself in so many various forms, you will see at once, the necessity of knowing the true causes, if possible, which assisted in producing the disease. Let me, therefore, implore you, not to be alarmed in administering medicines in fevers, or infact in, any other disease where good and sound judgment is required, you need not fear, if you will but pay good attention, and have confidence in yourself: I allude to such diseases as are *common* amongst us, because there are cases which require a *very* excellent physician: and under such circumstances, the heads of families need not be told the absolute necessity of having such a one. To give an evidence of the insufficiency of mere theories, with which boys come from colleges, I will take the liberty of stating an occurrence of early life, which transpired with myself—in the practice of medicine. In the state of Virginia, my first patient was an old gentleman of distinction, Col. Willis. His unbounded confidence in me, when taken sick, induced him to employ me in preference to his old physicians. The Col. was a man of full plethoric habit and had been taken with violent bilious fever. I bled him copiously; puked and purged him, with small doses of emetic tartar, to determine to the surface, or in other words to produce a moisture on the skin, and thereby lessen the fever. But all my remedies were unsuccessful; for the truth was, I did not know his constitution—or habit; and to describe to you my feelings on this occasion would be impossible—and here vanished all my theories, for want of a little sound judgment and practical knowledge. To the information given me, however by a faithful servant who had attended on him more than thirty years, I was indebted for his recovery. He stated that while he was in Philadelphia with his master, he had had a similar attack, and was attended by Doct. Rush: that the Doct. had given him warm brandy toddy—for said he, "my master always loved a little brandy, and most generally enjoyed himself." I took this seasonable hint from honest Bob, whose information had destroyed all my college theories, and taught me to scrutinize the constitution and habits: for in little more than fifteen minutes after I had given him some warm toddy, he broke out into a fine sweat, and soon entirely recovered. I afterwards related the anecdote to the Col. himself, who, after laughing heartily at the joke, assured me that Bob was certainly right. I shall close these general remarks on *Fever*, by giving you the key to medicine, or the art of distinguishing the true state of the system without which it would be impossible to administer medicine with certainty of success.

THE PULSE.

This is indeed the key of medicine; for without authentic and minute information on the subject of the PULSE, it is impossible for you to proceed to administer medicine to the sick with any certainty of success. But I shall describe it to you so plainly, and in words of such common use: that any person of common sense can understand this great *secret of medicine*, in the art of judging disease.

The meaning of the *pulse*, is the beating or throbbing of

an *artery;* there being no pulse whatever in the veins. The meaning of an artery, is a large blood vessel, branching out into smaller ones, which carry the blood from the *heart* to the ends of the body; in other words, to the points of the fingers and toes—where they join with the vains, which bring the blood back again to the heart: as I said before, the arteries throb or beat, and the veins do not. By pressing your middle finger hard on the vein, you will feel the artery beat under it destinctly. Every time the heart beats, it throws a column of blood into the arteries; then again the heart contracts or draws up, and a fresh portion of blood is forced on into the arteries. Reflect for a moment, on this wonderful machine, the heart; it goes with greater regularity than any watch, and at the rate of about *four thousand one hundred and fifty* strokes every hour. The swelling and contracting of the artery, then, constitute what I mean by the *pulse;* and therefore you may find the pulse in any part of the body where the artery runs near enough to the surface: for instance, at the *wrist*—the *temple*—bend of the *arm*—under the lower end of the *thigh*—under the *lower jaw*—and on the top of the *instep of the foot.* In different persons, although in perfect health, you will find the pulse differ very much: the usual standard of health, however, is from 75 to 80 strokes in a minute.—In *Children,* it is much quicker: and in *old persons* it is more slow and weak. Owing to the decreasing energies of the heart as you advance in age, it becomes less and less capable of propelling the blood through the arteries, which occasions the medical term *debility,* meaning *weakness.* By running, riding, walking, jumping, eating, drinking, speaking, joy, anger, &c. you increase the pulse: and in like manner you *diminish* the pulse, by fear, grief, depression of spirits, want of food, frequent stools, flux, or any thing else that tends to weaken the system. In feeling the pulse, you must make allowance for all these things: and always wait until all momentary emotions of the mind and passions have subsided and passed off.

1st. A full, tense, and strong pulse, terms used by physicians, is when you find that the *artery resists the pressure* of your fingers—*feels full*—and *swells boldly under their pressure.* If added to these, the beating be rapid and quick, the pulse is called *full and strong:* if slow, it is called *weak* and *fluttering*, and an irregular pulse.—

2d. A hard and corded pulse, is that in which the artery feels like a *string drawn tight:* and when you press it with your fingers, it gives *considerable resistence.*

3d. The soft and intermitting pulses, give their own meaning by name, and are very easily distinguished from each other; as in cases of great weakness, languor of circulation, or on the approach of death.

4th. When the stomach and bowels are oppressed, it frequently produces an intermitting pulse, which sometimes also arises from an agitation of the mind. A *vibrating pulse,* acting under the fingers like a thread, as if the artery was smaller with quick pulsations but very weak and irregular, may be considered as producing a *highly dangerous state of the system:* you will know this pulse by its being accompanied with heavy and deep sighs, difficulty of breathing, and a dead and heavy languor of the eye. By being attentive to the instructions given above, no man can be at a loss to distinguish the different states of the pulse, by which different diseases are indicated, as well as their different stages.

AGUE AND FEVFR.

This disease generally makes its visit in the fall season of the year; and those who live on the rivers or low lands, are more than others subject to its ravages. There are three stages of this disease, which are in substance the same thing, differing only in the intermission or length of time in which they make their attacks.

The first—is that which comes on every twenty-four hours:—this is called by Doctors *Quotidian.*

The second—is that which comes on every forty hours: this is called *Tertian.*

The third—comes on every forty-eight hours, and is called by physicians, *Quartan.*

I have merely mentioned these stages, in order that I might describe the disease more plainly, for the remedies and the treatment for the cure are the same; and the only difference between them simply is, as to their severity and time of coming on. If very severe, the remedies should be the most active:—on the contrary, if mild and gentle, remedies less active and powerful will answer.

I have said above, that there are three stages of this complaint—the *cold*—the *hot*—and the *sweating*. In the first, there is much *yawning* and *stretching*, the feet and hands become cold, the skin looks shrivelled, you seem to lose the use of your limbs by weakness, your pulse is small and frequent, you dislike to move, and finally take a chill succeeded by a cold shake. This shake continues about ten or fifteen minutes, according to the severity of the attack. In the second stage, as the chill and shaking go off, a pain in the head and back comes on, succeeded by flushings of heat. You now beg n to burn with heat and thirst, and desire that the covering be removed, that you may feel the cool air. Your face is read, your skin dry, your pulse becomes regular, hard and full. In severe attacks, where the blood determines to the head, I have frequently known delirium for a time. In the commencement of the third and last stage, the intense heat begins to subside, moisture begins to break out on the forehead, gradually extending itself over the whole body, the fever abates, thirst diminishes, breathing becomes free and full, desire to make water which deposits a sediment in the urinal or pot:—you then feel considerably relieved as the sweat increases, which soon restores you to your usual feelings and sensations, except great weakness and extreme prostration of strength.

REMEDIES.

In the cold stage, take warm teas of any kind, provided they are weak—such as sage, balm, hysop, ground ivy, &c. &c: make hot applications to the feet; and if you will apply a ***bandage***, wound round the right foot and leg, from the toes to the groin, and another *bandage*, wound round the opposite or left hand and arm, from the fingers to the shoulder, drawing both pretty tight, so as to *compress the muscles* without impeding the circulation of the blood, the shake will be much shortened by it; but you must not omit to loosen these bandages gradually, as the shake is going off. In many instances, the Ague and Fever can be entirely cured, by taking immediately, from *fifty* to *sixty* drops of *laudanum*, with a few drops of peppermint, in warm tea of any of the kinds mentioned above, on feeling the *commencement* of the chill; and as soon as the *hot stage* approaches, continuing to drink the warm tea plentifully, with a little acid of any kind in it.—If during this hot stage, the fever runs very high with considerable pain in the head, the loss of some blood would be proper. The object being, however, to bring on as early as possible the *sweating stage*, put into a pint of the tea or warm water, from four to five grains of tartar emetic, and give two or three spoon-fuls occasionally, so as to produce slight sickness of the stomach, which will promote and aid the sweating stage. My practice in this disease is, on its first appearance to give a puke of tartar emetic—for dose refer to the table. After cleansing the stomach, I give an active dose of calomel and jalap—and if that is not sufficient, I follow it with some mild purge, such as salts, castor oil, or senna and manna. Supposing, then, that the stomach and bowels are freed from their impure contents, the skin moist; and the body kept moderately open by gentle purgatives, it will then be proper to give the *dog-wood bark*, the *wild cherry-tree bark*, and *poplar-tree bark*, I allude to the large swamp poplar. These three kinds of bark are to be boiled in water, until their juices are extracted, and the water then given cold to the patient: and in such quantities as the stomach will bear. This disease is sometimes succeeded by a low, lingering, and constant fever: this must always be removed, before the extract of the different kinds of *bark*, just mentioned is given; nor ought it ever to be given in any paroxism of fever, *however slight*—because in such cases it invariably does material injury. From causes depending on the constitution at the time of taking this disease, it is sometimes extremely difficult to cure; and persons who have had it for more than *twelve months*, have placed themselves under my care. In these cases, when the various remedies above noticed have failed, I have used with *great success* the cold salt bath, as directed under the head of cold bathing. When a bathing machine cannot be had, a strong brine poured over the naked body in the morning when rising, is the best expedient that can be used; always taking care to wipe the body perfectly dry with a coarse towel: after which it might be well to return again to bed for an hour, before taking the morning meal, immediately before which, any common bitter such as *tansy* in spirits may be taken. When the disease is of long continuance, elixir vitriol is a good remedy, and may be given in doses of eight or ten drops, in a wine or stem glass of cold water, during the days in which the cold bath is used. I do not think it necessary to take the barks, as before described when an *ague-cake* or *hardness* termed by physicians, an enlargement of the spleen, has taken place; in such a case, use a tight broad bandage round the belly, with a padding of wool or cotton immediately over the *hard cake* in the side, and take care two or three times a day, to rub the place well with a coarse woolen cloth or a flesh-brush. This is called *friction* by physicians, and friction will be the more properly kept up by wearing flannel next the skin.

It will be proper here to state, that in some cases where the dog-wood bark, the wild cherry-tree bark, and the swamp poplar bark, prepared as I have mentioned, disagree with the stomach, which is sometimes the case from long sickness, the tea or decoction may be rubbed on the skin of children or delicate persons, and will produce an excellent effect. Another method of operating by the skin, with children and delicate women, is as follows; have a jacket made to fit the body, line it with the kinds of barks mentioned, which can easily be done, and cause it to be worn next the body. Both these modes of operating by the skin, have been known to produce fine tonic or strengthening effects, in cases of obstinate and long standing.

I shall now conclude these remarks, by giving the method of treating this disease by the Spaniards in the Island of Cuba. I there witnessed its unbounded success: and in no instance in which the remedy was fairly tried, did I ever know it to fail of success. Make a good sized cup of strong *coffee*, sweeten it well, and mix with it an equal quantity of *lime* or *lemon juice*. This juice may be had at any of the stores, doctor's shops, &c. the dose to be taken just before the shake is expected to come on, and must be drank warm, and on an *empty stomach*. This simple and always practicable preparation, may be relied on as a most valuable remedy. But the Spaniards of the Island of Cuba, are not the only persons acquainted with this powerful and efficient remedy. It is noticed in Doctor Pouqueville's travels in the MOREA, as follows:—"I have often seen intermitting fevers subdued entirely, by a mixture of strong *coffee* and *lemon* or *lime juice*, which is a successful remedy all over this county. The proportions are three quarters of an ounce of coffee, ground fine—with two ounces of lemon juice, and three of water: the mixture to be drank *warm* and *fasting*."—I quote from memory, but with a perfect assurance of being right.

It may be well before quitting the subject of Ague and Fever, to mention for the information of my readers, the late practice of physicians—which is as follows: as soon as the chill has somewhat subsided, take a good dose of calomel—see the table. Next, when the fever goes off, and you commence sweating, take two grains of *quinine*, which is the extract of *peruvian bark*. This quinine or extract of bark, must be mixed with a tea-spoonful of Epsom or other salts, and taken in water as you would other salts. Take this dose every *two hours*, until you take five doses; but you must omit to put in the salts, so soon as the bowels have been freely moved; because a continued looseness of the bowels would carry off the *bark* before it could operate on the system. Should the fever not go off in six hours, take a dose of castor oil to carry off the calomel—and then, as soon as the fever has left you, take the *quinine* or *extract* of *bark*, as before directed.

BILIOUS FEVER.

Bilious Fever, is nothing more nor less than the Ague and Fever just before described, under something of a different modification or character:—that is to say, in ague and fever, there is at certain times an entire intermission or stoppage of the disease; whereas, in Bilious Fever, there is nothing more than an abatement or lowering of the fever for a time. The analogy or likeness between them is so strong, that in both cases the patient is taken with a chill: and the little difference that does exist between them in the outset, consists in the simple circumstance, that the pulse in Bilious Fever is more *tense* and *full*. If, however, the attack of Bilious Fever, be *severe*; the skin becomes very hot after the chill, and sometimes of a yellowish hue; there is likewise great pain in the head; the tongue changes from white to brown, as the fever increases, the eyes acquire a fiery color and expression, and the whites have a yellow tinge; the light becomes painful to the patient, and he requires the room to be darkened; his bowels are very costive, and his urine highly colored: by these symptoms, any man of common sense may be enabled to distinguish *Bilious Fever.*

REMEDIES.

This formidable and dangerous disease, may in most instances be easily subdued, if you will divest yourself of irresolution, and timidity in the commencement of the attack:—I make this remark, because I have witnessed many instances, in which timidity and over-caution in the treatment of this disease, have proved fatal to the sufferer.—You are to depend on the *lancet;* and in the next and most important instance, on purging well with large doses of *calomel* and *jalap*. On the first appearance of this disease, give a good *puke of tartar emetic*, so as to cleanse well the stomach—taking care to make its operation fully effective, by giving *warm chamomile tea.* When the fever comes on, *bleed freely*, and regulate the quantity of blood drawn, by the symp-

M

toms and the severity of the attack: then give or administer, if to an adult or grown person, *twenty grains of calomel* and *twenty of jalap;* and if this is not sufficient, repeat the dose with thirty grains of calomel, and work it off if necessary with *castor oil—salts*—or *senna* and *manna;* [for dose see table of medicines.] By these active purgatives, given in time, you will in nine cases out of ten, give relief in a few hours; nor keep your patient lingering perhaps for weeks, and at length lose him. The administration of small doses of calomel, say of eight or ten grains, has been productive of all the injury that has disgraced the profession respecting the use of calomel, for several years past. A large dose always carries itself off; whilst a small one remains in the system, and frequently does much mischief, if neglected to be carried off by castor oil, or some laxative medicine; therefore let me urge you as you value the recovery and life of your patient, to give active and powerful *purgatives of calomel.* The only danger in this disease, arises from giving tonic or strengthening medicines, before the stomach and bowels are completely cleansed by an evacuation of their contents. If the fever should still continue, notwithstanding the administration of the foregoing medicines, my plan is to follow Dr. Rush's famous prescription, of ten grains of calomel and ten of jalap; the frequency of which prescription with the Doctor, procured him among his students, the ludicrous nickname of "*Old Ten in-ten.*" But the fact is, that this dose, after the stomach and bowels have been thoroughly cleansed, acts well upon the skin, and as a purge, drives the sweat from every pour, thereby lessening and finally breaking the fever.

During this fever, generally speaking, the skin is obstinately dry, and it therefore becomes important, that a determination should take place to the surface—in other words, that a moisture or sweat should take place on the skin, for the purpose of breaking the fever: therefore the nitrous powders should be given. The directions for making them are: to *sixty grains of salt petre*, add *sixteen grains of calomel*, and *one grain of emetic tartar.* Mix them well together by pounding them very fine; divide them next into *eight powders*, and give *one of them* in a little honey or syrup, every two or three hours. Emetic tartar made weak with water, and given at intervals, will produce the same effect; antimonial wine, and sweet spirits of nitre, mixed in equal quantities, and a tea-spoonful given occasionally, or *every hour*, will have the same effect; for antimonial wine is nothing more than emetic tartar mixed with wine, and sweet spirits of nitre is made from salt petre. Ipecacuanha, in doses of one or two grains, repeated every two or three hours, is also a good remedy to produce sweating. In this disease you will sometimes have an obstinate, severe and tedious case; in which you will find that the most active purgatives will not answer your wishes and expectations. Here the warm bath combined, will be found excellent, in relaxing the system and taking off the strictures of the vessels: and when you make use of the bath, be particular in making it of a temperature pleasant to the patient. Always follow the bath with injections or glysters, made of warm soap-suds; or molasses and water, pleasantly warm but not hot, to which may be added a little vinegar; these injections will cool the bowels, and remove from the larger intestines any offensive matter.

When the fever is on, the sponging or wetting the body with cold vinegar and water, will reduce the heat of the body, and be a great source of comfort to the sick person. If there is a pain in the head, cold applications of vinegar and water, will be of much benefit in relieving the violence of the pain. On the decline of this fever, *night sweats* sometimes occur: in these cases, use *elixir vitriol*, and gentle *exercise* in the open air. In Bilious fevers, a want of sleep and watchfulness often occur; the warm bath and a pillow of hops, and the room kept dark and all things quiet, will no doubt procure the desired tranquility; and if no inflammatory action or considerable fever exists, a dose of laudanum may be administered. The misfortune in the country is, that many persons who come to sit up with the sick, talk so incessantly as to prevent the sick person from having the repose necessary for promoting a speedy recovery:—and it may be important here to remark, that whenever laudanum or opium is given, the person must be kept undisturbed and perfectly quiet.—When the stomach is irritable, warm mint leaves *stewed in spirits* and applied to the pit of the stomach, will be proper—and then if the irritability should continue, the application of a cataplasm of mustard seed, or a large blister, will infallibly relieve irritation, and quiet the stomach.

I have now taken a comprehensive view of this disease, and given plainly and simply the remedies, and shall close with the following remarks. If the calomel taken in this fever salivates, you should not be alarmed or uneasy, but consider it a source from which you have derived safety to your patient; for when Bilious Fever is dangerous, the sooner salivation takes place, after the stomach and bowels have been thoroughly cleansed, the safer for the patient. It is to produce this effect, that physicians give small doses of calomel every two hours, say from one to two grains, in any kind of syrup; for, when salivation is produced, you may consider the danger of the patient at an end, the rest depending altogether on care and good nursing. After good purging, without salivation, I have found geed nursing and kind attention, the best and most salutary medicine. Cooling drinks slightly acid, will be proper: and when the fever is subdued, cold chamomile tea may be given as a drink; or a bitter made with dog wood-bark, poplar bark, and Virginia snake root, may be given as a cold tea, in small quantities, as the stomach will bear.

NERVOUS FEVER.

This fever carries in its title or name, its true character; because it affects the whole nervous system, and produces a tremulous motion of the body and limbs; the system seems to be sinking; there is a clammy, cold, and unnatural perspiration or sweat on the skin, and the pulse is extremely weak. Next, the sweat subsides, and the skin becomes dry and hot to the touch; and at the same time, the arteries of the temples and neck throb and beat with considerable action. The sleep is very much disturbed and unrefreshing; the countenance sinks or seems to change from its natural expression of feature, to a ghastly appearance; the tongue becomes dry, and frequently trembles, when put out, and with the teeth and gums, soon become covered with a dark buff-colored scurf; the spirits flag, and the mind broods over the most melancholy feeling, without knowing the cause; the sight of food is very unpleasant and sometimes disgusting, the stomach being generally much debilitated and weak; the difficulty of breathing becomes very considerable, and sometimes the hands are glowing with heat, whilst the forehead is covered with sweat. The symptoms, considered very dangerous are a constant inclination to throw off the cover; a changing of the voice from its usual tone; great vigilance or watchfulness; picking at the bed-clothing; inability to hold or retain the urine; invoiuntary discharges from the bowels; hiccupping; a muttering as if speaking to one's self; a wild and fixed look, as if the eyes were riveted upon some particular object; if these latter symptoms occur, there is little to expect but that the case will terminate fatally.

This fever originates from *putrid animal* and *vegetable matter* mixing with the air or atmosphere we breathe, such for instance as the decaying of vegetable and animal matter arising from stagnant mill-ponds, or any other ponds; or from filth and dirt, and want of personal cleanliness; or from any thing else that tends to weaken the system materiality. This disease also arises from *Bilious Fever* mentioned before: which, when of long standing, sometimes changes into *Nervous Fever;* and I have known it to remain in the system ten days before it broke out violently, having come on so slowly and gradually as to produce no alarm.

REMEDIES.

The *lancet,* or in other words *bleeding,* in this disease is certain death: no inducement whatever could prevail on me to bleed in Nervous or Typhus fever. Bleeding has been recommended by some physicians, when inflammatory symptoms appeared in the first stage of the disease; but I positively assert, that it is wrong, and denounce such doctrine, as dangerous to the last degree: the fact is, that in nineteen cases out of twenty, bleeding in this disease will result in death. There are two important considerations to be noticed in this fever; the first is—when it originates in itself as the first cause, and the second is—when it turns or sinks from Bilious fever, to a *Nervous* or *Typhus*. In the *first* case, give a puke of tartar emetic, or of ipecacuanha—[see table for the dose:] which mix with warm water until it is dissolved, say in six or eight table spoonfuls. Next give a table spoonful every ten minutes, until copious vomiting is produced, encouraging the puking *after it has commenced*, by drinking freely of warm chamomile tea, or warm water—the object being to cleanse the stomach. Then attend to the bowels with *laxative* medicines, such as rhubarb, cream tartar, epsom salts, &c. so as to free or throw off the contents of the bowels, which, when in a costive state, increase irritation and fever. You must however, by no means produce heavy purging; it is dangerous; and your own good sense will show you that it is a disease of debility or weakness. The object is merely to keep the bowels gently open, say by one or two stools a day, which will be quite sufficient. I always give glysters made of thin gruel of corn meal, strained, with a tea spoonful of hog's lard in them: they are to be given milk-warm from a bladder or pipe, and carefully thrown up into the bowels—look under the head "*glyster*," and those who do not understand the matter, will find it explained.

In the *second place*, when this disease sinks from *Bilious fever*, to a *Nervous* or *Typhus fever*, you will find the last part of the symptoms to agree with the sinking state of the system, and requiring moderate tonies, or stimulons and strengthening medicines. The danger of this fever, is in proportion to the weakness which attends it; and therefore you will easily see the importance of early supporting the system by stimulants, such as good wine, warm toddy, &c.

This distinction of the sinking state of the system, must be obvious; and sufficiently plain to be observed by every person of common sense. But I will still explain it further, in order that no mistake can possibly be made, in the course to be pursued; and shall state accordingly the following directions. Stimulants—in other words, common spirituous liquors, such as whiskey, rum, brandy, &c. must be made palatable to the patient, which must be given regularly, and varied as to quantity, according to what the case may seem to require. If they increase the pulse *considerably*, so as to occasion restlessness, a difficulty and oppression of breathing, a dry tongue attended with thirst, a flushed face, in other words, *increased fever*, they are *improper;* and you must *discontinue their use.* On the contrary, if they produce refreshing sleep; a pulse slower, softer, and more regular; and the patient feels sensible of relief—you are to continue the use of stimulants sufficiently to support and strengthen your patient, adding at the same time generous diet, and a pill of opium at night to procure rest: [See table for dose.] Blisters applied to the extremities, or cataplasms made of mustand and strong vinegar, will be highly necessary in a sinking state of the system.

If the head is affected by *delirium*, keep cloths constantly applied to it, wet in the coldest water and vinegar, changing them as they become warm: and if the delirium should still continue, a blister applied to the head, after shaving off the hair, will be necessary. If purging takes place in this disease, which it sometimes does, it must be stopped by laudanum or opium, given in small but frequent doses, increasing or diminishing them as necessity may require: for if the purging should continue in this complaint, which is weakness or debility, your own good sense must teach you, that it would speedily terminate in death, from *increased debility* or *weakness.* The late remedy used by physicians, which is called *quinine*, or extract of peruvian bark, is a good remedy, from the fact of its taking up less room in the stomach than the *bark in substance.* This quinine or extract must be made into pills, with some kind of syrup; and must contain from one grain to one and a half of the extract, and given three or four times a day, as the system may be able to bear the doses. The extract is a powerful tonic or stimulant, and may sometimes be difficult to be obtained; in this event, the black snake root, commonly called the Virginia snake root, should be used; its virtues are not merely considerable, but highly valuable in this disease; combined with the dog wood bark, or even without it, and I recommend it in preference to any remedy. The form of administering it, is in *decoction*, or as a *tincture* —that is mixed with spirits of any kind. This root is perfectly harmless except, when high inflammatory action exists; that is to say considerable fever. In the secondary stage of fever, where the skin has been obstinately dry, I have used this little root with unbounded success, not only in this particular disease, but in all fevers; and also where the symptoms indicated rapid prostration and death. Encouraged by my success in its use, I earnestly recommend that it be adopted in fever generally, and particularly in those I have described.

The salt bath, made as directed under the head of bathing, similar to sea-water, is as valuable a remedy as can possibly be used, in that state of the system when from fever, the heat of the bedy requires lessening: or if you would prefer it, you may spong the body well with cold water and vinegar. These remedies by bathing or sponging the body, you will recollect, are only to be used when there are no chilly or cold sensations; for if there are such, they would probably prove fatal: and you are also to remember, that they are to be used with as little fatigue as possible to the patient. This disease is frequently marked with extreme weakness of the stomach, called by physicians *debility;* in this case, common *yeast* will be highly beneficial, administered every three or four hours—say two table spoonfuls; and if the stools are very offensive, you may add a tea spoonful of common charcoal to the yeast. By this, the offensive state of the bowels will soon be corrected; and to insure the perfect knowledge of the reader on this subject, I will remark, that if the *yeast* and *charcoal* produce good effects, the pulse will raise and become slower and fuller, and the burning heat of the skin will subside. Under these circumstances, the remedy should be continued. I shall now finish my remarks on Nervous Fever, which have been extended to a greater length than was at first intended, in consequence of the recollection that it is a very common malady in Tennessee. Dr. Currie, and many other eminent practitioners of medicine, have given the best testimonials and favorable results, in the first stage of this fever, from the use of the cold bath, or in other words, from throwing cold water over the body, wiping dry, and returning to bed immediately. From the experience of so many distinguished men, I yield to their judgment; but, from my own experience, I should prefer the salt bath; as before mentioned—or sponging the body with vinegar and water made milk-warm; this, however, is never resorted to, until the stomach and bowels have been freed of their contents: or medically speaking, which means the same thing, until the whole alimentary canal has been evacuated.

COLIC.

In this disease the belly is considerably swelled, and seems to be bound round tightly with a cord; and there is also a disagreeable feeling about the navel, belching of wind, costiveness, and frequently the most excruciating misery. I have had many cases, in which a cold clammy sweat has been produced on the forehead, by the intense sufferings of the person afflicted. This complaint comes on without fever, but if it continues, it will produce fever, and perhaps inflammation unless soon relieved. It arises from wind termed by physicians flatulence; from indigestible food that; has been taken into the stomach—from acrid bile—from hardened fæces, which mean the stool—by suddenly stopping the perspiration or sweat—or from getting the feet wet—or from exposure—or from worms—and lastly, from the application of poisons to the stomach, of a metalic nature—by which I mean metals under various forms and preparations.

REMEDIES.

If the colic is produced from wind, which you will know from belching, or from a rumbling noise, in the bowels, or from the ease you experience by a discharge of wind, a tumbler of warm whiskey toddy, made with warm water sugar and spirit—to which may be added peppermint, or strong mint tea, or tea made of ginger, calamus, dog-wood blossoms, give relief, The application of warm salt to the belly will give ease immediately, or until more powerful remedies can be given. If the stomach is much distressed, an application of garden mint made warm by stewing it, and applying it to the pit of the stomach is excellent. You will then immediately, if necessary to the relief of the person afflicted, give a simple clyster made after the following directions: a quart of thin gruel, made of corn meal and strained; to this, add a table-spoonful of hog's lard, and another of common salt, which must be thrown up about milk-warm, into the bowels. For further directions as to clystering, look under that head for instructions, as to the apparatus to be made use of. If the pain still continue, and the person be corpulent or fat, *bleed and give the warm bath* immediately. If you have no bathing vessel or tub large enough to put the body in, apply cloths dipped in hot water and wrung out, as warm to the belly as they can be borne. If the above remedies fail, give a table-spoonful of castor oil, and in it put fifteen or twenty grains of calomel: and if there is yet no relief, give one grain of opium and ten grains of calomel, and continue the clysters. But, if the pain does not yet abate, laudanum must be given in large doses, both by the mouth and by mixing it in the clyster. The doses of laudanum must be increased gradually until relief is obtained; and I have given as much as a table spoonful before I could affect my purpose. If the misery be excruciating, to a grown person I begin with fifty or sixty drops in mint tea—and when relief is obtained, I give a good dose of castor oil, and clyster to open the bowels: this, practice has generally been successful. The practice of the Baltimore Institution, as directed by Dr. Patterson when professor there, was in *desperate cases* to give a simple clyster as before mentioned, omitting the salt and lard—reducing the quantity to half a pint of gruel, and putting into it fifteen or twenty grains of *emetic tartar* and injecting it into the bowels. This remedy I tried in Virginia, in two or three desperate cases of colic, with perfect success; but it should never be used, unless the situation and violence of the case demands its administration: it is an active and powerful remedy, and may be relied on in urgent cases. Persons who are subject to this dangerous complaint, should be very cautious as to their diet or food, abstaining from every thing that disagrees with them; and above all, they ought to avoid costiveness, or in other words they ought to go to stool every day at a certain time, and solicite nature to perform her duty—for by so doing, a *habit* of evacuation will be at length produced, which will overcome the most obstinate costiveness: and to produce a stool, a piece of hard soap about half the length of the finger, may be introduced into the passage. In all obstinate cases, which seem not to yield to common remedies, examine the passage of the fundament with the finger, so that if there be any hard lumps of excrement, they may be removed—for while they remain, all your purges and clysters will be useless.

A spirituous infusion of the berries or of the bark of the *Prickly Ash*, is made use of in Virginia, in violent colic and is a good remedy. This tree is a native of Jamaica, and other tropical countries, as well as of the United States, and grows to the height of sixteen feet, and is about twelve inches in diameter. It somewhat resembles the common ash, and the bark is covered with sharp prickles. The fresh juice expressed from the root, affords certain relief in *colick*, and what is called *dry belly-ache*. The important fact was discovered in the West Indies, by watching a female slave who collected the root in the woods, and gave two spoonfuls of the juice to a negro suffering under that colic called dry belly-ache, at intervals of two hours. It occasioned profound and composed sleep for twelve hours.

when all sense of pain and suffering had vanished; and the cure was completed by giving an infusion of the expressed root in water by way of diet drink.

CHOLERA MORBUS
OR
PUKING AND PURGING.

This disease is generally produced by the food becoming rancid or acid on the stomach; and if from an over quantity of bile. the purging and puking will show it, by the discharges being intermixed with a dark bilious matter. This disease is also produced from breathing damp air; or from being exposed to inclemant weather; or from getting the feet wet:—but mostly from eating *such food as disagrees with the stomach and bowels.* The mind has a powerful influence in this complaint; and I have frequently observed in my practice, that the disease was produced in many cases of females in delicate health, by the passions of the mind, as well as by sudden stoppages of the menstrual discharge. The disease generally commences with sickness of the stomach—painful griping, succeeded by heat and thirst, quickness and shortness of breathing, with a quick and fluttering pulse. When the case is dangerous, the extremities become cold—the perspiration or sweat is clammy and cold—there is also cramp, and great changes and irregularities of the pulse, which, when accompanied with hiccupping, are strong evidences of the approach of death.

REMEDIES.

Apply to the stomcah and belly, cloths steeped in warm water or in spirits in which camphor has been dissolved; or you may apply a warm poultice made of garden mint stewed; or a poultice made of mustard and strong vinegar will be found of great service applied to the stomach; or a blister of cantharides or spanish flies: and in extremely dangerous cases, where it is not practicable to draw a blister in the usual way, do not hesitate to *scald the part* with boiling water—at the same time applying hot rocks or bricks to the feet. Give hot whiskey toddy, or that made of any other kind of spirits; let it be strongly mixed with peppermint, or ginger, or calamus; and let chicken water or thin gruel be freely taken by the patient. Give clysters made by pouring boiling water on the inner bark of slippery elm, or those made of flax-seed tea, either of which must be thrown up into the bowels milk-warm. [See under the head of clystering for the manner of administering this operation.] The first object in this dangerous complaint is, to cleanse the stomach and bowels of any offensive matter—after which, the giving of thirty-five or forty drops of laudanum in mint tea will be proper; and if these should not arrest the progress of the disease, make a clyster of a table spoonful of starch, and a half pint of warm water, in which put a tea spoonful of laudanum, and throw it up the bowels, as directed under the head "*clyster*". If this does not give relief in fifteen or twenty minutes, repeat it again—and again.

If the person who is attacked, is of a full habit, that is fat, stout and vigorous, the loss of some blood by the arm, and the warm bath will be necessary. If the attack be moderate, a good dose of calomel will generally put a stop to it—for this will evacuate the bowels, operate as a stimulous, and remove the diseased action.

Very frequently this disease appears as a symptom of fever; and then of course you are to treat it as you would any other kind of fever. In all cases, after using laudanum to relieve your patient, particularly, when you have used it to any extent, it is proper and necessary to give *after relief*, a good dose of castor oil. Persons who are subject to this sudden and dangerous disease, should be cautious as to what kind of food they indulge in; and should be very particular in avoiding the causes which produce it; because by imprudence, the disease may return with double violence and danger.

The rapidity with which *Cholera Morbus* proceeds, requires the remedies to be promptly applied; for the disease is generally speaking highly dangerous, and soon terminates the life of the sufferer, unless relief is speedily obtained. A few hour's suffering, in severe cases, weakens the patient surprisingly; and therefore you will easily see the great importance of nourishment, of a *light stimulating*, and *strengthening* kind being given. Besides attention to nourishing diet, wine with any kind of bitter ought to be given, or cold chamomile tea three or four times a day, the dose, a wine or stem glass full, or elixir vitriol, ten drops three times a day, in a tea made of black snake-root or Virginia snake root: besides all which, flannel ought to be put on next the skin of the patient. But, in concluding my remarks on the treatment of this complaint, I must urge the particular necessity of the warm bath, and clysters, as almost certain means of relief, if properly and timely administered.

RHEUMATISM.

This painful and excruciating disease, in which the poor sufferer drags out a miserable and wretched existence, is quite frequent throughout the western country—and particularly in East Tennessee. I shall communicate respecting this disease, in which I have had much experience, such remedies as will if properly managed, succeed, in entirely removing it from the system, unless *anchylosis* of the joint has formed; for in such a case nothing can possibly be done with it. Anchylosis means a *stiff joint;* this state of the system is exhibited generally, under the form of *chronic rheumatism* of ten or fifteen year's standing. In every case, where the patient can in the slightest manner move the joint, I have no hesitation in saying that the cure can be made, if attentively and properly managed, according to the various methods of treatment laid down, which are as follows. Embracing the general mode of treatment as used by physicians, and the method I have invariably followed with unbounded success, in Virginia & Tennessee, hundreds are now living in both states who can attest or prove, that they have been entirely cured of this disease by me, of many years standing, after they had become entirely helpless, and unable to walk or move without assistance. There are two diseases, or rather two different stages of this disease: one of which is called *inflammatory* and the other *chronic*; the first is accompanied *with fever*—and the other, the last, is nearly or quite *without fever*, and of long standing.

Rheumatism is brought on by exposure to the cold and wet; by sleeping in damp places; by remaining too long on the damp ground; by sleeping in a current of air at night, immediately under an open window; by exposure to the night dews; by taking off a warm dress, and putting on a thin one; by being greatly heated, and becoming suddenly cool, thereby checking the perspiration or sweat.

There is a disease called by physicians *Rheumatic Mercurialis*, which means Rheumatism produced by the improper use of *mercury;* that is by permitting the mercury to remain in the system, without giving the proper remedy to carry it off, which is flour of sulphur. This flour of sulphur is nothing more than *brimstone purified*, and pounded or ground very fine like flonr; it is the true and certain antidote against mercury; as you will find explained under the head Sulphureous Fumigation—or a sweat produced by the use of sulphur.

First. *Inflammatory Rheumatism* is to be releived, in the first stage by bleeding; as you will perceive by the fullness of the pulse, and by the person afflicted being of a robust and full habit of body; here it will be necessary to bleed freely from a large orifice. If the heat is great, you must proportion the loss of blood according to the violence of the symptoms; and you must repeat the bleeding on the second day, if you find it necessary from the violence or continuation of the inflammatory symptoms—which can easily be distinguished by the pulse, the feelings of the sufferer, and lastly by suffering the blood to cool. If the blood, when cool, has on its surface, a *buffy* coat of a yellowish hue, it denotes a highly inflammatory state of the system; but, in bleeding, you must take care not to go so far as to produce debility: and, therefore, after the first bleeding, which must be regulated entirely by the violence of the attack, it will be proper to give an active purge of calomel and jalap, twenty grains of each, mixed well together, and afterwards with any kind of syrup. This should be carried off by gruel, or warm balm, sage, or dittany tea, if possible to produce gentle moisture or sweat on the skin. If then, the disease does not begin to yield, give another purge of ten grains of calomel and ten of jalap, mixed well and given as before directed. This will produce purging, and a copious perspiration or sweat. You will find now, that by moderate purging, so as not to debilitate or weaken the patient, the complaint will begin to subside, or perhaps entirely cease. These mild purges must be of epsom salts, glauber salts, senna and manna, or castor oil. If your patient at any time gets weak from purging, give warm toddy made of any kind of spirits; or if you wish effectually to check the purging, give twenty or thirty drops of laudanum or a pill of opium: [See the table of dose.] This will arrest or put a stop to the purging; and if there is any griping, put the laudanum when you give it, in some strong mint tea. When the joints are very painful, and the skin red swelled and inflamed, *cup* over the parts. [See under the head of Cupping for this operation.] which is very simple and easily performed. Cupping freely will be a useful remedy. The inflamed or swollen parts, should be kept wet with cloths dipped in vinegar made milk-warm: and at night a poultice made of rye flour, mixed with vinegar and warm water, will give much relief. If the inflammatory symptoms are considerably removed, a pill of opium or a dose of laudanum,[see table for dose.] will procure the rest or sleep so much desired in this afflicting complaint. The parts which are painful should be well rubbed with a liniment made of two table spoonfuls of laudanum, two of spirits of hartshorn—mixed over a slow fire in four table spoonfuls of butter without any salt in it: this being put into a bottle and corked tight, must be used three times a day, at the rate of a tea spoonful each time, and the parts kept well covered with flannel. These remedies should be used *separately* or *to-*

gether, as they may afford the afflicted person relief. The diet should be very light and cooling; this being a matter of great importance. By strict attention to this, you will be enabled to get quickly relieved, and save the taking a vast deal of medicine. In fact, while inflammation prevails, the less the patient takes of nourishment the better; and solid or animal food are both to be avoided. No spirits, wines, or stimulating drinks whatever, are permitted in this state of the system: and even when the afflicted persons is getting better, he must take only such nourishments as are necessary to support the system and recruit its powers—for by imprudence in diet a relapse may take place, of a dangerous and languishing nature

Second. *Chronic Rheumatism*, as distinguished from that called inflammatory rheumatism, has little or no fever with it. Chronic means when the fever or inflammatory action, has nearly, or sometimes in fact *entirely* subsided. It is sometimes brought on as a mere consequence of inflammatory rheumatism—and sometimes it proceeds from cold and exposure, or from violent exercise, or from the system being predisposed to it by some old disease; for it frequently steals on so gradually, that the patient hears with it until the pain seats itself in some particular joint, or part giving the most excruciating pain. When fairly seated by length of time, it usually prevents the sufferer from using his limbs, and from the misery attending it throughout, large lumps or swellings are produced by it: these are the symptoms by which you will know *chronic rheumatism.*

This slow, obstinate, and painful disease, must be treated as follows. First—the bowels are to be kept open by the simple laxative of sulphur. A tea spoonful must be given of a morning, mixed with honey, on an empty stomach—and one at night, if necessary to keep the bowels open. One or two purges a day will be sufficient avoid the damp ground, and also getting wet while taking sulphur; because it opens all the pores of the system, and under these circumstances becomes dangerous. This medicine is truly valuable in this disease, and too much can hardly be said in its favor: nor is there any danger in it, if you will but keep from the wet and damp. You may occasionally vary the treatment, by giving epsom salts in the room of the sulphur, but it must be in moderate doses. The next object in curing this complaint is, to keep up a gentle moisture on the skin, in other words, a gentle sweating; and for this purpose I shall give you a remedy which is very simple; and which in itself has cured hundreds, both of rheumatism and pains generally. Take one ounce of *gum guaiacum* and two drachms of *saltpetre,* put these two articles after pounding them together, into a quart of old whiskey, and give a table spoonful in a little cold water, three times during the day. This dose is for a grown person. If the stomach be weak, lessen the dose in proportion—and so on for a delicate or weakly person. It acts as a powerful stimulant—produces gentle sweating. &c. By continuing in the use of this simple remedy, in which there is no danger, I have effected cures in cases of long standing, several of which were considered hopeless.

The principle to be pursued in removing this complaint is very simple: it is either by *moderate* or by *profuse,* which means large sweats. Take a blanket, or any thing which will prevent the steam from passing off, and put hoops into it, in the same manner that you would into a partridge net, so as to keep the blanket, or whatever else you use, on the stretch. Let the bottom hoop be large enough to cover a tub, or whatever other vessel you use: let the next hoop be something smaller, and the next one smaller still, and so on up to the top one, which must be large enough to admit the head through. This machine, or whatever else you may please to call it, must be long enough to cover the body without touching it, *except at the neck,* where it must fit so close as to prevent any steam from escaping, which might affect the nose, face, or any portion of the head. In this institution, the patient being enclosed in the case—*naked;* let him sit or stand, with hot rocks placed under him; on which so as to confine the steam to the body, let the following extract be gradually and very slowly poured. Four or five days before you wish to give this bath, take a quart of whiskey, and put into it half an ounce of saltpetre, one ounce of seneka snake root well, bruised, and half an ounce of sulphur in a quart bottle. This liquor must be pored very slowly, or rather dropped through an apperture in the blanket on the rocks; by which a powerful sweat will be produced, which must be continued for a quarter of an hour, if the patient be not too weak to bear it so long. When the patient is in this bath, if any faintness or sickness takes place, the bath is to be stopped, the patient wiped dry, and immediately put to bed: and if much debility or weakness seems to exist, you must stimulate with warm toddy, made of any kind of spirits, with warm water and sugar. In my practice in Virginia, for five years, I used this steam bath with unbounded success; and in some cases which I considered absolutely hopeless, cures were produced. By the effects of the vapor or steam bath, as just described, I was induced to try its effects in two cases of *Inflammatory Rheumatism*, in which one of the patients was unable to move without assistance for six months previous. all the usual remedies in that stage of the disease having been tried without any benefit. John Sypold, a man of about thirty-five years of age; of a full habit, a resident of Montgomery county Virginia, was hauled to me in a woggon nine miles, laboring under inflammatory rheumatism. His situation was truly wretched, from the most severe and excruciating pains. I determined, with his consent, and after explaining to him my doubts, as to the final issue of his case, to try the following experiment, I bled him freely from both arms; and his situation was such as to require five persons to assist me in getting him into a wooden case I had constructed for the puspose. His pain was so severe, as scarcely to admit of his being turned over; but as soon as the steam was put in operation on him, he became tranquil—and in ten minutes a profuse sweat broke out on him, which produced great relief. He had continued in the bath fifteen minutes, when I proposed to have him removed; but the pleasantness of his sensations induced him to desire me to let him remain; he said that those were the only moments in which he had experienced a relief from pain in six months. After continuing in the bath for half an hour, he descended without assistance covered with sweat: his body was then rubbed well with coarse towels, and his joints also with the liniment I have before described, made of hartshorn, laudanum and butter without salt. I gave Mr. Sypold the bath three times, making each time shorter. In two weeks he was entirely relieved from pain, and in three months he walked to Lynchburgh with his waggon, a distance of sixty miles, and returned without experiencing the least return of his disease. Hundreds have since been relieved by me in Tennessee, of this disease, by this remedy of the bath, as just described—and in chronic cases, by the simple use of gum guaiacum as already mentioned. I shall now proceed to give the common remedies, as used by physicians in this complaint, many of which are valuable, and afford speedy and salutary relief.

In all local affections, distinguished by stiffness, and want of power to move the joints without considerable pain, rub the part well with the liniment before mentioned—or with opodeldoc—or whiskey, in which red pepper or mustard has been diffused or soaked—and with these, or either of them, rub the joints or places affected with a brush, continuing the rubbing for some time, the longer the better; and use inwardly the gum guaiacum as before directed. The poke-berry bounce, made by putting the ripe berries into whiskey, and using a wine glass full of it every day is of service. The seneka snake root is also valuable in this disease, by boiling an ounce of it in a quart of water, over a slow fire or on coals; stewing it down to a pint or less, and taking a table spoonful of it occasionally through the day: you may increase the dose as the stomach will bear it. Fat lightwood steeped in spirits, and taken in small quantities, is also serviceable. Tea made of sarsaparilla, and drank freely, is a good remedy: or take a large handful of rattle snake root and bruise it well—put it into a quart of spirit and let it steep by the fire for several days; and of this take a wine glass full every morning,

The stage which I have lately described, which is *chronic rheumatism,* the patient is frequently, by having had the disease a long time, reduced to great weakness: if so, he should use some bitters to strengthen the system; such as dog wood bark, wild cherry tree bark, and poplar bark, in equal quantities in whiskey, or spirit of any kind—old if possible: or if spirit disagrees make a tea, and use it three times a day—a wine glass full: or cold chamomile tea the same quantity; or take eight or ten drops of elixir vitriol, in a wine or stem glass of cold water, three times a day. In this state of the system, horse reddish and mustard will be proper to use with your food. Your diet should be as usual—no change is necessary in chronic rheumatism. Exercise is important, if the patient can possibly have it—and flannel should be worn next to the skin. The warm salt bath, as described under sea, or salt bath, will be of great utility in this state of the disease; or you may use it by pouring over the body three times a day, strong salt and water, made milk-warm. If the above remedies should not relieve, after a proper and patient trial of them, recourse must be had to the French remedy, called *sulphureous fumigation.* [For instructions see that head.]

INDIGESTION

OR

DYSPEPSIA.

This common and most afflicting disease, so much disturbs and deranges our moral and physical nature, that it is difficult to determine which suffers most from its attacks, the *mind* or the *body*. From the variety of shapes which this complaint assumes, it is very difficult to describe it in a plain and comprehensive manner; in fact, it is so frequently associated in colse connexion with other diseases to which it bears a strong resemblance, particularly, those of the *liver* and *bowels*, that in many cases, it deceives the most experienced and intelligent physicians. This complaint like the gout, may be said to be no respecter of persons: and from the prince to the begger, you can see misery inflicted, without discrimination of persons or ranks, by this demon of human suffering, *Indigestion*; under whose influence the body is tortured for years, and the mind continually wrecked in a troubled sea of the most unhappy and melancholy feelings.

This disease originates in a great variety of causes; among which it is often found associated with a diseased state of the *liver*. Persons who have used spirits of any kind to *excess*, or stimulants of any description, such as spices or highly seasoned food, and those also who have used tobacco to great excess, by which the coats and functions of the *stomach* have been impaired and debilitated, are liable to indigestion. A costive habit, acquired by permitting the bowels to remain too long without evacuation, will bring on this formidable malady; and, persons who are long confined to any stationary, or sedentary business, without taking the necessary exercise, are generally subject to this disease called Indigestion. When the complaint is firmly seated in the stomach, it is marked by eructations or belchings of wind; gnawing and disagreeable sensations at the pit of the stomach; risings of sour and bitter acids into the throat, occasioned by the food not being properly digested; great irregularity of appetite, which is sometimes voracious and at other times greatly deficient; and a sinking and oppressive debility or weakness of the stomach. In addition to these symptoms of indigestion, on gratifying the appetite at any time, the stomach in a short time afterwards, becomes oppressed with sensations of *weight* and *fullness*; the head becomes confused; the sleep very much disturbed; the bowels very irregular and costive; the urine high colored; and the poor victim commences taking medicines for relief, and brooding in dejected silence over thousands of unhappy retrospections of past life, and countless melancholy anticipations of the future, in which death in all its attendant and imaginary horrors, stands conspicuous and appalling. Nor are these the only miserable indications of indigestion; I have known many persons whose tempers and dispositions, have been materially affected by indigestion; so much so indeed, that they were incapable of describing their own sensations: and who, when ridiculed by their friends, in merely pleasant raillery, as hypochondriacs, have wished their sufferings were ended by a close of their existence!

If the *liver* is connected with this disease called Indigestion, a dead and heavy pain will be felt in the right side: the water deposited in the urinal or pot, will have, on cooling and settling, a brick-dust colored sediment, which if permitted to remain any length of time will adhere in rings of a reddish hue to the inner sides of the urinal; a pain will be felt in the top of the shoulder and back of the neck; the feet and hands will frequently get asleep, from want of regular and energetic circulation; the complexion will become of a yellowish hue or tinge; great and general uneasiness of the whole system will be felt; and sometimes, when the liver is greatly diseased, occasional puking will come on—in which last case, a diseased state of the *liver* being evident, I must refer the reader to that head.

REMEDIES.

In the removal or cure of this disease, great reliance is always to be placed on the systematic regulation of your diet as to the *times* of taking food—the *quantity of that food*—and the *qualities* to be taken; and any person laboring under *Indigestion* will soon discover, that regularity and temperance, in fact *abstemiousness* in eating and drinking, will be productive of as many benefits to the sufferer, as want of system and intemperance will be of *serious injuries*, and dangerous consequences. I am decidedly of opinion, with regard to dyspepsia, that by withdrawing the causes of irritation from the stomach, and applying such remedies as will have the effect of lessening irritability of the general system, unless the patient be entirely too much exhausted, *nature* would effect a *cure* without the aid of that farrago of medicines generally swallowed in this complaint: and I wish it here to be distinctly understood, that unless those who are tortured with *Indigestion* absolutely relinquish all excesses of the *table* and the *bottle*, no cure can be hoped for or expected.

DOCTOR JAMES JOHNSON, of the Royal College of Physicians, has correctly and elegantly described the remedies for indigestion, in nearly the following language. There is a great error committed almost every day in this disease, which is by flying to medicines at once, whenever the functions of the stomach and liver appear to be disordered, and the food imperfectly digested. Instead of taking purgative medicines day after day, we should lessen and *simplify* the *food*, in order to prevent the formation of such things in the body, as will assist to *produce* and *increase* the disease; but in attempting to induce a patient to adopt this rule; I am aware that great prejudices are to be overcome. The patient feels himself getting weaker and thinner; and he flies immediately to nourishing food, and tonics and strengthening medicines for a cure: but he will generally be disappointed in the end by this plan. From *four ounces of gruel* every six hours, under any states of *indigestion*, he will derive more nutriment and real strength, than from *half a pound of animal food*, and a *pint of the best wine*. Whenever he feels any additional uneasiness or discomfort, in mind or body, *after eating*, the patient has *erred* in the quantity or quality of his food, however restricted the one or select the other. If the food and drink irritate the nerves of the stomach, they must be reduced and simplified down even to the gruel diet above alluded to. I have known dyspeptic patients gain flesh and strength, on half a pint of good gruel, taken three times in twenty-four hours, and gradually bring the stomach step by step, up to the point of digesting plain animal food. On a *biscuit* and a *glass of water*, I have known persons who were afflicted with this disease to dine for months in succession; and on this small portion of food, to obtain a degree of strength, and a serenity of mind, beyond their most sanguine hopes. You will perceive, that in all the different forms of Indigestion, diet is the *first thing*, and the principal cure in this disease; and rely upon it, for I assert it from sad experience in my own person, that it is absolutely vain to expect a cure, unless you have courage and perseverance to reap the fruits of such a system as I have laid down to you in diet, and not to change it, however strongly you may be tempted by the luxuries of the table, and the seductions of convivial society, and when you have escaped the miseries of this worst of human affliction, you must be extremely careful how you deviate from the right diet which has restored you to health; for no disease is so liable to *relapse* as Indigestion. An unrestrained indulgence in a variety of dishes, or vegetable and fruit, or a debauch in drinking, will be certain of making the poor dyspeptic patient pay dearly, in suffering and wretchedness of feelings, for his straying from the correct path of temperance and propriety. The least over-exertion of the stomach, caused by its being overloaded or too highly stimulated, will be certain to cause you to be on the stool of repentance for some time afterwards. As soon as you have the least reason for supposing that you are laboring under Indigestion, commence first with an active purgative consisting of *ten grains of calomel, ten of rhubarb* in fine powder, and *ten of aloes* likewise finely powdered. These three articles are to be mixed well together, and made into pills, with honey or syrup. After this purgative medicine, which is intended to clear the stomach and bowels of all their unhealthy and injurious contents, which always when present, keep up a constant irritation in the stomach and intestines no more very active purges are to be given—because the frequent and almost constant employment of active purges, always do more harm than good, by unnecessarily weakening the system: one satisfactory evacuation by stool in the course of the day is quite sufficient; and by more than this, the stomach and bowels are *teased*, thereby producing *debility*—the real parent of morbid irritation. When this state of the body is avoided, and the stomach and bowels at the same time kept sufficiently *easy* and *clear*, and the *temperate abstemiousness* I have advised strictly followed, the poor sufferer under *Indigestion*, may *hope* and *confidently expect* an extinguishment of the flames of his torture.

A little rhubarb root chewed at night—or the following simple pill will be of service. Take of rhubarb in powder half a drachm, of castile soap one drachm, and of ipecacuanha in powder half a drachm, mix them well together in honey or any syrup, to which add a little powdered ginger, to make the mixture pleasant to the stomach: make it into *thirty pills*, one of which you must take every morning, noon and at night; this will give a *tone* to the stomach and bowels, but as an alternative; and keep them *gently open*—this is an innocent and most useful pill, and will afford great relief, with proper exercise and diet. A tea spoonful or a table spoonful of common *charcoal*, pounded very fine, and taken three times a day in a tumbler of cold water, is an excellent remedy in this complaint. This article is made in a proper manner, by taking a lump of common charcoal made of any kind of wood, and *burning it over again* in an iron ladle or skillet, to a *red heat:* then suffering it to cool —and pounding it as before directed. This coal powder, ought to be immediately put into a bottle and corked tightly, in order to exclude the action of the air on it—and whenever any of it is used as before mentioned, the cork ought immediately to be returned to the bottle. The quantity of the charcoal used, must be regulated so as to produce moderate operation by stool. I have known hundreds relieved by this simple and innocent remedy, when the diet has been properly attended to, after many other remedies had been tried in vain. Physicians call this pounded charcoal, *carbo ligni*, in their learned prescriptions; which I have often found very powerful in relieving diseases of the liver, when other remedies had totally failed. Epsom salts and magnesia in equal quantities, ground fine in a mortar, and given in doses of a tea spoonful in a glass of cold water, every morning on an empty stomach, is also a fine remedy in Indigestion or Dyspepsia—and if necessary at any time to have the bowels gently opened, will always be found beneficial and effective.

When the stomach and bowels have been kept free from irritation for any length of time, by the mild treatment I have laid down; when the tongue becomes clean; when the sleep becomes more refreshing; and when the mind becomes tranquil, the spirits something animated, and the head clear, fresh beef made into a weak soup, may be ventured on, with a little well boiled chicken; by this diet you may gradually try the powers of the stomach, and know by your feelings how much they will bear without injury. If it produce uneasy feelings, such as before described, to either the mind or body—or to both—within the day or night of this trial of *animal food*, it should be lessened in quantity. If that will not do, you must entirely relinquish it, and resume the old diet of *gruel*. When animal food can be taken, without producing any pain and uneasiness, you may gradually increase it according to your feelings. Begin with *one ounce* of animal food, and gradually increase the quantity, but with great caution. After a while you may venture on simple food, so that by degrees your stomach may acquire some strength and firmness, which it will now do beyond your most sanguine expectations; but you must always remember, to eat just such a quantity as will produce no *uneasiness* or *languor after eating;* no unhappy feelings of body or mind during digestion. It is quite unnecessary for me to enumerate all the kinds of food which it will be improper for you to eat; I have already explained to you, that the most simple food is the best. Milk and rye-mush is an excellent dish in this complaint; and I have known many persons, who, by using it six months together, without any animal food, have been entirely and permanently cured. No hot bread is to be used at all; stale bread and biscuit, the older the better, but without any butter, are very good in this complaint. How often have I been asked by my dyspeptic patients this question: Is it impossible to cure *Indigestion* without resorting to low and very abstemious diet? I have always said it is *impossible*—and I now repeat it, for the ten thousandth time; and those who think otherwise, will find, if they act up to their opinions, that after spending their money, and making apothecary shops of their bodies, that all the medical remedies in the world, *without very temperate and abstemious living*, are not worth one cent? Always have patience; there must be time for every thing, and particularly for the cure of Indigestion. Reflect on the length of time, and the great variety of causes which produce this disease, and you will soon see that it cannot be cured in a few hours, or in a few days. The stomach, like a weary traveller worn down by fatigue, requires *rest, tranquillity,* and *cooling diet,* to allay the feverish state of the system, produced by high and long continued excitement, and perhaps by *terrible excesses!*

Cold water is the only proper drink; and to persons who have been accustomed to the use of spirituous liquors, some gentle bitter may be taken, but in *very small quantities.* But in respect to drink, I am perfectly convinced that water alone is the best drink for persons afflicted with this disease of the stomach. After a complete change has taken place in the system, by a low, regular, and very abstemious diet, *for some months*—the patient will find, if it should agree with his stomach, which his own feelings will soon tell him, immense benefit from taking a *mixture,* compounded of equal quantities of the root of the poplar, the bark of the wild cherry-tree, and the bark from the root of the dogwood, with a small portion of black snake-root, made into bitters with old whiskey or very old rum. This bitters must stand four or five days before being taken; and then given in small doses, diluted with water, three times in each day—but if it occasions any *unpleasantness of feeling* or *sensation,* in the stomach or head, it must be *immediately discontinued.* Tonic or *strengthening* medicines are never to be given in the fever stages of *Indigestion,* or while the slightest *irritation* exists, or the consequence will probably be, an *inflammation* which will terminate fattally.

The *warm or tepid bath* should be frequently used in this complaint, taking particular care to rub over the stomach well with a brush in the bath, and a coarse towel immediately on leaving it. For bathing, and the manner of preparing the warm or tepid bath, look under the head Warm Bath. Injections or clysters of simple milk and water, luke-warm, or of warm water with a table spoonful of hog's lard mixed with it, thrown up into the bowels, occasionally, will be of much service in this disease: because they will remove any irritable matter which may remain in the lower intestines, thereby lessening one of the greatest enemies you have to contend with, which is *morbid irrita-*

bility. For clysters—look under that head. Clysters, constantly used with the warm bath, will obviate or do away the necessity of taking medicines by the stomach, and very much expedite the cure of the afflicted sufferer. In this disease, the acid or sour belchings may be corrected or removed, by the simple use of magnesia or chalk: a tea spoonful of either of which articles, may be taken in a wine or stem glass of cold water. The charcoal prepared as I have before mentioned, is also well adapted to removing this unpleasant and irritable state of the stomach arising from acid. I have now given a faithful, plain, and full description of this tedious and most afflicting malady, called *Dyspepsia* or *Indigestion*—together with an account of the most approved remedies for its removal.

CONSUMPTION.

Consumption spreads its ravages in the haunts of gaiety, fashion, and folly—but in the more humble walks of life where the busy hum of laborious industry is heard, it is seldom known. In the last stage of this dismal waste of life, although there are many means of alleviating, in some degree, its miseries, there is neither remedy nor cure for this disease—and yet so flattering is *Consumption*, even when very far advanced that the unfortunate victim frequently anticipates a speedy recovery, and is preparing for some distant journey for the renovation of health, when in a few days, perhaps a few hours, his wearied feet must pass the peaceful threshold of the tomb, and his body sink to everlasting rest; thousands are yearly falling in the spring-time of life by the untimely stroke of this most fatal of diseases, and although, medical men have for ages been endeavoring to put a stop to its ravages. I assert it without fear of contradiction, that in the last stage of consumption, there is no remedy within the whole circle of medical science, that will cure the disease, but I have no doubt the period will arrive, when this formidable enemy of the

O*

human species, will be subdued by some common and simple plant, belonging to the vegetable kingdom, which is at this period totally unknown; for I have always been impressed with a decided belief, that our wise and beneficent CREATOR has placed within the reach of his feeble creature *man*, herbs and plants for the cure of all diseases but old age, could we but obtain a knowledge of their real uses and intrinsic virtues. I wish it to be distinctly understood, with respect to what I have said of this disease, that I mean Consumption alone, and entirely unconnected with any other complaint. The cure of *Consumption* should always be attempted in its forming state, before it produces active symptoms of cough, or matter from the lungs, or inflammatory or hectic fever. I have often seen this fatal complaint cured by attention to it, in the first symptoms, but how often are they permitted to steal gradually on, creating no alarm or uneasiness, mistaking it for a simple cold, until it makes considerable progress, and the complaint becomes permanently seated in the system. *Consumption* can easily be distinguished from any other disease by the following symptoms, the patient complains of weakness on the least bodily exertion, the breathing is hurried, oppressed on ascending any steep place, the pulse small, and quicker than natural, a feeling of tightness as if a cord was drawn across the chest; slight, short, dry cough, becoming more troublesome at night; a spitting of white frothy spittle termed by physicians, mucus. As this disease advances, the spitting becomes more copious and frequent, and sometimes streaked with blood, of a tough, opake or dark substance, solid and of a yellow or green color, having an unpleasant or fetid smell when thrown on burning coals, or if this matter is put into pure water, it sinks to the bottom of the vessel, by this simple test, you can easily distinguish it from *mucus* which has no smell, and separates into small flaxes, and floats upon the surface of the water—thereby enabling you to judge as to the progress or formation of this complaint.

CONSUMPTION is considerably advanced when the following symptoms occur: a pain in the chest, and in the side, which is increased by exerting the voice by long or loud talking; pulse is quick and hard, generally from one hundred to one hundred and fifteen strokes in a minute; the urine or water is highly colored, and deposits in the urinal or pot a muddy sediment; the palms of the hands, and the soles of the feet, have a dryness and burning sensation; one cheek, and frequently both cheeks, have a flush or reddish hue, exhibiting itself about the middle of the day. This flush lasts one or two hours, when a remission takes place until the evening, when the feverish symptoms again return, accompanied frequently by a shivering or cold sensation, continuing until after midnight, then terminating in a profuse perspiration or sweat, occasioning great prostration or weakness. In the last stage of Consumption, the whole countenance assume a ghastly and cadaverous look, the white part of the eyes have a pearly and unnatural appearance, while the eye itself beams with sparkling animation and lustre; the cheek-bones are prominent, the mouth and throat resembles or looks like that of a child having the *thrush;* the legs swell, the nails are of a livid or purple color; frequent purging, ending in profuse sweating, cough hollow, difficulty of respiration or breathing, and the patient has a restless and disturbed slumb r; during sleep, a curious noise is made from the throat, like suffocation, occasioned by the collection of matter or pus, in the throat and mouth: when these last symptoms make their appearance, the period is last approaching, when the unhappy sufferer will lay his weary and aching head in the calm and peaceful mansions of the dead. The alarming increase of Consumptions in the United States, affords an ample field for medical research; the bills of mortality taken in the various cities show the immense number who die in the flower of life, by this merciless disease. In three years, the number of deaths in the British metropolis, is stated to be fifty two thousand, two hundred and thirty-seven; and among these, were, under the general head of Consumptions, seventeen thousand, five hundred and fifty-nine—making the number of deaths annually in London, by Consumption, three theusand.

The rapid progress made in our country by this fatal complaint, is sufficient to serve as a warning to every parent, and head of a family, in order to avoid those *causes,* which, sooner or later, end in this unmanageable disease. The causes which produce Consumption are, exposure to cold & damp air, using tobacco to excess, either by smoking, chewing or by using it in snuff to clean the teeth, acting as a powerful stimulant, thereby producing irritation; the use of spirituous liquors to excess; obstructions and inflammations of the lungs; the suppression of natural discharges, particularly the menstrual discharge or courses; scrofula, diseases of the *liver* and *stomach,* and unfortunately, receiving a hereditary disposition or taint to this disease from father or mother. The narrow chest and high shoulders, weakness of the voice, whiteness of the teeth, fairness of complexion, and light hair, have all been observed to accompany a predisposition to consumption. Much reliance however cannot be placed upon these signs, except where a number of them concur in the same person." While the empire of fashion bears so arbitrary a sway, and the followers of pleasure are bound by the fascination of example, and the contagious influence of that spirit, which insinuates itself into the bosom of each and every one of its votaries, so long will the sage precepts of wisdom be unheeded till the emaciated form, the glassy eye, and hectic blush, speak in language too strong for utterance, that the disease is established and the yawning grave stands ready to receive its devoted victim. I hardly know an object of more tender concern to the anxious parent, or the medical adviser, than a young and beautiful female in the pride and spring of youth, and strength of intellect, borne down by the invasion of a malady, which has so often selected for its sacrifices, the most amiable and interesting beings of God's creation. And when, moreover, all this can be traced to one single act of imprudence, one offering on the altar of fashion, who can forbear to utter a sigh, when they behold a lovely woman, laced to such a degree as to impede respiration, or breathing. As well might the hardy Russian or Laplander, amongst his snows, pretend to brave the severities of his icy climate in the flowing robes of tropical indolence, as a female to indulge in the Grecian costume or dress, under the influence of such a change as we experience during the winter and spring months. This predisposing debility for consumption runs in families, and may be traced from generation to generation—moving on the leaden pinions of unshaken time, without a remedy to arrest its course.

REMEDIES.

The cure for this formidable complaint is to be attempted by a removal to a warm climate at an early stage of the disease, and to attend to the preservation of an equal temperature in the atmosphere which the patient breaths, a sudden or frequent alteration of heat and cold is fatal to an irritable consumptive system, if possible consumptive persons should remove to a warm climate the moment a predisposition is discovered; a change to a warm or temperate atmosphere during the winter months, may be the means of removing the predisposing cause to this complaint; it is however, to be regreted, that this change is often delayed until a late period of this disease, when the strength is so much exhausted that sufferers can not take sufficient exercise to assist the climate in restoring health, it is then too late, and the unfortunate victim of this complaint had better remain at home, for by leaving it, he is deprived of the attention of the society of his friends, and exposed to much unnecessary fatigue and anxiety of mind. If the disease is so far advanced as to prevent the patient from going out of doors in the winter months, his chamber or room should be kept warm at an even temperature by a stove; the unpleasant smell which frequently arises from a stove in a close room, may be removed by burning tar upon it, this fumigation or vapour, constantly inhaled or breathed, is considered by physicians as a valuable remedy in *Consumption;* the usual method of inhaling the vapour or steam, is by putting a small quantity of tar into a coffee-pot or earthern vessel, which is to be heated and the fumes inhaled from the stem of the vessel, this simple but valuable remedy, allays the violence of the cough, and produces a free and copious discharge of mucus or matter, inhaling of the vapour arising from warm water with a little vinegar added to it, several times during the coarse of the day, will assist in promoting the discharge and tranquilize the cough. These valuable but simple remedies should not be omitted in this complaint. Bleak winds, night air, and exposure of every kind must be strictly avoided, the body should be well defended by wearing flannel next the skin, also the feet properly secured from the damp; frictions or in other words, rubbing the whole body with a brush or coarse towel from fifteen to twenty minutes in the morning, and at night, will be of great service in this disease; the friction to be continued twice a day, as long as the complaint lasts. As nothing tends more to aggravate the symptoms of a Consumption at an early stage than a desponding mind, brooding over real or perhaps imaginary calamities, every thing should be done to cheer the spirits, such as cheerful society, music, &c. &c. Be careful to regulate the bowels, if possible by diet, and by friction (as before described,) but if recourse must be had to medicine, let it always be mild, and in no larger doses than are necessary to discharge or move the bowels, for this purpose clysters of simple milk and water thrown up the bowels, or warm water with a tea spoonful of hog's lard will be proper, (for clystering and the method of administering them look under that head) *rhubarb* root chewed in small quantities at night will produce a motion, *Epsom salts* and *magnesia* mixed and ground fine in a mortar, dose a tea spoonful in half a pint of cold water—or a table spoonful of common *charcoal* pounded very fine in the same quantity of water, for the method of making and preserving this innocent but valuable medicine, read *Indigestion.* The consumptive patient should daily take as much exercise as his strength will admit of except when the weather is unfavorable, the best exercise will be riding on horse-back, but if this produces fatigue, substitute the use of some kind of carriage, or a swing, so constructed as to admit a chair in it, for the patient to recline or rest when fatigued: In my prac-

'tice I have used a large basket of a sufficient size to admit a small bed to be placed in it, the patient can lay at full length, and receive the advantages to be derived from the swing, without experiencing any fatigue, this basket is about six feet in length and two feet in width, having six handles by which it is suspended to the ceiling, with ropes, or in any convenient place, free from damp or moist atmosphere. In whatever exercise is taken, the greatest care must be observed to guard against cold in any manner whatever, for this important reason *tubercles* or ulcers of the lungs are formed in the winter in cold climates, and their progress to suppuration kept hack in the summer, and this is the cause why I urge your removal to a warm climate, at an early period of this disease, for when tubercles or ulcers become permanently seated in the lungs, the case may be considered incurable, but palliative remedies may be given with proper diet, and change of climate, as to prolong the life of the unfortunate victim of this disease;—I shall explain for the satisfaction of my reader, what is meant by the *lungs* and their structure. In anatomy it denotes the viscera or lobes in the cavity of the breast, by which we breathe; they are connected with the neck, and situated on the right and left side of the heart; being furnished with innumerable cells which are formed by the descent of the wind pipe into the lungs, those bronchial tubes communicate wi.h each other; and the whole appears not unlike a honey comb, the most important use of the *lungs*, is that of respiration or breathing, by which the circulation of the blood is supposed to be effected, the evacuation of the fæces or excrement, and urine, greatly depends on the constant action of the *lungs*, but likewise the sense of smelling is enjoyed by inhaling the air; and it is cheifly by the organic structure of these vessels, that mankind are enabled to speak;—lastly, they perform the office of excretion, and expel those useles matters, which if retained in the system, would be productive of fatal consequences. The treatment of consumptive persons must be regulated according to the manner in which this disease shows itself, an energetic course of practice by the physician in the first stage or symptoms of this disease may be the means of saving the life of his patient, or in other words preventing confirmed *Consumption* if there is a pain in the side, or breast, accompanied by cough with fever, the patient should be bled immediately, the quantity of blood taken must be regulated by the constitution, strength and habits of the person, *bleeding* should be continued every third day if the inflammatory symptoms continue to exist, regulating the quantity of blood, by the strength and feverish state of the patient. I have generally found in my practice that after bleeding moderately, the symptoms considerably abated, the fever diminished, less pain in the breast or side, cough relieved and the respiration or breathing much improved, after the inflammatory action is subdued, apply a blister over the breast, and side, if necessary from pain, this blister is to be kept discharging or running, and should it heal, put on another; the object being to continue a drain or running as much as possible (similar to a seaton or rowel) as you value the life of your patient, enforce a *rigid* and *low diet*, of the most simple nature, for hundreds die from imprudence in this respect who might be relieved if they could but have courage and firmness to live on *gruel* and *milk*, and avoid altogether animal or stimulating food. I have had an opportunity of testing the effects of low diet in *Consumption* and I feel fully satisfied, that it is highly essential in the cure of this disease. In the early stage of this alarming complaint, give an *emetic* or puke of *ipecacuanna*: [see table for dose:] and repeat this emetic, once or twice a week as the obstruction or case may require, this is to be continued through the disease, and much benefit will result from it, for I rely very much on emetics in my practice in consumption, for the purpose of moderating the irritation of the system and allaying cough and fever, give small doses of *tartar emetic* of half a grain dissolved in a small quantity of flax seed tea, balm or sage tea, slippery elm tea, marsh mallow tea, any of which may be used, the tartar emetic must be gradually increased and given at intervals until the irritation subsides, if the tartar emetic affects the stomach or bowels, add a few drops of laudanum to each dose. By a little caution the *emetic tartar* may be gradually increased with much benefit to the patient by lessening the fever, allaying the cough, and producing expectoration, or in other words, a free discharge from the breast, as an active and valuable expectorant; much benefit will be derived from the *Indian turnip*, this valuable plant is very common in the Western states, grows in meadows and swamps, six or eight inches high, purple leaves, three in number, roundish berries, of a light scarlet color; the root of this plant boiled in milk is a valuable remedy; or take of the peeled root one pound, and three pound of loaf sugar, pound them well together in a mortar so as to make a fine powder, and take a tea spoonful twice or thrice a day as the case may require; gum Arabic, or peach tree gum will answer, held in the mouth to allay the cough. Cooling medicines through the whole course of the complaint will be proper; particularly *nitre*, equal quantities of Epsom salts and magnesia mxed, pounded fine in a mortar, doses of a teaspoonful to be given in half a pint of cold water will cool the system and keep the bowels in a laxative state; the dose to be increased, if necessary to act on the bowels. In the advanced stage of this disease the patient is usually much weakened by night sweats, this should be checked by administering the following pills: copperas, (called by physicians, sulphate of iron) one grain, rhubarb one grain, gum myrrh two grains, oil of cloves one drop; these pills should be repeated three or four times, a day; and ten or fifteen drops of sulphuric acid, or the same quantity of elixir vitriol, taken every two or three hours, in a cup of flaxseed tea, when the febrile symptoms are severe. Pills composed of sulphate of copper one grain, ipecacuanha one grain made into a pill, and repeated every three hours, is a valuable remedy; infusion of wild cherry tree bark, made with cold water, tar water, and cold chamomile tea, are all good strengthening remedies in this stage of the complaint.

A purging attends this disease which is very exhausting, ending in profuse sweating, (as before mentioned,) for as soon as the one is stopped, the other too frequently comes on, producing thereby an extreme degree of weakness. When this takes place, use opium united with a small quantity of ipecacuanha or sugar of lead, if the disease is severe: [see table for doses.] An infusion of galls, or tormentil root with cinnamon and gum Arabic, will check the purging. About this stage of the disease, the mouth and throat are filled with sores, similar to the *thrush;* here astringent gargles of sage tea, with a little borax and honey, to wash the mouth and throat, will be proper, aided by tonic and astringent medicines, are the only hope of giving relief in this last stage of Consumption. My practice is, to give opium to a considerable extent; increasing or decreasing it, as the situation of the case may require. By this valuable medicine, we have it in our power to protract the period of life, and to lessen the distress of the patient. The inexpressible delight produced by opium, when the poor sufferer is prostrated, can scarcely be described. It always soothes the irritations of the cough, and mitigates all those symptoms which *cannot* be removed. The influence it exercises over the mind and imagination of the patient, no human language can describe. In some constitutions, opium disagrees with the patient, and produces restless and irritable feelings. When this is the case, recourse must be had to other sedatives or soothing remedies: for instance, to *garden lettuce;* which is fully equal to opium in producing a mitigation of pain, and in allaying inordinate action. For the manner of preparing this valuable remedy which every one is in possession of, see the head *Garden lettuce.*

ICELAND Moss, has also, for some time past in Europe, been resorted to as a valuable palliative in Consumption; and more recently in the United States, it has required considerable reputation in this disease. But like all other boasted remedies, its powers have been probably over-rated. It, however, not unfrequently proves highly beneficial, by strengthening the patient, diminishing the hectic symptoms, and allaying the cough. It has another important advantage. It strengthens the digestive powers, without producing a constipation or costiveness of the bowels. This medicine is quite innocent: the *Laplanders* use it in various ways, and among others as food. When employed as an article of diet, they bruise this moss, and steep it in several successive waters: by which means they extract its bitter qualities, and it then affords them a highly grateful food, of a soft and gluttonous consistency, similar to jelly; but the method of preparing it for consumptive persons is as follows. First, wash it well in clean cold water; then boil one ounce of the moss, with a quart of water over a *slow fire*—and while stewing, add of liquorice root, cut up very fine, *two drachms*, or about as much as the size of the middle finger. A tea cup ful of this medicine must be drank four times a day. Or—if the taste of this preparation is too disagreeable, you may boil a quarter of an ounce of the moss in a pint of milk for ten minutes, and take the milk for breakfast and supper—always taking care, that the quantity be not disagreeable to the patient's stomach. For a description of this moss, and where it may be had, [see Iceland Moss.]

Lichen or **Lungwort**, which grows on the bark of the whiteoak tree, and which looks like a shell or skin, is said to possess the same medicinal qualities as the *Iceland moss*. It is called *Lungwort*, (I had almost forgotten to remark) because of its strong resemblance in shape of the human lung. A tea made of a handful of the *lungwort* in a quart of boiling water, and used as a common drink, is not only a good palliative in consumption, but when made into a syrup with honey, is very beneficial in *hooping-cough*.

Doctor Hereford of Virginia, a gentleman of distinguished reputation as a physician, has made some interesting communications in the news-papers, relative to a plant called *liverwort*, which he presumed to be effectual in the cure of consumption. For a description of this plant, and the method of preparing it, [look under the head *liverwort.*]

The Doctor is certainly entitled to be considered the first who made use of it in the cure of consumption; and his communications on the subject, will entitle him to the thanks of posterity—if for no other reason, than that it has been found an excellent *palliative* remedy in this dreadful disease. So high was at one period, the excitement of the public feeling, respecting the virtues of this little plant, as a certain cure for consumption, and so great was the demand for it, that it was frequently sold at Nashville, for the enormous price of five dollars an ounce. After some time, it sunk greatly in price in this country, being discovered to be very plentiful in the mountains of Tennessee. Like all other Boasted remedies, which have been called *specific cures* in consumption, the liverwort is only considered a good palliative—a mere alleviator of the miseries of the disease.

CASES OF CONSUMPTION.

An anxious desire to communicate to my fellow beings, every useful information, respecting this most terrible of diseases (*consumption*,) induces me to extend the subject to a much greater length than was at first intended: the information being derived, however, from a source of very high respectability and experience, cannot but be acceptable to my readers. The quotation is from the writings of Doct. J. E. Cooke, of Winchester, Virginia—a gentleman of distinguished abilities in his profession.

"My object in the following communication is to give some cases, calculated to shew that consumption is not so incurable as is generally supposed.

In the year 1808, or 1809, my advice was required for a young man aged 18, all of whose brothers and sisters had died of pulmonary* affections. As he was the hope of the family, the approach of the disease was observed with great anxiety.

He was bled, and blistered frequently on the chest, one plaster being applied as soon as the blister from the preceding one was well. He took an emetic of ipecacuanha occasionally, perhaps twice a week, and every day a pill of one or two grains of the same medicine. The diet was low—he soon recovered and became perfectly well.

In 1818, a young lady of pale complexion, with cough

Disease of the lungs.

and expectoration of purulent matter, applied for advice. She was bled five or six times in the first week or ten days —blistered repeatedly, and treated as above. She rapidly improved; and in some weeks declared herself well. There still remained however, a slight cough and *very small* purulent expectoration. She would not be advised, went into company, ate, drank as usual, relapsed, neglected herself for six months and died.

Another, some of whose relations had been affected with pulmonary diseases, had *hectic fever, cough, purulent expectoration*, and *night sweats.* Under the same treatment she recovered almost entirely, but as soon as she was able to partake of the enjoyments of life, yielded to the temptation, and relapsed. She returned to the treatment above mentioned, recovered again, was again negligent, and again relapsed. In this way she nearly recovered and relapsed several times; but finally, under a severe attack, during which, the quantity of purulent matter expectorated was enormous, she died.

In consequence of the marked effect of the treatment, I was strongly induced to believe, that if a person would resolutely continue the practice as long as I thought necessary, entire recovery would follow. This opinion was advanced in conversation, and by medical men was reprobated. I could not produce a single case in which complete success had attended the treatment, excepting the first; to which, being in the first stage, objections were easily made.

In the next case that occurred, I determined, if possible, to carry the plan into complete execution. A man upwards of thirty, had pains in the chest, cough, and purulent expectoration, was emaciated, and little or no hope entertained by his friends of his recovery. He had so little expectation of it, that he was unwilling to enter upon the painful course proposed. I told him fully what he had to expect, and requested he would not commence. unless he was determined to continue it. He hesitated long, but was finally induced by his friends to submit. The course above mentioned, was fully carried into execution. He was bled repeatedly, whenever the pulse would admit of it; he was repeatedly, many times, blistered as above; took every night a pill of aloes and ipecacuanha, in equal quantities—which gave one or two passages a day; lived on tea and milk and butter-milk, with bread—avoiding meat, or any kind of fermented drink.

When at the lowest, many persons expected his death from the plan: he however, lived through it, and continued the treatment and spare diet, until he was able to ride about—he gradually became fat and healthy, and is at this day a large man.

One more case only I shall mention—L. L. a man about 30 years of age, when he applied to me, had been some time diseased, and was about going to sea as his last resource. He stooped considerably, his breathing was difficult and hurried, coughed and freely expectorated purulent matter. He was bled very frequently, the rule being to bleed whenever his pulse should become tense, and blistered continually as above mentioned. He took at night, ipecacuanha and aloes, and sometimes calomel sufficient to move his bowels once or twice the next day. From one to two grains of ipecacuanha and as much aloes, answers the purpose generally. He took occasionally an emetic. His diet was tea, coffee, milk, butter-milk, bread and butter.

He commenced this course in September, and continued it till the last of January. When I last saw him in January, he sat as erect as any man could—filled his lungs repeatedly at my request, to the utmost extent without inconvenience or coughing—he had no cough that would have been noticed by any person, and no expectoration; in short, no person could have pronounced what had been the nature of his disease from the existing symptoms. I wished him to continue the diet and occasionally to blister.

This did not satisfy his friends who had been long privately complaining of the severity of the treatment. They now redoubled their objections; insisted he would be killed by such energetic means, &c. &c. Accordingly, they finally succeeded in inducing him to send for another physician. This was done without my being informed of it, till some time had elapsed. The physician without knowing any thing of his previous treatent or its effects, excepting from his nurse, but resting his views on the present debility alone though he could sit up and converse, advised a better diet. This agreeable prescription was followed—he soon became unwell, continually got worse, and died some months after, two days after having partaken of a meal of animal food.

Fully persuaded from the event of the other case, that his recovery was possible, the treatment was pushed with confidence, and I was flattering myself with the fortunate issue, when the case was thus taken out of my hands, and a long continued and carefully conducted experiment, of the utmost importance, broken in at the moment of ex-expected success.

About this time, the following case was communicated to me by a friend; and the result of it so incontestibly proves the justice of my opinion, that permission was obtained to publish it.

Dear sir.

According to your wish, I send you the following statement of my case. Most of my nearest connexions, of about my own age, died of consumption; *one* of my two sisters, and *nine* cousins, in two families. My father was saved from the same end, in his youth, by going to sea for many years, and his sister, by living forty years with the most scrupulous temperance, though very often spitting blood, and suffering from a severe cough. I was constantly threatened from the age of fifteen, but occasional bleeding, blistering, and a light diet, subdued the symptoms. In the intervals, I lived and took exercise as usual. My attacks became less frequent, till at last they left me, and from my thirty-third, to my thirty-ninth year, though with a slight habitual cough, I had been so free from all warnings, that I had forgotten there could be any danger. Late in the summer of 1810, my cough increased; I supposed it, however, to proceed from a cold; all my other attacks had been sudden and severe, and checked by decided measures, excepting one, when I was eighteen years old, which lasted nearly a year. I now felt no pain, had no fever, was constantly about, and lived as usual, till the cough became almost suffocating; I had, at the same time, some strong bilious symptoms and a light fever. I consulted professional men, and took medicine, &c. but grew rapidly worse. I suggested to them the possibility of its being my old constitutional complaint, but they would not allow it. I, however, was at last, bled and blistered, and though I found relief, I was so strangely infatuated as not to continue these remedies, but ate, drank, and used stimulating medicines. It was insisted, that, as I *had no pain*, my lungs were not affected, and I *must* have the hooping-cough, because it was in the neighborhood, though I had *had* it severely when a child, which all my friends, as well as myself could perfectly remember. My fever was violent, my strength entirely failed, and was on the point of suffocation ten times a day; I coughed all night; my bed was wet through with perspiration; I became almost a skeleton, from the bilious state of my stomach, an emetic was administered, after which my appetite entirely failed, though I still continued to *swallow* meat, wine, and the most stimulating medicines. A large boil appeared on my breast, after the blister I had insisted upon having applied; this circumstance I urged as an evidence of disease within, but it was not regarded. Whilst the blister continued to discharge, my cough was somewhat alleviated: but the day after it closed, I had a more severe and distressing chill, preceding the afternoon fever, than I had ever experienced. While the fever of that day was raging, the cough and suffocation threatened immediate death. The spasm became extreme, my senses failed, at last were entirely gone. In the struggle an ulcer gave way, and when I opened my eyes again, I was expectorating with the most agonizing cough, large quantities of matter mixed with blood. This was the first time I had expectorated any blood, though it had frequently been discharged from my head, which I had often urged as a reason for a different mode of treatment. I then saw, what was my exact situation; I wondered at my late blindness. I had watched my sister through the whole progress of her disorder, saw her endure the same agony, with the same result, and then sink rapidly into the arms of death. I, therefore, gave up all hope; I considered all aid as too late. However, to satisfy my mother, wife, and sister, I sent to a town at some distance, for a physician who had formerly been at the point of death with the same disease, and who had seen my sister during her illness. The pain in my side now, for the first time, came on, and as the ulcer increased, and new ones were formed and discharged on the opposite lobe of the lungs, my condition became insupportable; in whatever position I was placed in the bed, it was almost impossible to turn from it, on account of the lancinating pains, the extreme soreness within, and the suffocating weight which a word or a motion would produce. In an upright position, I was but little easier. The gentleman for whom I had sent, came, but made no change in the treatment, till after he had watched by me, almost the whole time, for two days and nights. He then said that an entirely opposite course, carried to the last extreme, might *possibly* save me; at least it would relieve me from the raging fever, and dreadful suffocation under which I then labored, and which every day threatened to be instantly fatal, and that I should sink more gradually and with less pain. I acquiesced. It was then January; the temperature of my room, both night and day, was kept by a thermometer, at 55 deg's of Fahrenheit, which was not sufficiently warm to be agreeable; if increased, my fever became extreme, and if colder, my cough insupportable. In the first four days after this treatment was commenced, beef soup, wine, coffee, bark and opium, which I had been taking to support me, were prohibited, though I had no appetite, and was rapidly sinking. Three tea-cups of milk and water, in twenty-four hours, with a little bread dried in an oven and pounded, with three wine glasses of tea made of Iceland moss, taken cold, half an hour before the milk was taken; a very small quantity of cicuta was substituted for the opium. I do not, however, attribute *much* to the cicuta. I was bled moderately three times in the first four days during the fever; I had bleeding from the nose every morning, for two months after this prescription, and frequently, also, from my lungs, in the most violent paroxysm of coughing, which was easily distinguished from the other, by its color, and the sensation when it was forced away. My breast was covered with blisters, put on every night and morning; these means, however, appeared too slow; accordingly, on the sixth day, on the right side over the most painful ulcer, sulphuric acid and the alkali were applied, producing, in a week, a sore which almost exposed the surface of the ribs. This plan was continued for three months without intermission, and afterwards, with some intervals of a week, for a year; rhubarb, sufficient to move my bowels, was given every night. The regular bleeding at the nose rendered venesection unnecessary for a month; and after its cessation, it was performed as often as was requisite for some time, amounting to thirteen times in the course of a few months. As soon as I was able to travel, if pain and fever returned, and blistering did not remove them, I was bled and lived on tea and bred; after eating even milk for five or six days, I was obliged to intermit it. For twenty-two days my physician continued with me every night till 2 o'clock, regulating according to circumstances, the bed clothes; my limbs were frequently rubbed. I was put on a wooden horse, or an elastic board, which was moved by an assistant; at first, I could not sit upon it more than five minutes, but in six weeks, I could ride with facility, and move myself with a staff with several bars through it to exercise my hands many hours in the day. My appetite was literally starved back again in five or six days; but this was the only good symptom. The same severe treatment was continued; I gained no strength, but was every day *apparently* at the point of death with suffocation; I would survive the struggle: and throw up matter and blood, with the hard points of tubercles, and then be, for a few hours relieved.

To all *appearance* I was now much worse, as the treatment had taken away my color, except during the fever; my emaciation was extreme, and my mouth and throat were extremely sore. All who saw me, except my family pronounced my case desperate and, that the *treatment* must be fatal. This however, was my last hope, and with our approbation the physician had the courage to persevere. The prospect grew darker, and seemed on the point of closing forever, when suddenly, on the eighteenth day after the commencement of the treatment, when I was in a state of *extreme* feebleness, expecting the afternoon paroxysm of fever and suffocation,, which would probably be fatal, the fever was protracted an hour later than usual, the cough was not so distressing, the expectoration was less, the suffocation did not continue so long, and the lancinating pains were not so great.

From that moment I mended slowly. The Doctor left me on the twenty-second day, for a week, and then returned and stayed fifteen days more. I now increased the quantity of my bread and milk, but a little excess, even of milk or oatmeal gruel, increased all the bad symptoms, and obliged me to have recourse to blisters or to be bled. The mere bulk of the most innocent liquid increased my cough; my stomach was now in so good a state, from the regimen I had followed, that I had no longer any bilious complaint. I kept a small piece of sugar candy in my mouth to check the inclination to cough, and suppressed it by *main strength*, by holding my breath at times; as the lancinating pain in my side was always brought on by it, even when they did not precede it, convincing me that I *gained* much by *resisting* the cough. In March, the ulcers healed, and all soreness except of the throat, was gone; though great tenderness, and frequently pain in my side, accompanied by fever would oblige me to be bled or blistered, or both, for a long time after; still the least excess, even in my simple food, re-produced my bad symptoms. I had an extreme sensibility of cold, arising from a constant perspiration, which never lessened till the next September. If checked by cold air, or light covering, the difficult breathing, pain, and fever, were the immediate consequences. I was, therefore; obliged to endure it, and let it wear itself out. All attempts to check it by bracing medicines were equally injurious. I rode much during the summer, but if I had not every accommodation, it did me no good.

I could not bear the wind or the heat. The *side-way* a motion of carraige: in a rough road, gave me so much pain in my chest, that I was obliged to get out, perpendicualar motion was agreeable on good roads. The slow and easy trot of a horse I could bear, but was then too much exposed both to sun and wind. I mended regularly for two years, living on milk, vegetables, and fruit which had previously undergone some preparation by cooking. I seldom took the smallest quantity of wine, or a mouthful of meat, without being obliged to have recourse to diet or venesection, the second winter I was confined to the house for nearly three months, and was very comfortable with such exercise as I could use within doors.

For several of the last years, I have had no serious return of the complaint. I live much as others do, but with caution; rarely drink wine, principally because it makes me bilious, rather than affects my lungs; sometimes I blister my chest; once in about two years I am bled: and resort to *starvation* for a common cold, which immediately cures it. I go out at all seasons and in all weathers, and much more rarely suffer from it, than my hardy neighbors, who do not, like me, guard against the weather. I do not believe that a consumption can ever be cured by *medicine only*, without attention to regimen, air, and exercise. But I think it never should be considered hopeless, because *it is a consumption*, or because it is *hereditary*."

DISEASES OF THE LIVER.

The liver is much more frequently the seat of disease, than is generally supposed, even by many physicians of reputation and experience. The functions it is destined to perform, and on the *regular execution* of which depends not only the general health of the body, but the powers of the stomach, bowels, brain, and whole nervous system, show its vast and vital importance to human health. When the liver is seriously diseased, it in fact not only deranges the vital functions of the *body*, but exercise a powerful influence over the *mind* and its *operations*, which cannot easily be described. It has so close a connexion with other diseases; and manifests itself by so great a variety of symptoms of a *most doubtful character*–that it misleads, I am well persuaded, more physicians even of great eminence, than any other vital organ. The intimate connexion which exists between the liver and the brain; and the great dominion which I am persuaded it exercises over the *passions* of mankind, convince me, and has long since done so, that many unfortunate beings have committed acts of deep and *criminal atrocity*, or become what fools term *hyhochondriacks*, from the simple fact of *a diseased state of the liver*. I am well aware, that the remark just made, in allusion to the crimes of mankind, will by many be considered new and daring: to these men I answer, that my business is with *truth*, regardless of consequences. But to proceed with my subject:—I have long been convinced, and it may be added from experience, that more than one half of the complaints which occur in this country, are to be considered as having their seat in a diseased state of the liver. I will enumerate some of them. *Indigestion—stoppage of the menses—disordered state of the bowels—affections of the head—lowness of spirits—irritable* and *vindictive feelings* and *passions*, from trifling and inadequate causes, of which we afterwards feel ashamed–and *last*, though not *least*, more than *three-fourths* of the diseases enumerated under the head *consumption*, have their seat in a *diseased liver*. I will ask you, reader, of the particular description from which I write, is not this a most frightful catalogue? But, I will add one more of these *general* indications of a diseased liver, before I speak of the *symptoms* of those *particular* diseases to which I at first intended to direct my attention. Under the head "*Intemperance*," I have spoken on that subject, in general and philosophic terms; but I neglected to mention under that particular head, that a diseased liver is frequently the *cause* of intemperance, and sometimes the *effect* of it: and I will now remark, that in either case, when the disease has arrived at a great height and strength, it is next to impossible to reform the drunkard, without absolutely operating on him for a *disease* of the *liver*, by medical remedies which will actually affect his physical system.—I will also remark here, that many of those men who are called confirmed drunkards, are only men laboring under a disease of the liver, *whose* influence they cannot possibly resist by any moral power they possess, without the means I have just mentioned: or medical aid—and this may be the reason why Dr. Rush once alleged, that drunkenness was a disease.

How often do we see men, who in their moments of sobriety, confess to their friends and families, their improper courses, with a full determination to refrain, and no doubt with every sincerity of heart, who, after refraining from liquor a certain time, become restless, fretful or irritable, and depressed in spirits; now, I do know, that in hundreds of instances, the love of liquor is not the cause of their becoming again intemperate. You will hear those men attempt to describe the wretchedness of their feelings when they abstain from liquor; they cannot do it. Now, reader must not this be a disease, with which the mere love of liquor has nothing to do?

There aro two strongly marked forms of *diseased liver*, requiring entirely different courses of treatment to effect a cure; one is called *acute*, and the other *chronic*. The first is known by inflammatory symptoms of fever, accompanied with slight chills, and very much resembles an attack of pleurisy, being characterized by pain in the right side, which rises to the point of the shoulder. On pressing below the ribs on the right side, you will feel the pain more severe. There is sometimes a sharp, and sometimes a dull heavy pain about the collar-bone; you have painful and uneasy sensations on lying on the left side, difficult respiration or breathing, dry and hacking cough, sometimes a vomiting or puking of bilious matter, your bowels are costive your urine or water of a deep saffron color, and the quantity made, quite small, great thirst, tongue dry and covered with a white fur, hard and frequent pulse, from ninety to one hundred in a minute, and sometimes intermitting, skin hot and dry; and after several days continuance of the disease, the skin and whites of the eyes put on a yellow color. On a close examination of the blood drawn from the arm, you will find its appearances somewhat singular. Before it begins to coagulate or congeal, and while the red part is settling to the bottom—and before the buffy or yellow coat is fully formed, it looks of a dull green color; but immediately after the full formation of the upper coat, it changes from a dull greenish hue, to a yellow.

In warm climates, the liver is more apt to be affected with inflammation than any other part of the body;—this is owing to an increased secretion of bile, from the stimulous or heat, and several other causes. The liver is the largest, and most ponderous or heavy of the abdominal viscera or entrails. In adults, by which I mean grown persons, it weighs about *three pounds*—and serves to purify the blood, by secreting or taking from it the *bile*. Its situation is immediately under, and connected with the diaphragm, generally called the midriff; this is a muscle which divides the thorax or chest, from the abdomen or belly. When inflammation of this organ takes place in hot climates, it is a highly dangerous disease; which, when spoken of by physicians, is called *hepatitus.*—When physicians only mean general disease of the liver, they call it in equally general terms, *hepatic derangement.* The disease of the liver sometimes terminates in the formation of matter in an abscess, which has to be discharged, of which more notice will be taken in the proper place.

CHRONIC: a term applied to diseases which are of *long continuance,* and most generally without fever. It is the opposite disease to the *acute.* When this stage exists, the complexion and countenance put on, or rather assume, a morbid or diseased appearance. You will experience, frequently, a giddiness or swimming of the head; a general weakness, and dislike to motion or exercise; frequent headache; indigestion; flatulence, or belchings of wind from the stomach, with acid taste in the throat and mouth; pains in the stomach; your skin and eyes will be of a yellow color, similar to jaundice; your urine will be high colored, depositing a red brick-dust colored sediment in the urinal or pot, and frequently your water will be mixed with a ropy mucus, and when left some time in the vessel, will form a pink streak round its inside; and your stools will be the color of clay. By attending to these evacuation, their color will be almost a certain characteristic or mark of this disease: observe, however, that when you chew rbubarh root, it will always give your stools this light yellow color; you will experience a dull heavy pain in the region of the liver, extending to the point of the shoulder, and a great loss of appetite; your whole system will be oppressed with an unusual sense of fullness; on examination by pressure, there will be felt an enlargment and hardness of the liver; and in some cases, there will be experienced great oppression of respiration or breathing. I must remark, that the symptoms which I have here described, as indicative of the chronic stage of this disease, will always depend very much on the *length of time* the disease has been making its ravages on the system, for it may be compared to the midnight assassin, who steals on your hours of rest and security, with a noiseless foot—and deals you the deadly blow! The truth is, that chronic affections of the liver, is a far more common form of disease in the United States than the acute. A disease of the liver, of the acute form, is produced by all causes which produce inflammation or fever. The chronic form of this complaint, is generally produced in the United States, by the excessive and imprudent use of spirituous liquors. A residence of any continuance in hot countries, or even in warm climates, where a free and unrestrained course of living is indulged, is almost certain to produce the disease; intermittent fevers of long continuance, are also apt to produce chronic stage of the liver, but I am compelled to say, if I must speak with candor, that I believe more than two-thirds of the whole number of liver complaints in the U. States, may be traced to Intemperance.

REMEDIES.

For an *acute inflammation of the liver*, you are to depend principally on the prompt and immediate use of the lancet, by bleeding the patient freely, according to his age, his strength and the violence of his pains. After the bleeding, give an active purge of calomel and jalap—[see table for dose.] If this does not diminish the pain, bleed again and give an active dose of calomel at night, and a dose of epsom salts in the morning.—After the first copious bleeding, I have generally, by giving an active purge of calomel and jalap, succeeded in lessening the violence of the complaint; but, if it still continued severe, I pursued moderate and frequent bleedings, with doses of calomel at night, and epsom salts in the morning, and decreased the bleeding gradually until I stopped it. Apply, also, a large blister over the liver, which will assist in mitigating and lessening the pain in the side. Also, cup freely and daily over the liver; it will be of great benefit by drawing off the blood from the interior. [For cupping look under that head.] Small doses of emetic tartar in this stage of the disease, given occasionally in sage or balm tea, from one to two grains, will determine to the surface, or in other words produce moisture on the skin, and thereby relieve the feverish symptoms. In this stage of the complaint particularly—and indeed through the whole course of the disease, the warm bath will be found one of the finest remedies. Indeed too much reliance cannot well be placed on warm bathing, accompanied by friction—by which I mean, rubbing the body well with a brush, immediately after leaving the bath: the truth is, that this friction ought by no means to be omitted by the patient, I can from experience vouch for its beneficial effects.

After following the course of practice which I have here laid down, and the disease still continuing obstinate, which it frequently does when it has been of long standing you *must* depend on *mercury*. When I speak of this medicine, do not be alarmed or frightened at its name; for, with the rules which I lay down (read under the head mercury,) it will be as easy to manage this medicine as a dose of epsom salts: and the various injuries which result from this valuable medicine, (for without it, it would be impossible to practice medicine with any kind of success,) arise from its abuse: in fact, the injuries sustained by its use are owing to a *want of care*, and administering it on every trifling occasion, when medicines not so active would answer a much better purpose.

There are various preparations of mercury; but, at the head of this article for removing this disease, stands *calomel*; and thousands of empiricks or quacks of the United States, who publish in every news journal, some long-named remedy to cure disease *without* the use of *mercury*, are the very fellows who use it most in some disguised form: and indeed it becomes in this way truly dangerous; for the patient, regardless of weather or exposure, having no knowledge of what he is constantly using, destroys instead of benefits his health—or, in *removing one disease*, lays the foundation of *another still worse in its consequences*. This medicine is the only sure and positive remedy that can be relied on for the removal of the diseases of the liver, when permanently seated in that organ: and so powerful and necessary is it for the correction of its disorders, that it is called by a distinguished physician—the *key of the liver*. In administering this medicine, there are various ways of introducing it into the system, which must be done according to the stage of the disease, and the symptoms of the chronic form. If violent, active mercurial preparations must be used constantly, and steadily given. If the symptoms are gradual and not dangerous, the medicine must be in proportion to the state of this disease, and of a milder form of mercurial preparation. By reading under the head *mercury*, you will there see the different forms in which this mineral is prepared—and that it may be given to act *promptly* or *mildly* on the system. My course of practice on this disease, has been to employ the use of calomel from an early stage of the disease, after having purged the bowels well, frequently by its use alone or combined with jalap. I generally administered in small doses, say from one to two grains every three hours until salivation took place; or to act with more mildness, about the size of a nutmeg of mercurial ointment, (*oil of baze*) was rubbed over the region of the liver, every night until salivation was produced. I make use of the words, "oil of baze," because they form the name by which the country people usually ask for the article in the shops. When this takes place, you will know it by the following circumstances. You will spit freely; the salivary glands will become enlarged, and the throat sore; the gums tender, and the breath have an offensive and peculiar odour, &c.

In rubbing the ointment over the region of the liver, if any pain or uneasiness is produced by it, which is sometimes the case, you must rub it on the inside of the thighs. In some constitutions, calomel disagrees with the patient; I have had such cases frequently. When this is the case, and your patient's situation requires it, recourse must be had to a milder preparation of mercury—the *blue pill.* For the method of making this pill, look under the head of *Mercury.* The usual method of administering this mild and elegant preparation is, by giving a pill twice or three times a day, morning, noon, and night. If the symptoms are less urgent—twice a day will suffice—and if *very* mild and gradual, a pill at bed-time will be sufficient. Pursue this steadily, until the gums are affected, or a copperish taste is experienced in the mouth: this must be kept up gently until the disease is subdued, or some visible effect is produced upon the system. After the effect is produced, stop the use of mercury—and *give time* to see the advantage you may have derived from your course of practice.—The blue pill, although a mild preparation, is not without its inconveniences. It sometimes occasions griping, pain in the bowels, by which it will at times *run off*, without producing the effect intended. which is an approach to—or *salivation* itself—so as to induce a change or alterative effect on the liver. If this be the result, a small portion of opium or laudanum will check this griping, and prevent the pill from passing off without producing the effect intended and desired. Where there are uneasy and unpleasant sensations produced by these medicines, particularly when *Dyspepsia* or *Indigestion* is connected with a diseased Liver, which is very frequently the case in the United States, there is a considerable degree of morbid or diseased sensibility in the stomach and bowels, which can generally be removed by joining some innocent and gentle anodyne with them; but where this morbid sensibility does not exist, the anodyne ought to be omitted. When this slow and gradual mercurial taste can be kept up in the mouth for some time, without actually producing a free flow of spittle, or *salivation*, great benefit will be felt by the patient;—and I have always found, on an actual salivation being produced, the symptoms entirely removed, and a cheerfulness and a change of feelings so different, as at once to inspire that confidence of returning health, which can only be communicated by the prudent and careful use of this valuable specific. Persons who are prejudiced against the use of mercury, and there are many who entertain an unfavorable opinion of its use, whether from having observed its injurious effects from bad treatment, or from the terrible and unfounded tales which are daily circulated respecting it, I cannot say have never witnessed its innocently beneficial effects in diseases of the liver, in as many instances as I have. The fact is, that I have known those very persons travel one hundred miles to abtain relief "*without the aid of mercury*," from some published *quack medicine*, who always met mercury under some disguised form.

But—with those whose prejudices are not to be removed respecting the use of mercury, I shall give such remedies as are highly recommended in this complaint, by some of the most distinguished physicians of Europe and the United States. The late experiments made with the medicine I am about to recommend, have proved, by their influence in the practice, equal to mercury—in fact they prefer its use in the first instance: for, say they, "if it does not succeed, which is not apt to be the case; it leaves the system in a much better situation for the use of the last and certain remedy—mercury."

This medicine is *nitric acid*; and may be obtained at any doctor's shop, or wherever medicines are sold, at a very trifling sum. This article, in its pure state, is perfectly colorless, and transparent as pnre water. I have frequently received it from the northern cities of a light straw color; but this is not so good as that which is perfectly pure and transparent—and is, in fact, nothing more nor less than *aquafortis*. It is made of sulphuric acid, which is merely oil of vitriol—and nitrate of potass, which is no more than simple salt petre. Nitric acid, in its pure state, should be cautiously handled, or it will destroy your clothes, and stain your hands of a yellowish color which cannot be washed off. It is used by the country people generally, to color the stocks of their rifles. I suppose this caution will be sufficient. It becomes quite harmless, after being diluted or mixed with water. The method of using the nitric acid or *aquafortis*, is as follows. A quart bottle of water may be made agreeably sour, that is to suit the taste of the patient, and sweetened with sugar so as to make it a pleasant drink. Take as much of this drink from your bottle during the twenty-four hours, as your stomach will bear without inconvenience. Sixty drops of this nitric acid, will be sufficient for a quart of water. This medicine, like mercury, must be gradually continued, until some visible effect is produced on the system. This will be felt by an affection of the mouth and glands, and excite spitting, similar to mercurial preparations. In all constitutions of a scorbutic or scurvy habit, or those laboring under great weakness, the nitric acid will be a better remedy than mercury; because it acts as a tonic or strengthening medicine, at the same time that it tends to correct the scorbutic affection.

In several cases, in which I have had opportunities of trying the *nitric acid* in the form I have mentioned, it has always had beneficial effects, with the exception of the single case of a lady of delecate and irritable stomach: she was compelled to discontinue its use, from the *acidity* it produced on her stomach. This I endeavored to remedy, by gentle emetics or pukes, intended to cleanse the stomach of its impurities; and by afterwards giving magnesia, and charcoal, and such other articles, for the purpose of neutralizing or destroying the acid. All however did not succeed, and I was compelled to desist. From this practice, and general experience, I apprehended no other difficulty with regard to the beneficial effects of the *nitric acid* in chronic affections of the Liver, than the simple fact of the patient being unable to take it a sufficient time to produce the effect desired. In such cases as the above, therefore, much benefit will be experienced from the use of the *nitro muriatic bath.*

This valuable and grateful remedy, is by far too much neglected in the United States. The reason of this neglect I apprehend to be, because its application is considered to be attended with some trouble. I recollect a circumstance in point. I directed one of my patients, to bathe his feet every night on going to bed in this bath: "What doctor," said he "*every* night?"—"or every other night," said I.—he exclaimed—"How *much* trouble!" This is the reason, I have no doubt, why this simple but valuable preparation is so much neglected. But, to those, who like myself, have witnessed the surprising cures produced by its use, the trouble will be considered a matter of no consequence. I shall, for the satisfaction of my reader, relate a case.

Mrs. Stoner; wife of John Stoner, of Botetourt county, Virginia, was in the last stage of this disease. and had been attended by several distinguished physicians, who treated her case for consumption. At the time her husband called on me to visit her, his object was merely to procure the administration of some palliative remedies. to soothe her cough, and relieve her obstructed respiration or breathing, which had nearly suffocated her several times: he entertained neither hope nor relief, that any medical assistance could, by any possibility, permanently relieve her. In truth. from what I had heard of her case, I candidly stated to Mr. Stoner, that my visits would only be a useless expense; and advised such remedies as were calculated to allay irritation. Two or three days afterward, Mr. S. made a second application, and to gratify a tender and affectionate husband, and a numerous and highly respectable connexion, I consented to visit her. On my arrival, I found her situation, as I at first supposed, to be critical in the extreme, in fact, the last stage of consumption; hollow cough—breathing very difficult and obstructed—constant expectoration, or discharge of matter, occasionally streaked with blood—regular paroxysms of fever, accompanied with flushings at midday, and toward evening terminating in profuse sweats—diarrhœa or dysentery—in fact, her case was such an exact resemblance of the *last stage of consumption*, that the most experienced and skilful physician would have been deceived. I remained all night; and very attentively examined this, (as I at first supposed,) *hopeless case.* About midnight she requested some nourishment, which was immediately prepared, and of the lightest kind. She had hardly swallowed it, before it was rejected or thrown up:—and for the first time, I observed the extreme irritability of her stomach. On inquiry, she stated that from her first attack, the slightest food would oppress her stomach with a sense of burning and fullness, and become sour, accompanied with the most unpleasant sensations, until what she had eaten was rejected and thrown up. I now questioned her minutely, as to all the symptoms from the commencement of the disease; all her answers fully convinced me, that the *liver was the primary seat of the disease.* Fully impressed with this opinion, although debilitated in the extreme, and reduced to a mere skeleton, and so weak as almost to faint on the slightest exertion, I determined, even in this last and almost hopeless stage, to try the *nitro muriatic bath.* Fearful, that in the usual way, would be productive of fatal consequences immediately on its application, I hesitated some hours; but, with the consent of herself and family, having candidly stated to all parties *my serious* doubts, as to the success of the remedy in this stage of her case, I proceeded to the use of the bath in its mildest form, by suffering her hand alone to remain in it for fifteen or twenty minutes. In five minutes after her hand was in the bath, she complained of great uneasiness in the region of the *liver*, which gradually subsided after withdrawing her hand. This night she rested well. The following morning expectoration was greatly increased. This day I placed both her hands in the bath; there was immediately great oppression; her nervous system became much agitated; and here extremities were becoming very cold. I immediately removed her hands from the bath and *she fainted.* There was now much increase of pulse; and great oppression of breathing, almost amounting to suffocation. On a sudden, as if by a conclusive effort, she threw up about a pint of yellow bile, similar in color to the yolk of eggs. The oppression for this time ceased; her breathing become slow, easy, and regular:—and, by a continuance of this bath, gradually persevered in, and moderately increased to *sponging the whole body with it*—and lastly to using it as a *foot bath,* she improved daily—and in *eight weeks* I had the satisfaction of seeing her attending to her domestic concerns, in *tolerable health,* which gradually improved until she was entirely restored. The strength of the bath I used was about equal to weak vinegar and water. For the period of about six weeks, during which I was engaged in performing this cure, a relative of this lady, the Rev. Mr. Crumpecker, pastor of the Dunkard society, an individual whose character as a christian, a philanthropist, and a man of integrity, would do honor to any age or country—together with his friend, John Stoner, Sen. were absent on a visit to the State of Maryland. On their return, they were astonished to find Mrs. Stoner, of whom they had taken leave for eternity, in the vigor of comparative health and strength, and attending to all her domestic affairs. I mention the names of these gentlemen particularly, because when they peruse my report of Mrs. Stoner's case as treated by me with the *nitro muriatic bath,* they will confirm the fact of her entire recovery, from the use of this bath. It may be necessary to state, that Mrs. Stoner's diet consisted of milk and water, and mush and milk—and nothing stimulating—being entirely restrained from animal food.

The NITRO MURIATIC BATH is formed, by mixing equal parts of the *nitric acid* and *muriatic acid* together. You must pay strict attention to the following directions, or your carelessness will produce unpleasant consequences. When these two *acids* come in contact, that is to say, when they are poured together, without having been *previously* mixed with water *separately*, a *gas*, or volume of what appears to be *smoke*, will immediately fill the whole house. This gas has a very disagreeable smell, and is dangerous to the lungs. The proper manner of mixing them is—first, to fill a glass bottle about half full of cold water—next, you must put in one of the acids, and shake it up with water—then, you must put in the other acid, and immediately cork the bottle tightly, occasionally shaking the acids together. This will prevent the unpleasant smell I have mentioned, and retain the virtues of these medicines, if you keep your bottle well corked: the fact is, none other than glass bottles with stoppers of the same material, can keep these acids in.

Having stated to you how the *nitric acid* is made, it may be necessary also to communicate the method practiced in procuring the muriatic acid. It is distilled from nothing more than *common salt*, by means of *sulphuric acid*, or in other words *oil of vitriol*. It is less powerful than *nitric acid*, and is of a deeper yellow color. It ought always to be kept with *wax* over the cork, so as to prevent the fumes from escaping; they are very unpleasant and in large volumes suffocating. But when either of these acids is mixed with water, as I have before directed, and the other then added, they lose all unpleasant effects, and become nothing more than strong acid, like vinegar and water. You will easily perceive by these directions, that you may make the *nitro muriatic bath* weaker or stronger, as you may think proper. This bath is very easily made at any time; for, by mixing some acid from the *bottle* before mentioned, with water made pleasantly warm, to about the strength of vinegar and water, you *have the bath*. Bathe the feet and legs in this bath, from *ten minutes* to *half an hour*, according to the strength of the patient, immediately before retiring to bed. If the patient be very weak, bathing one hand a few minutes will be sufficient; if a little stronger, the whole body may be sponged with the acid: and if still stronger, the feet and legs to the knees may be bathed, according to the circumstances and the times just mentioned. A narrow wooden bucket or box—sufficient to admit the feet and legs, and to permit the bath to reach the knees, would be advisable: it would be a saving of the acid, the requisite strength of which can always be tested by tasting it. You may preserve the bath or acid in an earthern crock, or in any glass vessel, and by warming it again, continue to use it when required.

It is impossible to specify the time this bath should be used; this must depend on the effect produced, and the strength of the patient. The object is, to bring the system moderately and gradually under its influence; which is easily done, because it may be made so innocent, by applying it very weak, as to be borne in the most delecate state of the patient. I have witnessed persons being immersed in it to the chin for half an hour; while others, who were very weak and nervous, were strongly affected by the immersion of one of the hands. The great advantage of this bath is, that you may regulate its strength to any point necessary. I have no doubt it would be highly beneficial, in *Indigestion;* and in all depraved states of the *biliary secretions*, producing melancholy and despondency of mind, or in other words, *hypochondriasis*. The nitro muriatic bath, will be found also a valuable remedy to females. This bath, or the nitric acid taken by the stomach, ought always to be very much diluted with water; and if any very considerable effects are produced, the use of it ought to be stopped for a week or two, and gradually resumed again; whenever it produces *very uneasy* sensations, you must be guided by your feelings; nor are you ever to take any animal food, or use any stimulants of any kind, while using this bath, or the nitric acid in any way. If the bathing, or sponging the body, should not keep the bowels open, or in a laxative state, you must take some simple medicine, such as epsom salts, senna and manna, or aloes, or any thing else that will keep the bowels gently open.

In addition to what I have said, it may be remarked in

conclusion, that equal quantities of epsom salts and magnesia, ground very fine together in a mortar, and a sufficient quantity taken in cold water to keep the bowels gently open, always act beneficially in diseases of the *liver;* the common dose is from one to two tea spoonfuls, in half a pint of cold water.—Or you may mix equal quantities of jalap and cream tartar, ground fine in a mortar, and give doses of a tea spoonful. This last is a drastic purgative, and acts powerfully on the *Liver.* I have never used it in my practice, always prefering, as a mild purgative, the salts and magnesia. The low-ground sarsaparilla, found in almost every part of the United States, is also a very good remedy in diseases of the liver; it ought to be taken plentifully, cold, in decoction or tea, I must not omit to remark, and that *emphatically* and *strongly,* that the use of the *warm bath,* as described under that head, will be almost indispensable in the cure of all diseases of the liver, and in all *stages* of those diseases.

I cannot relinquish the subject of diseases of the *Liver,* without mentioning in terms of almost unqualified approbation, my candid opinions of the waters of the *Harrodsburg Greenville Springs,* situated in the county of Mercer, and State of Kentucky. These waters are well known to operate *powerfully* and *beneficially* on the LIVER; nor do I believe there has been many instances, if an absolute *consumption,* or an *induration* of the liver had not taken place, in which those waters have not been efficient in removing diseases of the liver. Their almost certain efficacy is so well known, that they are frequented by thousands of invalids, during the summer months, from every part of the United States. And, I would advise all persons laboring under complaints of the Liver—or under *Dyspepsia* or *Indigestion*—and who have become hopeless of the influence of medical prescriptions, never to omit, if it be possible for them to travel to those springs, to give those waters a fair trial. They are situated in a beautiful and healthful country, and the accommodations are always such, as to ensure the comfort and convenience of all invalids who approach them.

DYSENTERY
OR
FLUX.

This disease is always accompanied with *Tenesmus*, or a constant desire to go to stool, without being able to pass much of any thing from the bowels, excepting a *bloody kind of mucus*—which resembles that generally scraped from the entrails of a hog. These desires to go to stool, are usually accompanied with *severe griping*, and also with *some fever*. After a few days continuance of this complaint, your discharges by stool will consist of pure blood, and matter mixed; and from severe straining to evacuate, parts of your bowels will frequently protrude or come out, which soon becomes a source of great suffering. *Dysentery* or *flux* generally takes place about autumn; when the whole body has become irritable by a continuation of warm or rather hot weather, and has been suddenly exposed to cold or damp;—it is also produced by eating unripe or green fruit of any kind; by sudden suppressings or steppages of the perspiration or sweat; by the eating of some putrid or decayed food; and sometimes it arises, from some peculiar cause existing in the atmosphere:—when this is the case, whole neighborhoods and extensive tracts of country are affected by it fatally.

REMEDIES.

If your patient is vigorous, hale, and generally healthy—and there is considerable fever, the loss of some blood in the *first stage* of the disease will be proper. But if, on the contrary, the patient be a weakly and delecate person, the loss of any blood would be highly improper and dangerous. First:—cleanse the stomach by an emetic or puke of ipecacuanha; then give a purge of calomel; (see table for dose.) —Next:—if the disease does not abate, you must repeat the purging daily with castor oil: this is the best medicine you can possibly use in this complaint. As the stools are generally very offensive, you can easily correct them, by giving a tea spoonful of *prepared chalk*, in a little cold water, three times a day; this prepared chalk is nothing but common chalk freed of its impurities. Give clysters frequently through the day, made of slippery elm; which is to be thrown up the bowels *cold*. In case of violent pain, bathe the stomach with laudanum, and spirits in which camphor has been dissolved; and apply cloths wrung out of hot water to the belly; or blister over the stomach. If the belly is hard, and sore on being touched, grease it well with any kind of oil or lard:—here the frequent use of the warm bath will be of immense service. When the disease is very obstinate, administer a clyster morning and night, of a mucilage of cherry-tree gum—or peach tree gum, dissolved in water until it will be ropy and gluttinous—in which drop from fifty to sixty drops of laudanum, for grown persons; and so on in proportion to different ages. Throw this clyster up the bowels cold; (for the method of doing which, see under the head clyster.) The warm bath, and castor oil, in this disease may safely be depended on. If the desire of going to stool is very frequent and painful, introduce up the back side or fundament, (I must speak in plain terms,) a pill of opium of from three to four grains. It must be put up with much care and tenderness; because in this complaint the parts are always very sore—its remaining there will greatly allay the irritation of the lower gut, and produce much relief and immediate comfort; the proportions of opium in the pill, must be varied according to the age of the patient. The common black-berry syrup, ought to be prepared and kept in every family in this country, and used freely in this complaint. I frequently apply a remedy in this disease; which I claim as the discoverer; and which very often succeeds, when all others have failed: it is *flax seed oil*, to be given in the quantity of a table spoonful, twice a day to a grown person, and reducing the dose according to the age of the patient. It may be necessary to remark, that small doses of ipecacuanha combined with opium; say three grains of ipecacuanha to half a grain of opium, formed into a pill and given twice a day, after purging well with castor oil, will be an excellent remedy to check this complaint, by producing a moisture on the skin—and allaying the irritation of the bowels. The drinks should be of the mildest kind such as slippery elm tea—flax-seed tea—watermelon-seed tea—and diet of the lightest kind—such as jellies, chicken soup, lamb soup, &c. &c.

LAX,

OR

CONSTANT LOOSENESS OF THE BOWELS.

Called by physicians *Diarrhœa.* This disease is unattended with any fever, and not contagious or catching, as is the disease immediately before mentioned. It generally prevails among persons of weakly constitutions; persons advanced in years; and those who have lived *intemperately.* Many are naturally and constitutionally of this habit of body; and others are subject to its attacks, on the slightest cold or exposure, which at all affects their bowels. The appearances of the stools in this disease, are very different at different times: sometimes of a thick consistence—sometimes thin; at times of a slimy nature, and then again of a whitish color—changing the green, yellow, dark or brown, depending very much on the food, and the manner in which it agrees or disagrees with the stomach and bowels; sometimes, and that not frequently, it is produced by *worms.*

REMEDIES.

First:—give an emetic or puke, in the morning; and at night, for a grown person, give a large dose of castor oil with from thirty to thirty-five drops of laudanum in it—but, always lessen this dose, in proportion to the age of your patient. Next:—a stool is to be produced daily, by the use of the castor oil. When griping attends the complaint, warm garden mint *stewed,* and placed over the stomach and belly will give relief. When the disease has been brought on by cold, or sudden stoppages of the perspiration or sweat, use the warm bath, and take some snake-root tea, so as to produce a determination to the surface, or gentle moisture on the skin. . This troublesome complaint, frequently continues on many persons through life:—sueh persons should be particular as to what they eat, and avoid every thing that disagrees with their stomach and bowels—always taking care to defend their feet against the damp ground, and wearing flannel next to their skins. Friction—or rubbing the whole body, every day, with a brush—particularly over the region of the *stomach*, *liver*, and *bowels*, will be of much service. Old French brandy, taken in moderation, and well diluted with water, is not only a good remedy in this complaint when constitutional, but frequently a preventive against attacks. When *worms* are presumed to have any influence in producing this disease, which may be suspected from a fetid or offensive breath, the complaint is to be treated for worms:—see which head. When the complaint arises from *weakness*, opium will be found highly important in restraining its excesses, and removing the debility. By using the clysters of slippery elm, or those made of common starch and warm water, for directions how to use which, [look under the head *clystering*,] much benefit will result, by cooling the bowels, and allaying the irritation which always exists in this disease.

INFLAMMATION

OF THE

STOMACH.

This complaint can easily be distinguished from any other, by its distinctive and peculiar symptoms: it is, therefore, impossible to mistake it for any other disease, if the least attention be paid to the indications of its presence. There is always violent pain in the stomach, together with a sensation of heat and burning in it. There, is, also, a great increase of pain in the stomach, when any thing is swallowed; and an immediate rejection and puking of it up. Also, a sinking and loss of strength; great thirst and uneasiness; a continued moving of the body from side to side of the bed:—and as the disease advances, frequent hiccoughs, accompanied with coldness of the hands and feet. When these last symptoms occur, hiccoughs and cold extremities, they are extremely unfavorable, and will probably terminate fatally. Inflammation of the stomach is usually produced, by *corrosive poisons* taken into the stomach, or drinking extremely cold water, when the body is overheated; by receiving violent blows, or wounds in the region of the stomach; by the gout; by strong emetics; and lastly, by large quantities of *iced liquor* taken into the stomach.

REMEDIES.

This being a very dangerous disease, and the life of the patient depending on the bold and free use of the *lancet*, you are not to be detered from its use, by any apparent feebleness of the pulse. The proper practice is, to bleed freely every few hours, until the inflammation is subdued. As soon as you have subdued the inflammatory symptoms, by frequent bleeding, the patient is to be put in the *warm bath*, where he is to remain as long as possible. You are then to have a large *blister* prepared, which must be put over the region of the stomach, the moment the patient has left the bath; or, if there is no blister at hand, apply a large *cataplasm* or poultice of mustard and strong vinegar. Keep the bowels open, with clysters made of common starch, or slippery elm, or flax-seed oil, or thin gruel, or chicken water boiled strong. These clysters will assist to nourish the patient, especially as he will be unable to take the slightest nourishment on the stomach. When the inflammation is reduced, and the stomach will bear it, a pill of opium, (see table for dose,) will be serviceable. The diet should be of the lightest kind; such as jelly, slippery elm tea, rice, and light soups—a very little at a time, and administered with extreme caution, with small doses of laudanum. Small quantities of the best sweet oil, about a tea-spoonful at a time, given during the continuance of this complaint, will very much assist in allaying the inflammation. When this disease terminates fatally, it invariably ends in mortification; and this will nearly always be the case, unless the *lancet* is used freely in the first instance. A sudden change, from great misery to perfect ease, is conclusive evidence of *mortification.*

INFLAMMATION OF THE INTESTINES.

This complaint is extremely dangerous, and requires immediate use and very active measures to arrest its course. The symptoms are very distressing, and are always accompanied with sharp pains in the bowels, and particularly about the navel. The belly seems *tight* and *hard*, and so tender that the least pressure with the fingers, gives great pain; you will know it from colic by pressing the belly; in colic the pressure gives relief—but in inflammation of the intestines, the belly is so sore that the least bearing on it gives immediate and excruciating misery. Great weakness attends this disease, the pulse is small, quick, and hard;

the urine or water is high colored, and passed off with difficulty: and the bowels are very costive. Inflammation of the intestines, is produced by very nearly the same causes, as those which are productive of inflammation of the stomach; and is attended with very nearly as much danger as that disease. It arises from severe colic; from hard undigested food remaining in the bowels; from drinking cold water when the body is over-heated; by blows and wounds in and about the region of the bowels; by long and severe dysentery; by worms; and lastly by hernia or rupture.

REMEDIES.

The remedies are much the same, as those for inflammation of the stomach; the object being to arrest the disease instantly, and before, mortification can take place, which always when it occurs, terminates the matter fatally. The only *hope* of relief is from the immediate and free use of the *lancet;* for without its instrumentality, you may abandon every hope of saving your patient. Therefore, take blood immediately from the arm, letting the stream be large, so as to draw the blood off suddenly. You must repeat the bleeding frequently; as the urgency and critical situation of the patient may appear to demand it: cup the belly, and apply a large blister. Depend very much after the bleeding, on frequent clysters—to be made of slippery elm or flax-seed, (the elm is best for clystering,) and the warm bath; look under the different heads for information. The only medicine that ought to be given in this disease, is the best sweet oil, in doses of a table spoonful each, and that frequently. I have no authority for it; but I should in my own practice if attending a case of this kind, mix a tea spoonful of the *finest charcoal,* prepared as directed under the head of *Indigestion,* with each dose of sweet oil: and I should also mix charcoal with the clysters of slippery elm. A distinguished physician, recommends clysters of cold *lead water,* in this complaint, to lessen the high action, and subdue the inflammation. I would suppose, although I never tried it in this disease, that his remedy is valuable: it is made by mixing, very weak, the sugar of lead and cold water, and throwing it up the bowels with a clyster pipe. [Look under the head of clystering.]

After the violence of the disease is subdued, you must throw up the bowels as a clyster, fifty or sixty drops of laudanum in any simple mucilage, such as flax-seed tea or slippery elm. This clyster will allay the irritation, and may be given twice a day—early in the morning and late at night—diminishing the quantity of laudanum, according to the age of the patient. The diet should be of the lightest kind, and always cautiously given, to patients recovering from this dangerous disease: this caution is the more necessary, because the disease may, and frequently does return from very slight causes; especially where persons have been afflicted with it several times before. In truth, and to speak plainly, it is only by proper diet, and that of the most simple kind, with great care in preventing exposure, that such persons can remain secure. Flannel should be worn next the skin, and the warm bath frequently used, for the purpose of preventing the recurrence of this very dangerous, and often unmanageable complaint.

INFLAMMATION OF THE BRAIN.

This disease has destroyed some of the most distinguished men in Europe and America, among whom may be named, the celebrated Lord Byron, General Nathaniel Greene of the Revolution, and the late Doct. Dorsey of Pennsylvania. It arises from intense study; from exposure to the heat of the sun; and from every other cause which produces an overfullness of blood on the brain. The symptoms are, a very high fever—great pain in the head–the eyes look red and fiery—there is also great watchfulness—the patient is unable to bear the smallest light—there is also, generally, a heavy dull sleep, with frequent startings as if in alarm—the memory fails, and in the first stage of the disease, the patient dislikes to talk; but, as the complaint advances, the eyes assume a great brightness—the patient becomes furious and talks wildly, and generally on subjects which have left deep impressions on his mind when in health. The tongue becomes dry, and of a dark color—the pulse small, quick, and hard—and the poor sufferer is frequently seen, to put his hand or hands to his head.

THE BRAIN.—This organ is larger in man than in any other known animal. Its general weight is from two pounds five and a half ounces, to three pounds three and three-quarter ounces. I have weighed several at four pounds. The Brain of the late LORD BYRON, (without its membranes) weighed six pounds.

REMEDIES.

Bleed as largely in quantity, as the strength of your patient will possibly admit:—let the blood be taken as suddenly as practicable from the arm, by a large orifice or opening, so as to permit it to flow in a copious and bold stream. If the patient, by bleeding from the arm freely, becomes weak, and the disease is not subdued, shave the head, and cup freely all over it:—for the method of cupping, look under that head. Apply over the whole head immediately, the coldest applications that can be found, such as wet towels constantly wrung out of the coldest spring water—or ice if it can be had: these cold applications are to be constantly renewed, until the disease is subdued. Give, also, active purges, and that very frequently, consisting of twenty grains of calomel and twenty of jalap. If the symptoms are very violent, give a clyster, made of thin gruel, with thirteen grains of tartar emetic well mixed in it:—this clyster must be given once every day, as long as the disease continues severe. Your patient's head should be placed on high pillowing, and his body kept in bed, in as upright a posture as possible, so as to lessen as far as practicable the determination or flowing of the blood to the head. After the violence of the disease is removed by bleeding and purging, &c. apply constantly, poultices made of pounded mustard seed and vinegar, to the feet and ancles; or blister them, with cantharides or spanish flies, prepared in the usual manner. The feet and legs should, also frequently be bathed in the usual way with warm water:—this will divert, or draw off the determination of blood from the head. The diet and drinks should be of the lightest, simplest, and most cooling kinds. The room ought to be kept dark, and perfectly cool, nor ought the least noise to be permitted to disturb the quiet of the patient. When reason begins to return, and the fever to subside, be extremely careful to attend to these instructions:—because the slightest cause will bring on the disease a second time, with more violence than in the first instance, which will in all probability terminate *fatally*.

INFLAMMATION
OF THE
SPLEEN.

When there is an inflammation of the Spleen, considerable pain is felt in the *left side*, where the Spleen is situated. By pressing the fingers on the left side, a throbing sensation is easily discovered, and a pain is felt by the patient, extending from the side to the left shoulder, and not unfrequently through the belly. The most remarkable symptoms which attend this disease, and those which may be relied on, are puking of blood, great weakness, watchfulness, and not unfrequently, the mind is much confused. This complaint, like all other inflammatory diseases, is attended with considerable fever. It is brought on by long continued fevers, and by affections of the liver; and persons who have suffered much from long attacks of fever and ague, are liable to what they term *ague-cakes*, which are diseases of the Spleen, and which are apt to terminate, without the application of proper remedies, in *inflammation of the Spleen*. Where there is no inflammation, and the side is swelled, the disease is called *chronic*.

REMEDIES.

Purge well, and frequently, with calomel and jalap:—[see table for dose.] Also cup over the Spleen:—[for the method of cupping, look under that head:]—and, always, if the disease is of the chronic form, *blister* over the Spleen, in the usual manner. The *nitric acid* will also be found a valuable remedy; read affections of the liver, page 200, where you will find the acid treated on at large. A broad belt worn over the Spleen, with folds of cloth to press on it, will be a good remedy:—as will, also, rubing the side daily with equal quantities of spirits of hartshorn and sweet-oil.

INFLAMMATION OF THE KIDNEYS.

In this disease, there is always great pain in the small of the back, similar to that felt in colic, but seated much nearer the back bone and loins. There is also, in this complaint, a deadness and numbness of feeling in the upper part of the thigh; considerable sickness at the stomach; a great desire to make water frequently, which is done with much difficulty, and in small quantities at a time. The urine or water is of a deep red color, showing that there is great internal fever: the slightest motion gives pain; and, even in sitting upright in bed, the patient is extremely restless, always receiving mere ease by lying on the affected part. Sometimes one of the testicles is retracted or drawn up, so that you can scarcely feel it. The complaint is brought on, by great exertions in lifting; by violent and sudden strains; by exposure to cold when over-heated; by lying on the damp ground; and, by too frequent intercourse with women. Sometimes the disease is produced by hard substances, calculus, stone, or gravel, formed in the kidneys: and I have known two or three instances, of its having been produced in young persons, by that horrible practice called by physicians onanism.

REMEDIES.

Like all other inflammations, that of the kidneys requires the free use of the lancet; always repeating the bleeding from the arm, as the urgency and severity of the symptoms may seem to require. Cup freely over the small of the back; (for cupping, read under that head.) Apply flannel cloths wrung out of hot water, to the small of the back; and give clysters of warm milk and water in equal portions —which must be thrown up the bowels three or four times a day. All the drinks should be made warm, in which must be dissolved some kind of gum, such as that of the peach-tree, gum or any other kind of gum, that will produce a mucilage. Flax-seed tea will answer a good purpose, as will also a tea made of slippery elm bark; in both of which you may put a little spirits of nitre. The bowels are to be kept open by castor oil, and by moderate clystering. The warm bath must be frequently used, and applied for a considerable time at once, over the whole body; during which, the patient in the bath, must have his body well rubbed with a soft brush or woollen cloth: this bath must be repeated every day, and twice a day if necessary. The warm bath is a most valuable remedy, in this complaint, and must not be neglected. After the violence of the disease has been subdued, by the use of the lancet and warm bath, &c. as before noticed, to give ease, and quiet slumbers to the patient, administer a pill of opium, or thirty-five drops of laudanum: (for the different doses of which, proportion to the different ages, see table for doses.) Or a clyster at this time, made of flax-seed tea, with forty or fifty drops of laudanum mixed with it, will give great relief, by allaying both pain and irritation. A decoction or tea made of dried peach tree leaves, made by boiling a handful of the leaves in a quart of water, until it decreases to three half pints, is to be drank occasionally through the day—this is an excellent remedy, and has been known to succeed in this complaint, when the sufferings have been unusually severe. In some cases, inflammation of the kidneys cannot be removed, until abscesses or ulcers are formed:—this state of the case will always be known, by the pain becoming less severe; by great weight being felt in the small of the back; by chills succeeded by flushes of heat; and when by suffering the urine or water to settle in the urinal or pot, you can discover a mucus matter on the bottom. When this is the situation of the patient, the *uva ursi* will be found a useful medicine: for a description of which, and its medicinal qualities, read under the head *uva ursi*, sometimes called the upland cranberry, and sometimes the bearberry. The usual dose is, two or three times a day, half a pint of the decoction or tea, made of a handful of the leaves to a pint of water: or a tea spoonful of the pounded leaves, three times a day, taken in any kind of syrup.

INFLAMMATION OF THE BLADDER.

Immediately above the privates, in this complaint, there is very considerable pain; which is much increased, by pressing on the part with the fingers. There is, also, a constant desire to make water, which is voided with much difficulty, and in very small quantities. There is a constant desire to go to stool, and always some fever; also great restlessness, where the disease is produced by stone or gravel; or by stricture or contraction of the *urethra*, or canal which leads from the bladder; or by this passage being stopped up; or from the lodgement of hardened lumps in the lower gut, caused by costiveness or constipation of the bowels. In the last case, I have frequently known an instrument introduced, if the finger could not remove the solid and hard excrement, called by physicians, the fœces.

This disease is, also, sometimes produced by injuries received, such as severe blows, kicks, falls, &c. by taking the tincture of cantharides or spanish flies—and by that false and foolish delicacy, which leads some persons to hold their urine a considerable length of time. I recollect a case which terminated fatally by this *false modesty.* A young lady of respectability, was introduced to a merchant who was travelling from Philadelphia to New York, and placed under his protection to perform the same journey. The Poast-coach runs the distance, from ninety to one hundred miles in about eleven hours: this distance she travelled in excruciating torment from retaining her urine, and died from the effects of it, on the second day after her arrival at New York. She was in the bloom of youth, health, and beauty; and I mention the ease emphatically, as a warning to others, who from false delicacy, might do the same thing.

REMEDIES.

You must as in all the other cases of inflammation before mentioned, depend much on frequent bleeding, and the free use of the warm bath: and on all such medicines as will determine to the surface, or in other words, produce a gentle moisture on the skin Also get a syringe, and inject water made pleasantly warm into the bladder, which will remove the irritating causes: and, after washing out the bladder with warm water as just directed, make a decoction of slippery elm bark and let it become cool—with this decoction or tea, mix a very weak preparation of sugar of lead, which must be dissolved in cold water, and throw up this preparation into the bladder occasionally; this will lessen the inflammation, and assist in finally subduing it—but I caution you to make the solution of sugar of lead very weak.—You are *not to use a blister* in this complaint; because it would act immediately and particularly on the bladder, by suppressing the urine. Clysters of the mildest kind are to be given; they will always soothe, relieve, and reduce the irritation of the bowels, and the adjacent parts. If the pain is very severe, laudanum should be given—(see table for dose)—and the water frequently drawn off by a catheter: the fact is, that a physician should be immediately called; but, if necessity should urge the use of the catheter, by a person who is not a professional man, a description of the instrument, and of the precise manner of using it, both in male and female cases, will be found under the proper head.

DRINKING COLD WATER
WHEN
OVER HEATED.

The imprudent use of cold water when a person is over-heated, almost invariably produces *cramps* or *spasms* of the stomach, which usually terminate in death. In the year 1816, I saw five persons expire in less than ten minutes in the city of New York, from drinking cold water: in truth, the deaths became so frequent at the different watering places throughout the town, that placcards or printed bills, were ordered by the *city council*, to be stuck up on the different pumps, to caution all persons against drinking cold water when over-heated, or in too large quantities. Many deaths have occurred in the western country, during the harvesting seasons, from persons drinking large quantities of the coldest spring water, when over-heated and bathed in sweat. This dangerous and fatal practice, if it even does not produce immediate death, almost invariably lays the foundation of lingering and destructive diseases, which are extremely difficult of cure. That eminent and distinguished physician Benjamin Rush, describes the causes of so much fatality in these cases, in the following manner:—"When large quantities of cold water are suddenly taken into the stomach, under circumstances of an over-heated system, the person in a few minutes afterwards loses his sight, and every thing appears dark about him; he staggers in attempting to walk, and unless supported falls to the ground; the breathing soon becomes very difficult, and a rattling noise is heard in the throat; the feet and hands become cold, and the pulse cannot be felt—and generally in about five minutes, death is the consequence unless speedy relief can be obtained." *Ice'd toddy*, when taken under the same circumstances of being over-heated, has often been known to produce the same fatal effects:—and I have known many instances, in which ladies in full health, have been brought to the brink of eternity in a few minutes from eating *iced creams* when over-heated by dancing. The truth is, that very cold articles of food or drink, even when the body is moderately cool, sometimes, in peculiar constitutions, are productive of dangerous consequences:—cases which are not very violent, and which come on with *cramps* or *spasms*, should be immediately attended to, or they will also terminate fatally in most instances, *by inflammation of the stomach.*

REMEDIES.

"I have discovered," says Doct. Rush, "but one certain remedy in this desperate, and if not immediately relieved fatal disease:—this remedy, and it may be relied on, is *laudanum;* which has to be given in the quantity, of from a tea to nearly a table spoonful *immediately*, in violent cases before relief can be obtained." When laudanum cannot be had in time, a glass of strong *whiskey* or *brandy*, one of which is generally found forth coming every where may be given. Laudanum, however is so very easily made, and so frequently necessary in all families, that it ought always to be kept in preparation for use:—it will frequently save the expense of sending for a physician at an unseasonable hour, and oftentimes save life in sudden and desperate cases. [For the mode of preparing it, see under the head *laudanum.*] Every person about to drink cold water, when warm and in high perspiration, should observe faithfully the followidg rules. First—pour considerable quantities of water on the wrists:—and, next, wash the face, temples, and hands with water, and suffer them to dry. These measures from the coldness of the water applied, and the evaporation which succeeds, will abstract or draw from the interior of the body, and particularly from the vital parts, a considerable portion of heat; and prevent the sudden and dangerous action of the cold on the stomach, and other vital parts of the system. You are, also, when you drink, to take the water in small quantities at a time—in fact, not more than half a pint at once:—repeating the draughts about every five or ten minutes. It would be the safest plan, even with the above precaution, to mix some spirits with the water. Farmers engaged in harvesting their grain, should always let the water remain sometime in the vessel before using it:—many fatal diseases have originated, in an imprudent disregard of this cautious practice.

CATARRH

OR

COLD.

Colds are so common in all countries, and their modes of treatment so generally known, that not much need be said respecting them; further than to remark, that early attention will frequently prevent their laying the foundation of other complaints, which may in the end prove highly dangerous, and very difficult to remove. Persons of delecate constitutions are most subject to colds; and from the carelessness of such persons, in neglecting to avoid exposure, and to remove the early symptoms of disease, more than two-thirds of the whole number of *consumptive cases*, in all countries, arise and become fatal. Cold usually comes on with a dull heaviness of the head, which feels as if the nose was stopped up, which is generally the case. There is, also, at times, much sneezing, which is always followed by discharges of a thin watery mucus from the nostrils. You have soreness of the throat; cough; and chills stealing over you, with occasional hot flushes:—persons of very weakly constitutions have, also, a tightness and pain in the chest; Sometimes the symptoms are highly inflammatory or feverish; this is nearly always the case with very irritable constitutions—in which instance, the complaint must be arrested immediately. Here I repeat because it is all-important, that most of the *Consumptions* of this country, originate in *neglected colds*, brought on by exposure to the night air. by damp feet; by changing warm clothing for thin; by becoming warm from exercise, perhaps in a crowded ball room, and suddenly exposing the body to a cold current of air: and by many other imprudent courses of conduct.

REMEDIES.

Immediately before going to bed, bathe the feet and legs in warm water fifteen or twenty minutes; then wipe and rub them perfectly dry, and wrap them carefully in warm dry flannels. After lying down, take a large drink of warm sage, or balm, or hysop tea, or any thing else that will sweat you moderately. If the head is much stopped up with the cold, you may relieve yourself in a sitting posture, by covering the head with flannel or a blanket, and producing a steam beneath & surrounding the head; this can easily be done, by placing a hot rock in a crock or basin, and gradually dripping water on it, at the same time holding the vessel on your lap, and closing all the avenues by which the steam might escape from about your head, excepting one through which you are to breathe. This will give much relief in a short time. My practice in the commencement of a cold is, to give an emetic or puke, which in nine cases out of ten relieves the patient at once, and cuts short the advance of the fever:—[see table for dose.] When fever is very considerable, with violent pain in the head, indicating inflammation, the loss of some blood would be advisable:—after which, give a tea spoonful of *Antimonial wine*, every three hours, in any kind of drink; this will determine to the surface, or in other words produce a gentle moisture on the skin, and allay the feverish symptoms. The bowels should be purged moderately, by the daily use of Epsom salts, in small quantities, dissolved in cold water. If there be any pain in the chest or side, after employing the above remedies, put a blister over the part affected with pain, and keep it running as long as possible; (look under the head blisters.) The diet in colds should be light and cooling. Heating or stimulating articles, either of drink or diet, are highly improper, and always produce more or less fever. The best drink during the day, is flax-seed tea, with a small portion of acid in it.——After the feverish symptoms are removed, a troublesome cough sometimes remains:—this may be relieved by the use of *balsam copaiva*, in doses of ten or fifteen drops, on lumps of sugar, given three times a day; and a dose of paregoric, each night at bed time—[see table for dose;] or a small pill of opium—[see table.) The FRENCH have an excellent remedy for curing *cold*, which I have frequently employed with success, producing immediate relief. They apply a poultice of boiled onions to the sole of each foot on going to bed, after having bathed the feet and legs well in warm water:—and if the throat is sore, they apply the boiled onion poultice to it. This is a valuable application and may be much relied on. If the chest is much oppressed, the application of this poultice to the breast, will almost invariably relieve.——The following remedy, which is an excellent and efficacious one, has frequently afforded relief, in cases where colds had nearly settled down into confirmed *Consumptions*. Take one tea spoonful of flax-seed, half an ounce of liquorice, and a quarter of a pound of raisins:—put them into two quarts of rain water, and simmer the whole over a slow fire, until you reduce the quantity to one quart. Then prepare some candy made from brown sugar, and dissolve it in the liquor boiled down to a quart:—half a pint of this is to be taken every night on going to bed, mixed with a little good vinegar to give it a slightly acid taste; this will certainly relieve a cold, if used a few days. I have been more particular on this disease than at first view might seem necessary; but, considering it as intimately connected with, and in many instances the forerunner and foundation of *consumption*, I think I am justified in treating it with great attention.

DROPSY.

Dropsy is a disease of the whole system, arising from debility or weakness, and can easily be distinguished from other diseases, by the collection of water in some part of the body. By pressing the fingers on the flesh with some force a depression or pitting will take place, which can be seen some little time after the fingers have been removed: in other words, the flesh will have lost its elasticity, and will not immediately spring back on the removal of a pressure. Or—if the water is lodged in any particular *cavity* of the body, it may always be heard distinctly, on any sudden change of position, or rapid movement of the body. Among physicians, it is called by different names, according with the different parts of the system, in which the water may be deposited. When the water is seated in the cavities of the *head* or *brain*, the disease is called by physicians *hydrocephalus:*—when seated in the cavity of the *chest*, it is called *hydrothorax:*—when in that of the *belly*, *ascites:*—when seated in the *scrotum* or *bag* of the privates, it is called *hydrocele:*—and when the water is effused in the *cellular membrane*, which is the thin and delecate skin found among the muscles or flesh of the body, and which is the same that butchers blow up in their veal and mutton, the dropsical disease is called *anasarca*. There is strong resemblance, between dropsy of the *testicle* or *stone* in men, and *ascites ovarii* in women; the latter being small collections of dropsical fluid, in the *ovariica*, which are two oval flat bodies, which are about an inch in length, and half an inch in breadth, situated about an inch behind the womb, and which are supposed to contain and supply whatever the female brings to the procreation or formation of the fœtus or child. This is proved from analogy, by the simple fact, that an animal deprived of the *ovaria*, as in the case of spaying swine, looses all power of conceiving, and all venereal desire. I omitted to mention, that *hydrocephalus* or dropsy of the *brain*, is a disease common to children, and will be treated of under the proper head. I have in the first instance, and contrary to the impressions of some medical men, given it as my decided opinion, that *dropsy is a disease of the whole system:*—and my reader may be assured, that I am sustained in that opinion, by many of the most distinguished physicians in the United States.

REMEDIES.

More diseases of dropsy have been removed by bleeding, and more relief has been obtaind from it than from any other known remedy; for which reasons, it is now considered as satisfactorily proven, that this complaint is more frequently inflammatory than was formerly supposed. For this very important information, we are indebted to that highly distinguished physician Doctor Benjamin Rush. Bleeding must be entirely regulated, as to frequency and quantity, by the relief it affords to the patient. In my practice, I always use it freely; and never omit, at the same time, to purge freely with calomel and jalap:—[see table of dose:] or jalap alone. If these purges operate without pain, and the stools are fluid or watery, and your patient is not much weakened by them, it does not matter how many stools are produced daily; because the remedy is an efficient and a proper one. One ounce of cream tartar, in half a gallon of water, drank during the day, will be of much service: in truth, all articles which will increase the flow of the urine, or water from the bladder, called by physicians *diuretics*, are very useful in this complaint. The following cures, which I shall notice in the words of an experienced and distinguished man, give evidence of the correctness of some of my *introductory* remarks, among which are the following:—"The discoveries of each succeeding day convince us, that the Almighty has graciously furnished man with the means of curing his own diseases, in all the different countries and climates of which he is an inhabitant; and, there is scarcely a day, month, or year, which does not exhibit to us, the surprising cures made by roots, herbs and simples, found in our own vegetable kingdom, when all foreign articles have utterly failed." &c. &c.—The truth is, that the wise and beneficent CREATOR of the *Universe*, has made nothing in vain; and the time will come, when the apparently most useless and noxious plants, will be found eminently useful in the cure of diseases, which have hitherto baffled the profoundest skill, and the most powerful energies of genius. The following are the words of the author just alluded to. "I am knowing to two extremely distressing cases of dropsy, being entirely relieved by means of the bark of the *common elder*. One, a woman advanced in age, in the last stages of this disease, who lost a brother some short time previous, by the same complaint. The other, a young woman, who had been for eighteen months confined to her bed, during four of which she was unabled to lie down, and who is now wholly free from *dropsy*, and recovering strength in a most surprising and unexpected manner. A great many other cases, less aggravated, have been cured by the bark of the common elder; I have used it myself, with universal success—and its immediate adoption by the afflicted, is truly important and deserving attention. The receipt is as follows:—Take two handfuls of the inner bark of the white common elder; steep them in two quarts of Lisbon wine twenty-four hours—if this wine cannot be had, Teneriffe or Maderia will answer: take a gill every morning fasting, or more if it can be borne on the stomach. The bark and leaves of the elder, have long been known as powerful evacuants. I ought to have said in the proper place, that the young woman I have mentioned, used the elder—barked—wine, at the instance of one of the most distinguished physicians of Boston; who had previously tried every known prescription without success, and that the use of the elder entirely cured her;" The following remedy, handed me by a most respectable man, who resides in Roane county, Tennessee, Mr. William Mead, will undoubtedly be worthy of trial, and I therefore submit it to the reader

"Take two or three handfuls of rusty nails, and put them into half a gallon of good apple vinegar:—then boil, or rather simmer the vinegar down to a quart, and strain it well through a linen cloth:—next, add to the vinegar a quart of molasses, a handful of chamomile flowers, and a handful of lavender from the garden. Boil or stew this mixture down to a quart. The dose for a grown person, is a large table spoonful, to be increased gradually to one and a half: the dose of course, must be smaller for younger and more weakly persons." The character of Mr. Mead for integrity and veracity, and his solemn assurances that the prescription has often been eminently successful, induce me to place it on record. The oxide of iron, in other words rust of iron, would probably answer a better purpose than the nails mentioned by Mr. Mead.

SCURVY.

This disease is frequently of a highly putrid nature, and generally afflicts persons who have lived a considerable time on salted provisions, or unsound and tainted animal food. Those are also subject to it, who have been long confined without due exercise; those also, who have been unable to obtain vegetable food for a considerable period. Cold moist air, bad water, the morbid influence of depressing passions, such as grief, fear, &c. and the neglect of personal cleanliness, will also produce scurvy. With regard to cleanliness, I must speak in plain terms. Neglect of personal or bodily ablutions, in other words washing, among females at particular periods, are in reality the causes of very many cases of scurvy: and here I am compelled to say, that such are the cleanly habits of the French of the better order, male and female, I have never known a single case of scurvy among them, although much accustomed to their society in Europe: they are in the constant practice of using the warm bath. The disease called scurvy, can always be known by the softness and spongyness of the gums, which, even on being gently rubbed with a soft sponge, will invariably bleed. Ulcers next form around the teeth, and gradually eat away the lower edges of the gums, by which the teeth become loose, and sometimes fall out. The breath is always offensive, and smells badly; the face is usually of a pale yellow color, and considerably bloated; the heart palpitates or beats rapidly and irregularly, on slight exortiou; the legs and feet swell; small ulcers or sores, break out on different parts of the body, and more generally on the legs; pains are felt over the whole body; the urine or water is highly colored; the stools smell very badly; the strength becomes very much reduced and bleeding takes place from the nose, ears, gums, and fundament. When these last symptoms take place, the sufferer is near the termination of his earthly career:—and it is no less singular than true, that the appetite remains good to the last, together with a perfect retention of memory.

REMEDIES.

All acids are valuable medicines in scurvy:—such as common vinegar with fresh vegetables; in fact, a bath made of vinegar and water, in which the whole body can be frequently bathed, will be of essential service: as will also the plentiful use of ripe fruits. Sour krout, or pickled cabbage, is so excellent a remedy in scurvy, that a Dutchman whose name I have forgotten, received a large premium from the British government, for introducing it into the English Navy. Where there is much debility, the moderate use of good old wine will be proper; as will also the use of the nitric acid: (see diseases of the liver, where you will see this medicine plainly described, together with its effects,) by which the bowels will generally be kept sufficiently loose, at the same time that the system will be strengthened. If, however, the bowels should be found, dissolve a table spoonful of cream tartar in a pint of boiling water, and when cold, use it as a drink. I must not omit to mention, emphatically, that regular exercise is absolutely necessary in this complaint. You will find the following medicine, also, a good remedy:—dissolve three ounces of common salt petre, in a quart of good vinegar, and take one or two table spoonfuls three or four times a day—or less quantities if the state of your patient will justify it. When the gums are much swollen, with considerable ulceration, and the mouth, teeth, and breath, have a fœtid or bad smell, the mouth must be frequently washed with water, prepared as follows: boil red-oak bark in water, then strain the water well, and in it dissolve a lump of alum, to which add a tea spoonful of finely powdered charcoal, which is to be prepared by burning common smith's coal over again. I have omitted to state, that if the breathing is difficult, or there is much pain in the breast, a blister should be applied on the chest over the pain: you are *never to bleed in scurvy*: if you do, you will lose your patient. Pure fresh air, moderate yet sufficient exercise, and the warm bath of a pleasant temperature, with a sufficiency of vinegar in it, as before mentioned, will rapidly restore your patient.

PLEURISY.

Pleurisy is an inflammatory complaint, and requires remedies for the immediate reduction of the inflammation. The symptoms are, a sharp pain in the side, particularly when you draw your breath; the pain then shooting into the breast, back, or shoulders:—great difficulty in lying on the affected side; the tongue is of a white color; the urine or water of a high color; the face flushed and red; and the body very hot, denoting much fever. Sometimes this disease is accompanied with cough; and when this is the case, it is what physicians call a short dry cough. Sometimes the cough increases, and is accompanied by spitting up a tough phlegm; and the blood when drawn from the arm, when suffered to cool, has a coat or covering on it of a *buffy color*, which always denotes inflammation. This complaint is brought on by exposure to cold and wet; by sleeping on the damp ground, and getting the feet wet; by being exposed to sudden currents of cold air, when the body is over-heated; by the suppression of certain periodical evacuations, or in other words, by the obstruction of the menstrual discharges in women. The winter and spring, are the seasons in which this complaint is most prevalent. I will endeavor, for the satisfaction of the reader, to notice such symptoms as indicate a favorable termination of the disease; and, also, such as argue an unfavorable and fatal issue of the complaint. First—the symptoms are *favorable*, when there is a free perspiration or sweating; when there is a copious discharge, by expectoration or spitting freely; when the urine or water, deposites, on settling, considerable sediment or grounds, in the urinal or pot; when there is a spontaneous bleeding at the nose; or a gentle purging comes on; or the skin becomes warm and soft, with an abatement of thirst; and, when there is considerable relief from pain in the *head* and *side*. Second—the symptoms are *unfavorable* when there is violent fever, when the patient is delirious or out of his senses; when the pain suddenly stops, and the face or countenance changes its expression; when there is little, perhaps no expectoration or discharge by spitting—or if there is any thing spit up, it is of a dark color; and, finally, when there is a *sinking* and *irregularity* of the pulse: these symptoms are highly dangerous.

REMEDIES.

I have stated above that *pleurisy* is an inflammatory disease, and that it requires the immediate reduction of the inflammatory symptoms. You must, therefore, bleed in the first instance, as freely as the constitution and state of the patient will bear. If the fever still continues high, and the pulse remains *hard* and *full*; or, in other words, if the pain and fever, after the first bleeding should be relieved for a short time, and afterwards return with any violence, it will be proper to bleed a second time moderately. In fact, I have frequently been compelled to bleed three and four times, before I could reduce the inflammatory symptoms. After the first bleeding, apply a large *blister* over the pain, whether situated in the side or chest:—and if the blistor should not run sufficiently after being dressed, and the pain should continue, apply another *blister*. After the bleeding and blistering, give a large dose of epsom salts—and if any considerable pain is felt, put the patient in a *warm bath*, which will cover the whole body. I have, in more than fifty cases in the State of Virginia, relieved *pleurisy* by immediate and copious bleeding, and as early as convenient afterward, by using the warm bath. After the inflammatory action is in some degree removed, the seneka snake-root tea will be found a valuable remedy: (look for a description of this root, under that head.) Throughout this complaint, the bowels *must* be kept open, by the use of epsom salts, or senna and manna, or castor oil; epsom salts, however, will always be best, if they can be procured. Clysters of any simple kind, such as thin gruel milk warm, or starch dissolved in warm water will be perhaps equally as good for keeping the bowels open. [See under the head clystering, and how to prepare clysters.] When perspiration or sweating is not produced in moderation, by the remedies I have mentioned, equal quantities of antimonial wine and sweet spirits of nitre, mixed, and given in doses of a tea spoonful every two hours, will assist in producing perspiration. Toward the close of this disease, and after the inflammatory or feverish symptoms have subsided, and *not before*, if the cough should continue troublesome give a pill of opium at night, or a dose of paregoric or laudanum: (see table, for doses of these articles;) and, also, under the different heads, how they are made.—If the pulse should sink, and your patient become weak, stimulate him gently but cautiously with warm toddy wine mixed with sugar and water, and apply blisters to the ancles—and cataplasms or poultices to the soles of the feet, made of mustard-seed pounded fine, and mixed with vinegar. These measures sometimes become necessary, from sinking of the pulse, coldness of the feet, or extreme weakness: they always produce excitement and warmth in the system. This complaint requires the strictest abstainance from all animal food, and from every thing which has a tendency to produce fever. The patient should live on the lightest diet, and such as will keep down all fever and inflammation: in fact, there is no disease mentioned in this book, which require a more rigid abstainance from solid food than *pleurisy*. Nothing but toast and water, barley water gruel, or flax-seed tea, ought to be taken in this disease, and that warm and in very small quantities at a time; a little panado may be given as nourishment. Unfortunately, and want of experience, when any person is taken sick in this country, and refuses to eat for two or three days, great alarm is created immediately lest the patient should *starve to death:* and I have known several instances since I have been in the western country, in which the officious stuffing of patients with food, with the best possible intentions, has produced *death*, in spite of medical assistance. I wish all such persons as are disposed to *cram* their patients with food, when there is no appetite for it, and the stomach rejects it, to remember that *nature generally speaks the truth.* After recovering from this disease, great care must be taken to avoid all *cold* and *dampness*, and particularly exposure to the *night air;* because they almost always produce dangerous relapses. Flannel ought to be worn next the skin; and dressed buck skin, I am convinced from my own practice, worn in the same manner by delecate persons, is also an excellent defender from cold, and much superior to flannel.

GRAVEL AND STONE.

Gravel and stone, which originate in the same causes, are to be distinguished thus from each other. *Gravel* is usually understood to mean. *calculi*, (from the old word *calx*, a *limestone*, or *little sand like stones*, which pass from the kidneys, through the ureters, into the bladder. The ureters are small tubes, which run from the kidneys to the bladder, and convey the urine into the latter. The word *stone* speaks for itself; it is a strong concretion of matter, which enlarges and hardens by time, seldom found in the ureters or tubes themselves, but generally lodged in the kidneys or bladder; when the stone is in the kidney, it is because it is too large to be passed off by the tubes leading to the bladder —and when found in the bladder, it is from the simple fact, of its being too large to be passed off through the channel of the penis.————When a disposition to *gravel*, which I have just explained, exists in the urinary system, there will be occasional paroxisms or fits of *pain in the back*, which sometimes shoot downward to the thighs; and sometimes a numbness of one of the legs inside, accompanied with a retraction or drawing up of one of the testicles or stones in men. The pain I have just spoken of is often extremely violent, and is sometimes terminated by a discharge of small gravel stones from the urethra, with the water in the common way. The *stone*, however, which I have also described, and which is usually found in the *kidneys or bladder*, sometimes in both, is a disease of more serious and dangerous consequences altogether. When the *stone* has acquired some size, if situated in the bladder, there is a frequent and almost constant desire to make water; sometimes the water passes off, drop by drop—with much pain—and sometimes in a small stream, which occasionally stops short; in the last case, when the water passes in a small stream with sudden stoppages—there will be great pain for some minutes after, in the glans of the penis, in other words the head of the penis. In some persons, the violence of straining to evacuate the urine, make the *rectum* or lower gut contract and expel its excrements:—or if that gut be empty, this straining occasions *tenesmus* or a constant desire to go to stool. In discharges of urine, when stone exists in the bladder, there is very often blood to be seen in the water, and sometimes pure blood itself is passed off in small quantities. When the calculus or stone is formed in the *kidney*, in addition to the general symptoms of stone in the bladder, there will be felt a dead, heavy, dull pain, in the loin where the kidney containing the stone is seated; frequently accompanied by fits of shuddering, and creeping coldness, in and over the part affected; this shuddering and coldness of sensation, are sometimes so great, that sufferers have been known to blister the small of their backs, by exposure of the parts naked to the heat of large fires. In severe cases of calculus or stone, either in the kidneys or bladder, there is frequently experienced, during the time of passing the urine, sickness of the stomach, a desire to vomit, and much faintness.—Aged persons are most liable to disorders of the urinary passages; which do not in all cases arise from gravel and stone, or even from spasmodic strictures in those parts. These apparent disorders of the urinary passages, frequently occur in old persons, from the constipation and retention of feculent and fetid matter in the bowels, which ought always to be attended to by gentle purging, and particularly by frequent clystering:—(for clystering see that head.)—The *gravel*, and sometimes the *stone*, when the latter has not become much enlarged from the lapse of time, may much more easily be removed from the bladders of *females*, than from those of males. In women, the urethra or canal which leads from the bladder to the exterior, is always straighter, shorter, and wider, than in men—and may in many cases be dilated so much by artificial means, as to admit the gravel or stone to pass off with the water.—The extraction of the stone from men, by the use of the knife, is called by the physicians, *lithotomy*. This is a delecate, dangerous, and very painful operation; and I have uniformly advised persons much advanced in age, and who were afflicted with the stone, to employ palliative remedies for the pains attending it, rather than lithotomy.

REMEDIES.

When there is much difficulty in passing the urine, and that difficulty arises from strictures or obstructions in the *urethra* or canal which conveys off the water; and especially where inflammation of the bladder is apprehended, the catheter must be used: (for which see the head *catheter*.) When the complaint is painful and oppressive, in what are called paroxysms or fits of the gravel or stone, for I make no distinction between them as to remedies, and there is so much irritation as to lead to apprehensions of inflammation, *bleeding* should be immediately resorted to, followed by the *warm bath;* in which the patient should remain some time. In most cases, I have been enabled to allay the pain entirely, by bleeding in the first instance, using the warm bath next, and then giving a pill of opium or a dose of laudanum; (for which see head warm bath—and table of doses.) After these remedies, if considered necessary, the privates and belly should be rubbed and bathed, with flannel cloths wrung out of warm water, in which chamomile flowers have been boiled; after which the cloths themselves should be applied warm, and suffered to remain. The drink of the patient should be flax-seed tea, given as freely as you please. Should the pain still continue severe, give a clyster made of gruel, and strained, in which put two table spoonfuls of castor oil or sweet oil,—and forty drops of laudanum, This is to be thrown up the bowels pleasantly warm:—(see head clystering.) Old persons who are afflicted with gravel or stone, will find great relief from frequently using such clysters, and from taking in moderation, occasionally, laudanum or opium to procure rest: (see table of doses.) But, among all the palliative remedies ever yet discovered, I am compelled, from both *experience* and *incontesatble authorities* to believe, that, in all diseases of the urinary organs, and particularly in *stone* and *gravel,* the *uva ursi* of the mountainous regions of Europe, and possibly of this country, stands conspicuous and alone. The following cases of actual experiment, to which had I space, many more might be added, will prove conclusively that it is a sovereign remedy, if not dissolving the stony matter, at least in banishing the sufferings with which it is usually attended.

CASE 1st. At the age of thirty-two, Mr. B——having tried various remedies, submitted to an operation for the stone, with which he had been afflicted many years. When the usual passage was opened into the bladder with a knife, a rough stone of the mulberry kind was taken out. Although the operation was well performed, the incission perfectly cured, and the severe pains he formerly felt had ceased for a time—yet. after the lapse of some weeks, he again began to be afflicted with excruciating pains, and great difficulty in making water. The urine was accompanied with a discharge of matter, which had continued ever since the operation—and now, instead of decreasing as was expected, it had become more abundant, bloody, fetid, corrosive and inflammatory, and excited exquisite agony at every attempt to pass it off. After various remedies, ordered by the best physicians, had been tried in vain, the use of the *uva ursi* was recommended, and many cases in which it had been successful related to him by way of encouragement.—On the 10th of October, 1762; after taking some medicines by way of preparation, he began with *half a drachm* of the powder of the plant *uva ursi*, which had been brought from Vienna for the greater certainty; this dose he took twice a day, observing a temperate diet and abstaining from every thing considered pernicious. In three weeks his pains were appeased; the matter was greatly diminished in quantity, and was also of a much less acrid quality; and he voided his urine more freely. These circumstances gave him great hopes of being perfectly cured; nor were his expectations ill grounded:—for in ten weeks, he was entirely free from pain, made water easily, and was no more afflicted with fruitless provocations to urinate. And now, April 25, 1763, by persevering in this course, he is so perfectly free from all symptoms of the complaint, that he considers himself entirely cured.

Case 2d. A youth twelve years of age, of a tender constitution and delecate frame; having been frequently subject to coughs and other ailments, was suddenly attacked with severe pain in the region of the bladder. This continued for several days; during which time he frequently cried out as if upon the rack: his water, which was very mucus, dropping from him very painfully, gave strong suspicion of the gravel. The usual medicines were given; but in vain. He was next sounded by a skilful physician, and a *stone* was found in the bladder. About this time, De Haen's account of the *uva ursi* became public; and this was considered a fair case in which to give it a trial. After proper preparations, half a drachm of the powdered plant was given twice a day. For a week, no perceptible relief was obtained; but, in three days more the pain abated, and the water became less charged with matter. In short, by observing a regular diet, and by steady perseverance in the medicine, he is now so entirely well that an operation for extracting the stone by the knife is no longer thought of.

CASE 3d. A gentleman near forty years old, of a good constitution, living in a place supplied with water of a *bad quality*, became afflicted with the gravel to a very painful degree. He frequently passed small stones, of a sandy substance, which he could plainly perceive to fall from his kidneys, where they seemed to be generated, through the ureters into the bladder—always exciting, during their descent, intolerable misery. All the most celebrated medicines adapted to such complaints, were fairly tried. Little or no relief was obtained. The matter voided in his urine, gave suspicion of decay in the kidneys. The *uva ursi* was therefore advised, and continued in the dose of half a drachm twice a day; by which, with regular and abstemious diet, the patient in *three months* became perfectly well.

I consider the foregoing cases, to which, as I have before remarked, many others might be added from excellent authorities, entirely conclusive as to the medicinal virtues of the *uva ursi:* for a particular description of which, together with some other cases of cures in *stone* and *gravel*, I most strongly and seriously refer the reader.

SUPPRESSION, OR STOPPAGE

OF

URINE.

This is a disease, which is frequently produced by inflammation of the *urethra*, or canal which conveys the water from the bladder:—it is also sometimes produced, as I have mentioned under "Inflammation of the bladder," by falls in various ways, and by that false delicacy, which induces a bashful and inexperienced person, to retain the urine an usual and dangerous length of time. It is also produced, among those who have worn down their manhood in indiscriminate debaucheries in early life, and sometimes among those who are naturally of delecate and weakly constitutions, by taking too large quantities of the *tincture of spanish flies*, for purposes which I forbear to name. It also, sometimes, arises from the necessary application of *blisters*, and not unfrequently from costiveness, or *constipation of the bowels*.

REMEDIES.

Draw some blood; this will relieve the system. Then put the patient in a warm bath, which must be continued from a quarter to a half hour. Next give a warm clyster, made of starch and water, in which must be mixed three table spoonfuls of castor oil. For the warm bath, and clystering, look under the heads. If it becomes necessary, after these remedies, give a dose of castor oil by the mouth. If all these means fail of producing a flow of urine, the *catheter* must be skilfully and cautiously used:—for which look under the head. Throwing cold water on the belly and thighs, will sometimes afford relief, when all other remedies have failed. A clyster of warm water, in which tobacco leaves have been steeped for a few minutes, is an excellent remedy; it must, however, be used with great caution; being very powerful in its effects, it must be made weak—and should by no means be repeated, unless under the direction of a physician. Its immediate effects are—a general relaxation of the whole system, accompanied with prostration of muscular power, faintness, and sickness of the stomach — profuse sweat breaks out over the whole body; and if the remedy succeeds, the urine is immediately evacuated.

GREAT FLOW OF URINE.

This complaint is called by physicians *diabetes*. The word *diabetes* is derived from two Greek words, which signify—to *pass through:* and, I mention the fact merely to show, how little connexion there usually is between the *derivation of words* and their *real meaning.* The quantity of water usually discharged in diabetes, is more than double the portion of liquid taken in both drink and food. The attacks of this disease are generally slow and gradual:—I have known instances, in which it has been more than two years in making its advances on the constitution. The symptoms of diabetes are:—larger and more frequent discharges of water from the bladder than common; the urine is clear and transparent as spring water: and having a sweetish and sickish taste, like sugar and water—accompanied by a faint smell, as if mixed with *rosemary* leaves. These symptoms generally occur without pain—and are usually attended with a voracious or greedy appetite. When this disease occurs on young persons, or is attended to in grown individuals at any period, it can very frequently be removed:—but, when suffered to proceed for any length of time, or when it attacks persons in advanced age, or those who have indulged to excess in spirituous liquors, it is extremely difficult of removal. As this disease increases on the constitution, for I certainly consider it a constitutional complaint, the whole body becomes emaciated, and gradually wastes away; the mind becomes dull and melancholly; the patient has a strong aversion to motion and exercise; there are frequent darting pains in the privates, accompanied with a dull and heavy pain in the small of the back; nearly constant thirst, which it seems impossible to satisfy; the bowels are costive, and the pulse irregular; as the disease advances, fever takes place, similar to that in hectic and consumptive cases, the feet begin to swell, and death in a short time usually closes the scene. The favorable symptoms in this disease are the following;—the appetite becomes more natural, and the thirst diminishes; the urine is voided in smaller quantities, and the desire to make water less frequent; the water assumes its natural color, and regains its usual smell; the skin becomes more flexible or soft, and suffused or covered with gentle and natural sweat; the mind gradually becomes more cheerful, and the desire for exercise increases: when these symptoms manifest themselves, there are always great hopes of speedy recovery. The bodies of many persons who have died of *diabetes*, have been accurately examined by skilful anatomists:—and the results have always shown diseased state of the kidneys and their vessels, and consequent derangement of their secretions—in plain language, and I am supported in the opinion by the celebrated Rush, and several other physicians of note, *diabetes* is a *consumption of the kidneys.*

REMEDIES.

Emetics or pukes are frequently to be given in this disease, and much dependence may be placed on them for a cure. Ipecacuanha is perhaps the best puke that can be given:—[see table for dose.] Blisters are to be applied to the small of the back, and kept continually running: and a Dover's powder is to be given at night, which will produce a determination to the surface, or in other words a gentle sweat: to prepare these powders, look under the head *Dover's powders.* Use the warm bath frequently, and have the whole body rubbed well twice a day with a flesh brush, or coarse towel; the rubbing should at least continue half an hour to benefit your patient: Flannel must be worn next the skin. The tincture of cantharides, cautiously administered, is a valuable remedy, and should be given to a grown person from eight to ten, and twelve drops, every four or five hours in a little cold water, or in water in which some gum has been dissolved:—wild cherry tree gum will answer. Astringents may be serviceable in this complaint, and should be tried agreeably to the following directions. Alum dissolved in water, and occasionally given throughout the day, as the stomach may bear it without inconvenience or unpleasant feelings, will be serviceable:—or sugar of lead, given from a grain and a half to two grains, twice a day in cold water, for grown persons, has afforded much relief and expedited the cure:—for the dose of alum or sugar of lead, see table for the doses adapted for different ages. When it is possible to obtain chalybeate water, or in other words spring water impregnated or mixed with iron, you should direct your patient to use the water freely. East Tennessee abounds with those springs, on almost every branch or rivulet. As there is an acid of the stomach, which frequently accompanies the complaint, it will be proper to give your patient weak lime water, or chalk, or soda powders: look under that head, and you will see how soda powders are made. If fever is present in this disease, which is sometimes the case, the loss of a little blood occasionally will be proper. Your patient is to use no strong drink of any kind; to eat no vegetable food, but live on animal food; to avoid cold and exposure of every kind; and to defend the feet and body well against the damp air—and, in good weather, to take moderate exercise. In my practice, I use the uva ursi tea, and have derived great benefit from it: I therefore recommend it with the utmost confidence. By the use of emetics, with this tea, and frequent bathing in warm water if commenced at an early period, a cure may be speedily expected. Read under the head uva ursi, for a description of this plant, how it may be obtained, and how to use it. The bowels are to be moderately purged, and kept open by castor oil; or by rhubarb, either by chewing it, or taking it in powder. Rhubarb is preferable to castor oil in this disease, and should be used if it can be obtained. Look under the head rhubarb, for an explanation of its qualities and (see table for doses.) Doctor Samuel Sair, lately read to the Acadcmy of Medicine in France, an interesting memoir on this subject. He refers most cases of incontinence or involuntary flow of urine, or *diabetes*, to a want of equilibrium in power, between the body of the bladder and its neck; in other words, when the muscular power of the neck of the bladder, is so much weakened, or relaxed, as not to retain the urine against the contractible power of the bladder itself. With this view of the subject, he imagined that if he could stimulate the neck of the bladder, and *not the body* of it, he could succeed. He introduced, by means of a catheter, some tincture of cantharides, so as to touch the urethra in its prostatic part, and also the neck of the bladder:—by this process, he cured three patients who labored under this disease. When this remedy is to be resorted to, the aid of a skilful physician will be required.

ERUPTIONS OF THE SKIN.

The close connexion which exists, between the stomach, skin, and bowels, is evidently demonstrated by the simple fact, that in many instances where the bowels is internally disordered, the skin exhibits external evidence of disease. The many eruptions which show themselves on the face, hands, legs, and bodies of individuals, are positive proofs of the deranged state of their systems internally.—and by removing the primary or first causes, you invariably remove those eruptions, which are in general mere *effects*. You should therefore, always endeavor to ascertain, whether those diseases of the skin are not produced from some impure state of the blood, from a foul stomach, from costive bowels, or from some constitutional disease derived from parents. If either of those causes produce eruptions of the skin, you will easily see that they are to be removed by internal remedies—I mean those which strike at their roots:—for, if you should succeed in driving in the eruptions of the skin, by merely external remedies, you will always produce fever, and almost invariably seat some fatal disease on the vital organs. Whenever diseases exhibit their effects on the skin, you may be assured that they are *efforts of nature* to *relieve herself* from oppression; and, the real business of a physician is to *assist nature*, and *never to retard or stifle her operations.*

REMEDIES.

The first great and important rule, in all eruptive disorders of the skin, is to open the bowels and keep them in a laxative state, by cooling medicines, such as Epsom salts, or equal quantities of cream of tartar and sulphur. If the stomach is out of order, there being a close connexion between it and the skin, a gentle emetic will sometimes be necessary to cleanse the stomach, and to assist nature in throwing the whole disease on the surface, where it may expire and fall off in scabs. Tea, made of sassafras, or sarsaparilla, should always be used as a common drink. Whenever fever takes place, which is sometimes the case, draw some blood from the arms, and give an active purge of calomel at night, followed by a dose of Epsom salts in the morning. Common starch rubbed on the skin, in all kinds of eruptions, is a cooling and pleasant remedy; and the application of it on going to bed, will produce much relief from the itching, and consequently easy and refreshing sleep. Persons who are subject to eruptions of the skin, should live on light and cooling diet; avoid salted provisions, and every thing of a heating nature; avoid spirituous liquors, and use cooling acid drinks—and, by all means, keep the skin clean by frequent warm or tepid bathing.

SAINT ANTHONY'S FIRE.

This disease, is called by physicians, *ery sipelas:*—it is of an inflammatory character, and always attended with some fever.—The skin burns and itches very much, and usually turns to a scarlet color. It generally commences in a red spot or blotch, and quickly extends itself over the whole body. Sometimes the face swells very much, and becomes inflamed: there is also, head ache, sickness at the stomach, and, not unfrequently, violent fever attended with delirium.

REMEDIES.

This disease is attended with inflammatory symptoms, and like others of the same character, must be treated by moderate bleeding, cooling purges, and cooling drinks. Bathe the feet and legs frequently in warm water; and remain in your room, so as not to be exposed to damp cold air, by which the disease might be struck inwardly. Every two or three hours, give equal quantities of antimonial wine and sweet spirits of nitre, in doses of a tea spoonful, in a stem or wine glass of cold water. If the head ache is very severe, the loss of some blood, a blister between the shoulders, and poultices made of mustard seed and corn meal, will give relief—Sprinkling the body with fine starch, or with wheat flour, will greatly assist to cool and allay the irritation.—A tea spoonful of sugar of lead, put in three half pints of cold water, and used as a remedy by washing the body, is also a valuable application.

TETTER

OR

RING WORM.

This is a disease confined to the skin, for which medicines are seldom given internally. It first appears as an inflammatory eruption or small magnitude, not larger than the finger nail, and gradually extends itself in a circle, which sometimes embraces the hands, sometimes the face, and not unfrequently large portions of the body. Unless relieved, it at length becomes extremely painful, and is attended with an itching sensation, which is greatly increased by the least warmth or exercise.

REMEDIES.

Puccoon root called by some persons Blood-root, and by others Indian paint, steeped in strong vinegar, and applied as a wash to the parts affected, is a most excellent remedy —perhaps the best one known in this disease. The Blue Dye, made by the country people to color their cloth, has been sometimes known to remove it, when many other remedies had failed:—this must be owing to the indigo and urine the die contains I do not recollect, however, one single case in my practice in Virginia, in which the puccoon-root and vinegar failed. In France, the application of the fume of sulphur is always resorted to with success, in all diseases of the skin:—(read under the head sulphuric fumigation.

SCALD HEAD.

In this disease, the whole scalp or skin of the head is covered with small sores, which discharge very offensive matter. These sores eventually turn to little *scales* or *scals*, while fresh ones continue to break out at the roots of the hair, and follow the same process of turning to scales and falling off. This disorder is infectious or catching, and is often taken by children, in consequence of wearing the hat or cap of a person affected with it. Sleeping in the same bed, or combing with the same comb, when a child has constitutionally a scrophulous taint, will also communicate the disease—which is sometimes tedious and difficult to cure.

REMEDIES.

First, shave off the hair as close as possible; then cleanse the sores daily with warm soap-suds—and put on the following ointment, which must be spread on a bladder, and worn as a cap. Take two table spoonfuls of tar, and a sufficient quantity of suet or lard to make an ointment; to these add a table spoonful of powdered charcoal, and two tea spoonfuls of sulphur. The bowels must be kept open with epsom salts, and a tea made of sarsaparilla and sassafras drank freely; these measures will purify the blood. Once or twice a week, bathe the whole body in warm water of a pleasant temperature. Doctor Chapman of Philadelphia, one of the Professors of that University, recommends highly the following remedy. Take of liver of sulphur, three drachms; of Spanish soap, one drachm, of lime water, eight ounces; and of rectified spirits of wine, two drachms:—mix them well together, and use the whole as a wash. Where the remedies I have mentioned *fail*, look under the head sulphuric fumigation, for a certain remedy in all diseases of the skin.

TOOTH ACHE.

This disease does not always arise from decayed teeth; it is frequently the offspring of *nervous affections* of *cold*, of *rheumatism*, and not unfrequently among females, of *stoppages* of certain evacuations. I have known many sound teeth to be extracted unnecessarily, and on account of diseases which were afterwards discovered to be seated in other parts of the body; and, I therefore earnestly recommend, that great caution be used in discovering the causes of tooth ache, before a tooth is suffered to be drawn. Tooth ache, in very many instances, arise from a disordered state of the stomach and bowels. In these cases, the suffering is generally severe, and must be removed by attention to cleansing the stomach and bowels. Many instances have occurred in my practice, where persons have requested teeth to be drawn to remove tooth ache, when all their teeth on examination were found to be sound. In these cases, I have always relieved them by a good purge. Among women more than one half of the suffering from tooth ache, may be fairly traced to some bodily habit, or some nervous sympathy, to which the female constitution is peculiarly liable—and which may be removed by other means, than the extraction of the teeth. Persons who have written before me, on the subject of tooth ache, have spoken of the disease as peculiar to, and confined to the teeth alone; when the fact is, that common sense and experience, will teach any man the palpable absurdity of such doctrine, and convince him that *tooth ache* is very frequently a *common symptom of other diseases* which are to be sought out and removed before relief can be obtained.

REMEDIES.

When tooth ache is presumed to arise from nervous affections, the nervous system is to be strengthened by gentle tonics, nutritive and cooling food, and moderate exercise in the open air. When it proceeds from cold or from rheumatism, consult these two heads for directions to remove it: and when it arises from stoppages of the menses in females, see and consult that head, *among the diseases of women.* Extracting teeth ought always to be the last remedy resorted to; it is a painful operation, and oftentimes a dangerous one, when attempted by an unskilful and clumsy hand. When a tooth is discovered to be defective, and that there is inflammation at the root, which is the cause of the pain, let the inflammation be reduced by blistering the surface of the check. or by scarifying the gums, with a lancet, and the tooth pluged with gold leaf, or silver or tin foil. Tooth ache is frequently owing to the nerve of the tooth being exposed to the air from decay: in this case, it is always advisable to avoid the extraction of the tooth, and to have it pluged as I have just told you, with gold leaf, or with silver or tin foil. These articles can always be obtained pure. There are cases, in which the diseased tooth will not bear the wedging pressure of being plugged with gold leaf; in these instances, pure tin or lead ought to be used. These last mentioned articles, however, wear out in a few years; and it is a truth well known, that tin will corrode, rust, or turn black in a short time, from the action of the acids generally used in food. Gold in its pure state, is always preferable for pluging a tooth; it will sometimes last twenty years.—If the disease arises from inflammation, the practice of holding hot and stimulating articles in the mouth is highly improper: you will know when it arises from inflammation, by the following indications—you will have head ache, which will be attended with fever. Take a full dose of epsom or glauber salts, and repeat the dose if necessary. Apply to the face cold mush and milk poultices; or those made of meal and vinegar, as cold as possible, and if the inflammation runs high, and is attended with fever, the loss of some blood will be proper, together with the application of a blister over the pained part. Great suffering about the teeth, is frequently caused by certain nervous pains, to which females are sometimes constitutionally liable:—these cases are to be treated with simple remedies, and scrupulous care, until the original causes are removed—and you may apply to the face, some irritating tincture, such as cayenne pepper, tincture of Spanish flies, or volatile liniment. I have said before, that tooth ache sometimes arises, though not very frequently, from *rheumatism:*—when this is the case, the whole side of the face will be pained together with the sound as well as the decayed teeth. There will also be felt, a dull heavy pain, extending along the jaw bone; and a stiffness of the neck, sometimes attended with pain in the shoulder. The following is a good remedy. Put a piece of lime, the size of a walnut, into a quart bottle of water; with this rinse the mouth two or three times a day—and clean the teeth with it every morning until the pain ceases. But in rheumatic affections, of the kind just described, see under the head rheumatism.

The *tartar or scurvy of the teeth,* is a very destructive disease; it greatly injuries the teeth, and frequently destroys them, before you are aware of the danger. Tartar is an accumulation of earthly matter, deposited on the teeth from the saliva or spittle. It collects on the teeth of some persons, much faster than on those of others; this is owing to the natural or constitutional state of the fluids, of the mouth. When first deposited on the teeth, it is soft and very easily removed with a tooth brush; but, if suffered to remain, it acquires hardness by time, and thickens about the necks of the teeth. The gums become irritated and inflamed by it; the sockets are next destroyed—and the teeth being left bare, without any support, are pressed out by the tongue, or fall out. The importance of removing tartar from the teeth, must be obvious to all:—and the operation ought always to be performed by a skilful person, called a *Dentist*—or by a physician. To prevent the accummlation of tartar on the teeth, and to restore the healthy state of the gums, nothing more is requisite than a stiff brush, and pounded charcoal, mixed with an equal quantity of peruvian bark. The use of all acids for the removal of tartar, is a base imposition. Acids will, indeed, make the teeth look beautifully white for a few days, dissolve and remove the tartar, and stop the tooth ache; but, in a few months, the teeth will become of a dead chalky white, next turn dark colored, then begin to decay and crumble to pieces, and finally leave their fangs in the sockets, exposed to pain and inflammation. Milk warm water, and the tooth powder I have mentioned, will not only preserve the teeth, but correct in a great degree the offensive effluvia arising from decayed teeth and unhealthy gums.

ITCH.

This filthy disease is infectious, or in other words catching; and is frequently produced by want of cleanliness: it is confined to the skin, and first shows itself between the fingers, in small watery pimples—gradually extending to the wrists, thighs, and waste. There is a constant desire to scratch, which is much increased after you become warm in bed. Cleanliness, and early attention to this dirty disorder, will prevent its being communicated to a whole family: children are apt to take it at school, and to communicate it to those with whom they sleep. Travellers are apt to take it, from sleeping in beds that have been previously occupied by persons who have it:—therefore, a good caution in travelling is, to have the sheets and pillow-cases changed. Frequent instances occur in travelling, where persons of much respectability have taken the itch, and been much mortified by it, from want of this precaution.

REMEDIES.

Take one drachm, or sixty drops of *sulphuric acid*, which is *oil of vitriol:*—mix it well with one ounce of hog's lard, or fresh butter without salt will answer. After it is well prepared by good rubbing, anoint the parts affected until cured; this is an innocent and certain remedy for the itch. Or you may make an ointment of a table spoonful of sulphur, and a table spoonful of lard, or butter without salt, and put in the ointment a table spoonful of the essence of lemon, or a tea spoonful of the oil of lemon, which will give it a pleasant smell. This ointment must be rubbed on the parts affected, three or four nights on going to bed. Sulphur is nothing more than common brimston purified and pounded fine. Or, you may take one drachm of red percipitate, and rub it well in a mortar with an ounce of hog's lard, or butter without salt, and anoint the parts affected; this last is a valuable and certain cure.—A strong decoction or tea of Virginia snake-root, known generally as black snake-root, will frequently cure the itch when used as a wash. Tobacco leaves steeped in water, and used two or three times a day as a wash, will effect a cure; but this remedy must be used with caution on children. Water dock grows in wet ditches mill ponds, and sides of rivers; and flowers in July and August. The root boiled in strong decoction or tea, and used as a wash, is a good remedy for itch: the narrow and broad leaved dock, found in yards and fields, will answer the same purpose. Mercurial ointment, sometimes called oil of baze, is frequently rubbed on the joints for itch: this is highly improper, because it frequently salivates, and produces pains in the joints and bones for life.

EATING SNUFF.

Nothing is more difficult to be accounted for, even by men of acute and profound observation, than the strong attachments of the human species, to practices which are absolutely at war with nature, and hostile to every principle of enjoyment and happiness. How the use of tobacco, under any form, could ever have become a luxury among mankind, especially considering its *nauseous* and *disgusting* qualities, is an enigma not to be solved on common principles. We can easily account for our attachments to food, and even to those luxuries of life which have any thing tempting in their use, by referring them to instinctive impulses to the preservation of life, and our native propensities to heighten the enjoyments of existence: but—to account for our attachments to habits and practices, which are absolutely *disgusting*, *offensive*, and *highly injurious to health*, and which almost invariably lead to *immoral* and *dangerous* excesses, we are compelled to refer them to the degeneracy of our species, and the entire corruption of their moral tastes and feelings.

The use of tobacco in any way, unless as a medicinal application to the system, the instances of which will be found under the head *tobacco*, is dangerous to health, to happiness, and to morals;—in support of the truth of this doctrine, it would be idle to adduce proofs; those who use tobacco, are conscious of its defective effects, and those who do not, may hourly witness its dreadful consequences on the health and morals of society. We are all well acquainted with the effects of chewing and smoking tobacco, and taking snuff in the common way; but we have something yet to learn and disclose, respecting the hitherto unheard of practice among the females of our country, of *regularly eating Scotch snuff!* It appears, from what I have been informed on veritable authority, or I certainly would not believe it possible, that the practice among our *ladies*, of eating daily *considerable quantities of Scotch snuff*, arose in the first instance, from their using it as a *tooth powder*—yes, most courteous reader, a tooth powder! If this is any thing more, than a mere pretext for the filthy and disgusting practice, which *taints* the breath with a *fetor worse than assafœtida:* deranges all the physical sensations, and the whole nervous system; imparts to the rosy cheek of youthful beauty, the delightsome complexion of a *cake of bees-wax:* subverts, ruins and finally destroys the digestive powers of the stomach; and, renders that stomach a filthy reservoir of *dregs* and *crudities* which taints and corrupts the whole system—the *eaters of Scotch snuff* may be induced to abandon the destructive practice, when I point out to them a much better tooth powder—which is nothing more nor less, than powdered charcoal, mixed with peruvian or dog-wood bark.

In speaking of the evils which arise from eating snuff, I have not enumerated the half of them; the fact is that language itself would fail in classing and giving them names. We all know perfectly well, that the stomach is the *work-shop* of the whole human machine, and that when its functions are deranged or impaired, the whole system suffers in its remotest extremities. Hear what the celebrated Rush says, respecting the practice of eating snuff:—"I have known two instances of death from eating snuff. It is a habit which is increasing among the ladies of our country, with a rapidity only equaled by the ravages of ardent spirits, and which is no less ruinous to health and destructive to life. The practice of eating snuff, had its probable origin in using the Scotch snuff as a tooth-powder;—a fondness is soon acquired for it, and hundreds among us, especially among our females, *get drunk* upon it every day of their lives."—Doctor Rush's views of this subject are undoubtedly correct; but he has not said all that might have been alleged, respecting the consequences of snuff eating. He might have said, that those who are in the practice of eating snuff. may easily be distinguished from those who are not. He might have said:—here is a snuff eater; notice this complexion; it is a pallid sickly yellow; the skin seems to be under-coated with a layer of Scotch snuff, there is nothing of "the rose's bloom of opening unsullied beauty," on this lank, faded, and hollow cheek:—look at this eye, the owner is an eater of Scotch snuff;—do you see any thing of that healthful brilliancy, that sparkling fire of youthful beauty which inchants mankind, in that jaundice, sunken, hollow, dead and beamless eye? No: the vital energies have been worn out and exhausted by snuff eating; the animations of youth have been overpowered and killed by this excess; this is but the shadow of a human being!—Catch a scent of this *breath*,—is it pure and sweet, with youthful passion's tender bloom? Does it remind you of the gale of spring, that gently shake the blossoms from the orange grove?—Does its healthful purity bespeak the paradise of sweets from which it comes?—No: like the wind of night, that has swept the sepulchral shades of death, it comes with corruption and infection on its wings!—It reminds you of disease, debility, decay, and death, of every thing but *love!*—Doctor Rush might have said all this of the snuff eater, and forfeited none of his high claims to professional honors, integrity, and truth—I am decidedly of opinion, and I record the allegation without fear of contradiction, especially by those who know any thing of the subject, that of the two characters, the *drunkard* and the *snuff-eater*, the drunkard is the more worthy personage, if consequences be taken into consideration. Snuff eating invariably produces languor, extreme debility, aversion to the performance of the common duties of life, tremors of the nerves, capricious and disagreeable temper, and restless melancholy, and lowness of spirits, unless the person is immediately under the disgusting stimulant. But, this is not all; snuff eating always produces want of appetite, nausea, inordinate thirst, pains and distention of the stomach, dyspepsia or indigestion, tremors of the limbs and whole frame, disturbed sleep, emaciation or wasting of the body and limbs, epilepsy or fits, consumption and death.—Nor is this all; tobacco is an absolute poison—a very moderate quantity introduced into the system, or even applied moist to the pit of the stomach, has been known to produce instant death. The Indians of our own hemisphere, have long known of its poisonous effects upon the human system; and formerly used to dip the points of their arrows in an *oil* obtained from the leaves, by which faintness and death occurred from their wounds.

I was once acquainted with a young lady of the first respectability, whose kind and affectionate heart was possessed of every noble and generous sentiment, who was in the habit of snuff eating. She was taken dangerously ill. and it became necessary to give her an emetic or puke, and the fact was, that in the operation of the medicine, she threw up nearly half a pint of snuff from the stomach.—How young, blooming, and tender girls, can bear the use of snuff in this way, or indeed in any other way, after experiencing the wretched sensations always produced by it, is to me absolutely unaccountable, unless on the pinciples I have mentioned:—and I must also here confess myself unable to account for the fact, that the parents of these girls, knowing the evils of snuff eating, cannot merely over-look the practice in their blooming daughters, but absolutely *encourage* it by their example. I really trust, that the preceding remarks, and they are founded in experience and truth, will have some influence in restraining the practice of snuff eating, and in restoring many of the fair of our country, to the possession of their native charms and beauty.

APOPLECTIC FITS.

This disease derives its name from a Greek word, which signifies to *strike* or *knock* down; because those affected with it are suddenly prostrated to the earth, and deprived of sense and motion. A variety of causes have been assigned for *Apoplexy;* but, they may all be comprised in the following words—whatever determines, or *throws*, so great a quantity of blood on the *brain*, that it cannot return from that vital organ. It is not necessary to enumerate those causes, further than to remark, that among them are:—violent fits of passion, excess of venery, stooping down for any length of time, overloading the stomach, and wearing any thing too tight about the neck, great cold and intemperance.—Persons most liable to apoplexy, are such as have short necks and large heads. In attacks of Apoplexy in the severest form, the blood vessels are found bursted, and the blood poured out in various parts of the brain; and when Apoplexy attacks in milder forms, those blood vessels are found distended, or swelled with too large a quantity of blood. This complaint has deprived the republic of some of her greatest ornaments, among which were the Hon. Dewit Clinton, the Irish patriot Th: A. Emmet, and William

V*

Pinckney Esq. our former minister to London. Intense and protracted mental exertion, was probably the cause of the death of Messrs. Emmet, Pinckney, and Clinton; but, in most instances, Apoplexy is to be dreaded by corpulent or plethoric persons, such as I have before named, having large heads and short necks, epicures, gluttons, and those who use spirituous liquors to excess.

REMEDIES.

The chief remedy in Apoplexy is large and copious bleeding, which must be repeated if necessary. Cupping at the temples ought also to be resorted to, the great object being to draw the blood from the head and to relieve the oppression of the brain, as speedily as possible. The next thing to be attended to, is to give the most active purges:—[see table for dose.] Apply cold cloths wet in vinegar, and the coldest water constantly to the head. If your patient should recover by the means directed, in order to escape from a second and third attack, the person should scrupulously observe the following rules of living: he must eat vegetable food, drink no wine or spirits of any kind, avoid all strong and long continued exertions of mind; and after the full state of the brain has for some time subsided, the use of Chalybeat waters, such as those of the Harrodsburgh Springs in Kentucky, will be of much service. As this is a common and often fatal disease. I will make some further remarks on it. Many physicians have recommended, and put in practice, in this complaint, opening one of the external jugular veins. They imagine, that by drawing blood from one of these veins, they unload the brain and relieve its blood vessels from distention, and the danger of rupture. The fact however seems to be otherwise. Instead of unloading the vessels by this operation, the *pressure* which is necessary to be made on the vein for the purpose of drawing the blood, evidently retards the return of the blood to the heart—and, as a certain and *inevitable consequence* of this pressure, accumulation of blood in the arteries, and greater distention of the blood vessels immediately take place. To exhibit the force of this reasoning clearly, I will make an example of blood letting from the arm. The arteries of the arm convey, by the muscular power of the heart, all the blood in those arteries to the points of the fingers:—here the veins take up the same blood, to return it again to the heart.—Now—when we cord the arm tightly in order to draw blood from a vein, what are the consequences? Why;—we stop the course of the blood back to the heart, swell the veins of the arm next, and lastly distend the whole of the blood vessels of the arm: and, are not the same effects produced and the blood vessels of the head, by a strong pressure in cording the jugular vein? The above doctrine, as well as it can be explained from the words of the great Doctor Baillie of London, I am induced to consider correct. Instead of opening the jugular vein, in cases of emergency, I would recommend bleeding in the *foot.* In performing this operation after the bandage has been put on, the foot should be put in warm water: the fact is that warm water applied to both feet, in bleeding for apoplexy, would be attended with manifest advantages.

EPILEPTIC FITS.

This disease differs from apoplexy, by the former having convulsions, and frothy spittle issuing from the mouth. The ancients gave it the name of the *sacred disease,* because it affected the mind, the most noble part of the rational creature. These fits last from ten minutes to half an hour, depending on their violence; they always leave the sufferer in a stupor, attended with great weakness and exhaustion of the body. Epileptic fits arise from the following causes:—Original or natural defects; in other words, defects derived from nature; and severe blows in the head. When the disease arises from either, or both of these causes in combination, it is seldom if ever cured. But when it proceeds from any of the following causes, cures may be effectuated by medicine, proper diet, &c.—In children, when it proceeds from worms, cutting teeth, impure and acrid matter in the stomach and bowels, eruptions of the skin which suddenly strike in, and sores on the head which are too quickly healed up, relief may be obtained by medical means. Relief may also be had in the cases of grown persons, afflicted from the too free use of spirituous liquors, from violent excitements of those passions which affect the nervous system, from stoppages of the menses in women, and those who have not yet had their courses according to nature. This disease is sometimes, although not often, produced by great debility or weakness; and sometimes by onanism.

REMEDIES.

In fits of this kind; a few days previous to the expected attack, draw blood from the foot; and every night on going to bed, bathe the feet some time in warm water, so as to prevent too great a determination of blood to the head, as these fits generally attack persons during sleep. If considered necessary, give an emetic or puke to cleanse the stomach, followed by an active purge to act on the bowels: (see table for doses.) These fits generally occur about the change or full of the moon. The singular and surprising influence, which this planet is known to exercise in many instances over the human species, is absolutely unaccountable, and is even ridiculed by many physicians; but, I feel fully confident, from reflection and experience, that this planet has considerable control over certain diseases to which the human system is liable—one or two of which I will notice. The monthly courses of women at particular times, are evidently under its influence: madness, or mental derangement, is in many cases greatly increased at the changes of the moon: and it is well known to almost every person, that the periodical return of epileptic fits, is generallly about the full and change. These circumstances certainly denote some secret and mysterious agency, which is concealed from human knowledge. On a full examination of the different remedies recommended in epileptic fits, where they arise from circumstances which can be traced to some particular cause, please to refer to the different heads, remembering always, that when you expect to effect a cure, it can only be done by removing the cause. I have mentioned emphatically, bleeding in the foot, and the warm bath; these will remove the blood from the brain, when harsher means have failed. The bowels must be kept in a laxative state, by epsom salts, castor oil, or mild clysters:—(see table for doses and the head clysters.) By permitting the bowels to be the least bound, you subject the person to much risk of having a fit. An issue or a seaton in the neck, something resembling a rowel, and kept continually discharging, is a good remedy in fits. The use of tartar emetic ointment, is a remedy resorted to in the hospitals of Europe with success; I have tried it in two cases; it succeeded in one and failed in the other:—this, however, is the usual fate of those remedies applied in this disease. Seatons always lessen the fits considerably in number and severity, and the tartar emetic ointment sometimes removes the complaint; they are, therefore, both worthy of a fair trial. For the mode of preparing this ointment, and the manner of using it, look under that head—and for issues or seatons, see that head. All that can be done during the fit, is to prevent the person from injuring himself, by placing a bit of soft wood between the teeth, and unclenching the hands. The following remedies should be tried separately, and with moderation, where there is any hope of success:—plunge the whole body in a strong bath made of salt and water, a few mornings in succession, before an attack is expected; or you may give spirits of turpentine, in small doses, on an empty stomach; or, take the person afflicted through a gradual and moderate salivation with mercury. Doctor Currie, an eminent physician, speaks highly of the Digitalis or fox glove, as a remedy in this complaint; but it must be used with much caution. Five or six drops of tincture, increased two drops every five or six days, ought to be given: [see table of doses.] The bowels must be kept open with senna and manna. Doctor Wharton, of Shenaddoah county, Virginia, a man of distinguished abilities, administered it with great success: see page 184, Med. Recorder:—Persons who are subject to these fits, should avoid all strong and heating food together with all kinds of spirituous liquors. Hog meat should never be used as food in any way; nor should any thing difficult of digestion ever be eaten. Moderate exercise must be taken, and every thing must be avoided which is calculated to produce melancholy:—because the mind and passions have great influence on the nervous system.

PALSY.

Palsy is a disease, attended with the loss or diminution of the power of voluntary motion. It sometimes affects one part of the body, and sometimes another; but, in whatever part of the system it prevails, there will always be a numbness, and almost entire want of feeling, and a loss of power to move the part affected. This disease may rise from apoplexy; from any thing that prevents the flow of the nervous fever from the brain to the organs of motion; from luxurious and intemperate living: from the suppression of certain evacuations, such as are mentioned in epileptic fits; from spasmodic affections or cramps; from whatever causes a determination of blood to the brain; from too frequent intercourse with women, by which the nervous system is much weakened: from exposure to cold; from affections of the spinal marrow; from any mechanical compression; in fact, from whatever has a tendency to weaken and relax the system in an extreme degree. Dissections frequently show collections of blood, and sometimes of serous or watery fluid, effused or spread out on the brain; and what is something singular, the collections and effusions, are generally found on the opposite side of the brain from the parts of the body affected.

REMEDIES.

In no cases of the palsy should bleeding be resorted to, unless the patient is of a stout and full habit of body, and where the disease originated in the head, causes a great determination of blood to the vessels of the brain. In all other cases, bleeding is of much more injury than benefit. Where the person is of a full habit, and there is much determination of blood to the head, in addition to bleeding in the first stage of attack, active purges will be very beneficial. If, on the contrary, the person is of a delecate and weakly habit of body, is considerably advanced in life, or if the disease has affected the system for a time, bleeding and very active purges should never be used; it will be sufficient here to keep the lower bowels gently open, by mild and at the same time, stimulating clysters: (see the head clysters.) The fact is, that constipation of the bowels on the one hand, and excessive laxness on the other, are extremes equally to be avoided in palsy. Constipation or costiveness of the bowels, always oppresses the brain with an accumulation of blood, which must be relieved.—and too much purging with very laxative medicines, invariably weakens the system greatly, and as I have somewhere before remarked, produces morbid irritability. Palsy, with the exception of the cases I have mentioned, must be treated with tonic or strengthening medicines. Every second or third night take two grains of calomel, and three of ground ginger, in a little honey: these doses are to be continued, until there is a copperish taste in the mouth, or some soreness felt in the gums and mouth; here you are to stop taking them. During all this time, you are to have the affected parts well rubbed with a brush, for half an hour three times a day; and you are also, once a day, to bathe in strong salt and water made pleasantly warm. See the head warm bath, where you will find, that out of 996 cases of palsy, 813 were benefited by the warm bath. Blisters are also very beneficial in this disease, one of which ought to be placed between the shoulders, one on the inside of each ancle, and one over the part affected: they should all be kept continually running, by the application of some irritating ointment. An issue or seaton in the neck is also highly recommended, especially where the disease, has originated from apoplexy. I have found great benefit in palsy, by using on the affected parts, the following liniment. One ounce of spirits of heartshorn, one table spoonful of spirits of turpentine, one table spoonful of the tincture of Spanish flies, made by steeping the flies in whiskey. These articles are to be mixed in half a pint of sweet oil, and well rubbed on the parts affected three times a day. If these articles cannot be had, bathe the parts in whiskey, in which cayenne pepper has been steeped so as to make it strong of the pepper. Use horse raddish freely with your food; and take thirty-five drops of spirits of turpentine, on a lump of sugar, three times a day. As soon as practicable, take exercise in the open air, and when on the recovery, make use of water impregnated with iron, and use your bath cold instead of warm, in the manner of a shower bath:—see that head; the water should be mixed with salt. I will remark in conclusion, that electrifying or shocking in this disease, is very highly recommended:—as is also, the method of cure resorted to with great success in Austria, France, and Germany, which is the use of the *sulphur bath*, by which 673 cases were cured in the hospitals of Paris, and 484 in those of Vienna. See head Sulphuric Bath.

ASTHMA.

In this disease, from an extensive experience, I unhesitatingly say, that *asthma* when once firmly seated in the system, is a complaint that may be palliated but never entirely removed by medicine. When the disease attacks young persons, abstemious diet and due exercise are the best remedies for subduing its violence; but, an entire, and permanent cure of the complaint, is only to be expected from the spontaneous and powerful efforts of nature herself. In aged persons, where the disease is of long standing, great care and attention, are required to lessen the severity of the attacks; this is nearly all that can be done by the boasted powers of medicine, when the disease has become obstinate by age. Many physicians have asserted that asthma is a nervous disease; the contrary however, has been established, by many dissections in the hospital of Paris and other cities of Europe. Corvisart, Raumus, and Roston, besides many others, allege that asthma depends on a morbid or diseased *alteration* in the organs of breathing or respiration and circulation, by which congestions or collections of blood in the lungs are produced. Roston, particularly, gives in evidence of this opinion, the following facts:—he says in substance, that the bodies of many who had died of asthma, were opened immediately after death, and that in all of them *alterations* in the structure of the heart and arteries, were found combined with extensive congestive diseases of the lungs, proving that disorder of the heart and large blood vessels, have much greater influence in the production of asthma than is generally supposed. The symptoms of asthma are:—difficult breathing or respiration for a time, succeeded by short intervals of comparative ease, which are followed by attacks similar to the first, in many cases, amounting to almost suffocation; a great tightness across the breast, and in the region of the lungs; a wheezing noise in breathing, attended by a hard cough at first, which gradually diminishes in toughness, until a white stringy tough mucus is discharged from the throat and mouth, accompanied perhaps by a gentle moisture on the skin. Persons subject to periodical attacks of asthma, generally know the approach of those attacks, by the following symptoms and sensations:—depression of spirits amounting to melancholy; sense of fullness and distention about the stomach, attended with uneasy and restless feelings; drowsiness accompanied with head ach: and a sense of tightness or constriction across the breast. These indications usually occur about the close of the day, increase in severity during the night, and sensibly diminish toward morning.

REMEDIES.

Bleeding must never be resorted to in asthma:—although it is frequently practiced by physicians, it is altogether wrong, and must always be avoided. The reason is obvious, and particularly so, in the cases of persons advanced in age. Bleeding retards, in fact it *prevents* expectoration by the mouth and throat; in other words, it prevents hawking and spitting up mucus from the throat and lungs, which always gives relief in asthma. So soon as symptoms of an attack are felt, which I have just described, give a mild emetic or puke; this will always shorten the attack —during which the feet must be bathed in warm water, and the steam of warm vinegar inhaled, or breathed from the spout of a coffee-pot. Stew down over a slow fire, half an ounce of seneka snake root in a pint of water, after bruising it with a hammer, to half a pint: of this take a table spoonful every ten or fifteen minutes, and drink a small glass of warm toddy. I have frequently afforded relief in a short time, by merely bathing the feet and giving plentifully of warm toddy. The Indian tobacco is a valuable remedy in this complaint, used in the following manner. Take of the leaves, stem and pods, nearly as much as you can hold grasped between the fore-finger and thumb. Put it into a bottle of whiskey, and in five days the liquor will be fit for use; of which give a tea spoonful every half hour until relief is obtained: When this complaint attacks young men, for it is much more apt to attack men than women, they should rise early and take active exercise, particularly by ascending the highest and steepest hills and mountains, where they can breast the pure mountain breeze. These people should always rise from a hard bed instead of a soft one, and swallow a raw egg before walking.—To persons severely afflicted with this disease in advanced life, smoking the dried root of the Jamestown weed will be beneficial, as will also smoking the dried root of the skunk cabbage. Look under the head Jamestown weed where this plant is described; it must always be used gradually and with some caution. Baron Brady states, that he cured himself of asthma of 21 years standing, by the internal use of mustard seed, of which he took every morning and evening a tea-spoonful in tea or broth. Doctor Pitschaft says, he derived much benefit from the internal use of mustard, in pectoral disorders attended with cough, and excessive mucus expectoration.

SORE LEGS.

Sore legs frequently arise from the imprudent neglect of bruises; and, from trifling sores, which are permitted to become inflamed, and finally ulcerous. Sore legs, like consumptions, and other diseases which descends from parents to children, sometimes run in families for several generations:—when they run in families, it is generally in such families as are addicted to *king's evil, scrofula* or *scurvy*. Doctor Rush says, that he considers them, in many instances, as arising from general debility or weakness, operating on the whole system, but centering more particularly on the legs. Persons who have been afflicted any length of time with ulcerous sore legs, or indeed with ulcers situated any where els, if of long standing, should be cautious how they heal them suddenly, without purifying and preparing the system for the change:—because the sudden suppression of a habitual discharge, without this previous purification, almost invariably seats some new disease on a *vital organ*, or produces death by apoplexy.

REMEDIES.

The first and important remedy in sore legs. is to keep them perfectly clean, by frequently washing them with soap and water. Doctor Rush say, and I perfectly agree with him in opinion, that the great success of old women in curing sore legs, arises more from keeping the ulcers clean, than from any peculiar efficiency of their medical applications. Where sore legs have been of any long standing, it is of importance, as I have told you before, to attend to purging and purifying the whole system, with frequent doses of *epsom salts*. *Nitre* or *saltpetre*, given in doses of ten, fiteen, or twenty grains, three times a day in a little cold water, will be found a useful and cooling medicine. Pouring cold water on the sores three times a day, is an excellent application; but it must be done on an empty stomach. Poultices of light wheat bread and milk, applied as cold as possible, will reduce the inflammation, or fever: so will also, a poultice of slippery elm bark, pounded well and moistened before being applied. A wash of white oak bark, in old ulcers is a valuable remedy. I have succeeded in curing old sores, when every other means had been tried in vain, by the application of common tow to the ulcer, and kept wet with new milk. A salve made of Jamestown weed, will be found an excellent remedy; as will also a salve made of the common elder bark. When the sores are sluggish, and refuse to heal, a poultice made of common garden carrots will be found of great utility. Should proud flesh take place, after washing the sores with castile soap-suds, sprinkle a little red percipitate on the sores—or a little calomel—or a little burnt alum—or dissolve a little blue vitriol, (blue stone,) in water and wet the ulcers with it.

In sore legs of long standing, moderate exercise should be taken, and tight bandages applied, commencing at the toes and winding up the leg, which will give due support to the vessels. In such cases, tonic or strengthening medicines are necessary, such as bark, iron rust, &c. &c.—with a moderately nourishing food. The use of opium, see table for dose, will be a useful medicine in allaying the pain and invigorating the whole system. Rest in a lying posture, should always be particularly attended to, in all cases of sore legs: and the diet should be cooling, accompanied with pure air. Every thing of a heating and stimulating nature should be avoided, particularly ardent spirits. In some old ulcerations of the legs, nitric acid (aquafortis) very weak, is sometimes taken internally and also applied outwardly as a wash for the sores. charcoal will correct the smell, and purify the sores; or if made into a poultice is an excellent application to ill-conditioned ulcers. Water dock which grows in wet boggy soils, and on the banks of ditches, boiled to a strong decoction, is a good wash for old ulcers: and, an ointment made by simmering the root in hog's lard, is a valuable remedy, derived from the Indians.

PILES.

There are two kinds of piles, originating from very nearly the same causes:—one is called the bleeding piles, and the other the blind piles. The piles are small swelled tumors, of rather a dark appearance, usually situated on the edge of the fundament. Where there is a discharge of blood from these tumors when you go to stool, the disease is called bleeding piles; but, when there is only a swelling on the edge of the fundament, or some little distance up the gut, and no bleeding when you evacuate the bowels, the disease is called the blind piles. Both men and women are subject to piles; but women more particularly, during the last stages of pregnancy, in which the womb presses on the rectum or gut. In passing the stool, you can plainly feel these tumors, which extend from the edge of the fundament, to an inch or more upward, if you have them severe;—when these burst and bleed, the person is very much relieved; and when the pain is excessive, it is apt to produce some fever. Many persons are constitutionally subject to this disease through life. It is, however, generally brought on by costiveness, or having irregular stools. Piles is also produced, by riding a great deal on horse-back in warm weather; by the use of highly seasoned food; by sedentary habits, in other words, want of exercise; by the use of spirituous liquors to excess; and by the use of aloes as a purge, if constantly taken for any length of time to remove costiveness:—therefore, persons subject to costiveness, should particularly avoid aloes.

REMEDIES.

Cold water is one of the best remedies that can be applied in this complaint:—nor will any person ever be afflicted much with bleeding or blind piles, who will bathe the fundament well, with cold spring water daily, or with iced water to prevent, or to relieve the disease if formed. I have known many persons who have exempted themselves from this painful disorder, merely by bathing twice a day in the coldest water. For those, who from laziness or neglect, omit to use this simple and powerful precaution, I shall proceed to give the usual remedies. When there is a fever attending piles, it will be proper to lose a little blood, and to take a dose of epsom salts or castor oil: (for doses see table.) Purging and bleeding should be repeated, if the inflammatory or feverish symptoms do not subside. If the pain is violent, bathe the fundament with some laudanum, say a tea spoonful of laudanum, mixed in a table spoonful of cold water:—or set over a tub, in which some tar has been heated or set on fire, so that the steam may sweat the fundament:—this steaming should continue some time, and be frequently repeated. Sweet oil applied to the fundament is a good remedy; and cooling applications of sugar of lead is also good—made by putting a tea spoonful of the lead into a pint of spring water, and bathing the parts frequently with it. Mercuiial ointment, otherwise called oil of baze, is a fine remedy; and, by greasing the parts with a small quantity three times a day, speedy relief will be obtained in a short time. The root of the Jamestown weed, made into a slave, and the fundament greased with it, will also afford a speedy relief from pain. All persons subject to piles, should live on light diet of a cooling nature, avoid costiveness, and use plenty of cold water in bathing, as before directed.

PUTRID SORE THROAT.

In this infectious or catching disease, the respiration or breathing becomes hurried, and the breath hot and offensive. The swallowing becomes more and more difficult; the skin burning and disagreeably hot, without the least moisture; and the pulse very quick and irregular:—the mouth and throat assume a fiery red color, and the palate and glands of the throat much swelled. Blotches, of a dark red color, appear on the face about the third or fourth day, which gradually inercase in size, and soon spread over the whole body. On examining the throat at this stage of the disease, you will discover small brown spots inside of the throat, which soon become deep sores or ulcers—a brownish fur covers the tongue; the lips have small watery pimples on them, which soon break and produce sores, the matter of which is of an acrid nature. If this disease is not immediately relieved, it soon terminates fatally, from the fifth to the seventh day. As the disease advances, the following symptoms denote an unfavorable and fatal termination. Purging a black matter, of a very offensive and fetid smell; the hands and feet become cold; the eruptions becoming of a dark liver color, or suddenly disappearing; the inside of the mouth and throat assuming a dark hue; the pulse becoming small, quick, and fluttering; the breathing much hurried, with an almost constant sighing; and a *cold* and *clammy* sweat.—When putrid sore throat is about terminating favorably, the skin becomes gradually soft and moist, denoting the abatement of fever; the eruptions of the skin becomes of a reddish color over the whole body; the breathing becomes more free and natural; the eyes assume a natural and lively appearance; the sloughs, or parts which separate from the ulcers, fall off easily, and leave the sores of a clean and reddish color:—when these symptoms occur, as I said before, the disease is about terminating in a recovery of the patient.

This infectious and frequently mortal disease, made its appearance in Knox county, in the fall of 1827, and proved fatal in very many instances. Having a short time before arrived from Virginia, and being a stranger, my practice was necessarily confined to some cases which occurred at Knoxville. I immediately determined, to use a remedy which I had seen successfully administered, in the West Indies, in this disease; and the result of the prescription was successful in my own practice. Feeling it a duty to communicate the remedy to several gentlemen in the country, whose children were attacked with the complaint, I was informed it was unusually successful, in every case in which it was resorted to in the early stages of the disease.

REMEDIES.

In this disease, which is generally a dangerous one, unless treated with judgment, *bleeding* and *purging* are always fatal in their consequences, and you are scrupulously to avoid both. Many physicians have treated this complaint injudiciously, from the simple fact of not giving themselves the trouble to investigate its causes. It generally makes its appearance at the close of sultry summers; when the system has been much weakened by protracted exposure to intense heat, and when people have been for some time, exposed to breathing the putrid atmosphere arising from stagnant waters and decaying vegetation.

You are in the first instance, to give an emetic or puke of ipecacuanha: (see table for dose,) and the dose must be repeated in moderation the next day if considered necessary. This will throw off the acrid matter, which would otherwise produce injury by descending into the bowels—which are to be kept *gently open* by clysters:—(see under that head.] If it is necessary, a little castor oil by the mouth, or a little rhubarb may be given to assist the clysters in removing offensive matter:—use, then, the following valuable prescription, which is well known in the West Indies, whence I derived it. Take *cayenne pepper*, in powder, two table spoonfuls:—with one tea spoonful of *salt;* and put both into half a pint of boiling water. Let them stand one hour and strain off the liquor. Next put this liquor as pure as you can make it, into half a pint of strained vinegar and warm it over the fire. Of this medicine, give two table spoonfuls every hour. Make also, a strong decoction or tea of seneka snake root, and give of it two table spoonfuls every half hour. If any debility or weakness should come on, bathe the grown person or child in a strong decoction of red oak bark. If the weakness is very considerable, add one fourth of whiskey to the decoction, and give wine, or toddy made with spirits and sweetened with sugar, to support the system. Wash the mouth and throat frequently with the liquor made of pepper, vinegar, and salt:—and, apply to the throat, a poultice frequently renewed, of garlic, or onion, or ashes well moistened with vinegar, and enclosed in a small bag, so as to produce slight irritation of the skin. Volatile liniment will answer:—look under the head; but blisters must never be applied to the neck. I have never used the compound, but am strongly impressed with the opinion, that a tea spoonful of good *yeast*, mixed with the same quantity of *powdered charcoal*, and given three times a day, would be a good remedy in this complaint.

HEAD ACHE.

This affection is produced from a foul stomach, from costiveness, from indigestion, and sometimes from exposure to the rays of the sun. There is also a painful affection of the head, accompanied with some nausea, called *sick head ache*, which comes on periodically, or at particular times:—this last is sometimes called *nervous head ache*. It is not nervous head ache: it arises from want of acid on the stomach, or from an excess of acid. There is, indeed, a nervous head ache, which arise from the same causes as those which produce tooth ache in *female diseases:* and which may be produced, also, by grief or any of the depressing passions, and should be treated by gentle stimulants.

REMEDIES.

If produced from a foul stomach, give an emetic or puke; if from costiveness, give an active purge—(see table for dose;) if from exposure to the sun, read under the head Inflammation of the Brain. In sick head ache, a late remedy has been discovered, which may be relied on; it is *citric acid* which may be had at any drug store; in plain terms it is nothing but the *acid* of *lemons;* of which you have only to put a little in cold water, and to drink it. This remedy is believed to be an effective one; and was like many other valuable discoveries, the result of mere accident. A girl who attended a bar in London, was called on to make a glass of lemonade. She was so afflicted with sick head ache, as scarcely to be able to prepare it. On tasting the lemonade to know if it was good, she found that every sip she took relieved her head, and finally, she obtained entire relief, from drinking the whole glass. When sick head ache arises from excess of acid on the stomach, a tea spoonful of finely powdered charcoal, in a little cold water, will correct the acid:—a tea spoonful of magnesia will do the same. When head ache arises from debility, stimulants are required, particularly by delecate females. Wine *sangaree,* made with warm water, wine sugar, and nutmeg, is an excellent and gentle stimulant. I have in many cases, given a bottle of Maderia wine to a female in the course of a day, and produced much benefit from it in this disease—without the least intoxicating effect.—The best wine must always be used.

EAR ACHE.

Many persons are subject, on the slightest cold, to painful affections of the ear. These pains usually subside in a day or two, and the disease ends in a discharge of matter.—Sometimes great pain is produced, by some insect crawling into the ear of a person whilst sleeping: and it is not unfrequent, that an accumulation of wax takes place in the ear, and produces *deafness.*

REMEDIES.

Warm some fine salt, place it in a bag, and apply it in the ear; or—make a poultice of roasted onions, and apply it to the ear and side of the head—first putting into the ear a little fine wool, on which has been dropped a few drops of laudanum and sweet oil warmed. If the pain or deafness is occasioned by the lodgment of hard wax in the ear, inject strong warm soap-suds into the ear, so as to soften and finally dissolve the wax. If the pain is very severe, a blister behind the ear will relieve it; and if the deafness continue for some time after the pain has gone off, inject into the ear once or twice a day, a little strong salt and water—after which, keep the ear stopped with some wool, which must be moistened with spirits in which camphor has been dissolved.

MUMPS.

This complaint is so universally known, as to make a minute description of it unnecessary. It appears on the throat; sometimes on one side, and sometimes on both sides. It makes its appearance in a lump immediately under the jaw, which swells and becomes large and painful, and often renders the swallowing difficult. The cheeks and whole face generally swell at first, and continue swelled for five or six days. When the disease is any way severe, it is usually attended with fever:—children are generally affected with it, but it is not exclusively confined to them. When it attacks grown persons, male and female, great care shoud be observed in treating it. In men, the testicles frequently become swelled as large as goards, and extremely painful:—in women, without great attention, the disease is apt to settle in the breasts, which become swelled and very hard; in this case there is much danger of an accumulation of matter. These consequences, however, both to men and women, usually arise from want of attention, and from the taking of colds:—when due caution is exercised, there is very little danger from the complaint.

REMEDIES.

In simple cases of mumps, nothing can or ought to be done, but avoiding the taking of colds. Keep the face, throat, and head, moderately warm, by wearing flannel round the parts. Keep the bowels gently open, by a little castor oil or epsom salts; and always avoid the damp ground, and wet feet, or even damp feet. If the testicles swell, immediately lie down on your bed, and move as little as possible:—and also be bled from the arm, and purge freely. Apply to the privates, poultices of cold light bread and milk, which are always to be renewed as soon as they become warm. Dissolve a tea spoonful of sugar of lead, in a pint of cold water, with which you are to wet the poultices and also the testicles; which are to be suspended, or held up in a bag made for the purpose; a handkerchief will answer the same purpose, which is merely to prevent their *weight* from doing injury. Women, in cases of swelled breasts, must pursue the plan of bleeding and purging prescribed for men, and apply the poultices to their breasts to prevent the formation of matter in them. Poultices made of flax-seed, applied cold, are also effective in reducing inflammations.

SORE EYES.

This is so common a disease in the western country, that it requires to be treated of with much attention. The eyes are exceedingly tender, and subject to a great variety of maladies, some of which usually terminate in total blindness, unless speedy relief can be obtained. This delecate organ exemplifies in the wisdom of its construction, the boundless and incomprehensible power of an *Almighty God.* It may be called the mirror of the soul; the interpreter of the passions of mankind. At a single glance, it takes in the sublime beauties, and magnificent splendors of the visible creation; reaches by its mystic energies the bosom of unlimited space—and, at the next moment, by an effort of microscopic vision which is absolutely unaccountable, it expatiates on the mild tints of the opening rose-bud, and detects the analysis of a physical atom! The loss of such powers of vision, then, must be indeed a great misfortune.—and frequently, when I have reflected on the dangers of so great a loss, I have been astonished at the carelessness and inattention, with which diseases of this noble and distinguished organ are sometimes treated.

In a work like this, which is intended for popular use and benefit, it would be irrelevant and unimportant, to treat of such diseases of the eye, as require surgical operations; such must always be met, by the skill and judgment of a practiced physician.

Opthalmia is the general name, given by physicians to inflammatory diseases of the eye:—these diseases are either inflammations on the *coats* or *mombranes* of the eye, or they are inflammations of the *whole orbit* or *globe of the eye* it self. In *common opthalmia,* for there is such a disease as *venereal opthalmia,* the eyes exhibit considerable inflammations, owing to the fulness of the small blood vessels; there is also much heat and pain over the whole surface of the eye; and, generally speaking, an involuntary flow of tears. When the inflammation is suspected to be deeply seated, throwing a strong light on the eye will determine the fact, by producing sharp shooting pains through the head, accompanied with fever. When the pains of the eyes and head are not much increased by an exposure of the eyes to a strong light, we may safely conclude, that the inflammation is of a slight and local nature. It is my opinion, and I know it is contrary to the *common opinion,* if any judgment can be formed from the general practice of physicians, that inflammatory diseases of the eye, are very frequently connected with diseased states of some of *the other organs*, or with, *general* and *constitutional derangements of the whole system.*

Inflammatory diseases of the eye, are usually produced by severe colds; by sudden changes of the weather; by exposure to cold, raw and damp winds; by residing in very damp or very sandy countries; and by exposures of the eye to the vivid beams of the sun, on sandy or snowy wastes of country, for some length of time. In the salt mines of Poland, to which many convicts are consigned for life, and where the exclusion of day-light render torches necessary, not only the prisoners, but the horses themselves become blind, from the insufferable brilliancy of the salt rock. This simple fact, is sufficient to place all persons on their guard, against exposing the eye to a strong glare of light. In addition to the above causes, inflammations of the eye, are often produced from external injuries, such as blows and bruises; and also from splinters, dust or any other irritating matters getting into the eyes. Healing old ulcers, or sores of long standing—and particularly driving in eruptions of the head and face, will very often inflame the eyes Besides all these causes, the suppression or stoppage of some habitual discharge, such as the menses, bleeding at the nose, hemorrhoids or piles, &c. will produce inflammations of the eyes:—and, to close the catalogue of the causes of inflammatory diseases of the eye, *venereal opthalmia* itself is produced, by the action of the virus or poison of the *venereal disease*, on scorbutic or scrofulous habits of body. This last disease of the eyes, generally terminates in impaired vision, or total blindness:—You, who are yet tyros in the school of experience and humanity:—you, who are melting down your physical and vital energies on the corrupted bed of lust and debauchery, listen to this!

REMEDIES:

In all inflammations of the eyes, presumed to arise from a diseased state of the general system, from a foul stomach from costiveness of the bowels, from colds accompanied with fever, or even from local affections of the organic structure of the eye, the stomach is to be thoroughly evacuated and cleansed by gentle emetics or pukes, and the bowels by active and cooling purges. If the inflammation should be severe, some blood should be drawn from the arm occasionally, at the same time that very cooling purges are in operation. The diet should be of the lightest kind, and of the most cooling nature. Cold acid drinks are also proper, because they tend to lessen the inflammation, and to cool the whole system. The skin should be kept clean, and perspiration or sweating kept up continually, by the warm or tepid bath, after bleeding and purging have been sufficiently resorted to. Doctor Physic, who is probably among the greatest men of his profession, either of this, or any other age, expressly recommends, that in very severe inflammations of the eyes, blister plasters should be applied *over* and *around* them, which are to be kept shut; and, that between these plasters and the eye-lids, two or three doublings of gauze are to be placed, in order to prevent the *flies* or *cantharides* from entering the eyes. When the inflammation is considered merely local and external, and not deeply seated in the system or vital organs, poultices made of light bread and milk, and applied as cold as possible will be beneficial:—in fact, the coldest applications are to be kept to the eyes, such for instance, as the following:—Take twenty grains of sugar of lead, and ten grains of white vitriol—dissolve them in half a pint of pure rain water—and let the mixture settle for several hours:—then pour off the clear part from the top, and keep the eye constantly moistened with this water. If the eyes are very painful, you may add to the mixture a tea poonful of laudanum, to allay the irritation. Persons who are constitutionally subject to weak eyes, will find much benefit from bathing them frequently in pure water; and if the weakness is unattended by inflammation, by bathing them in weak spirits and water. In cases of *films* over-spreading the *cornea*, or stransparent part of the eye, so as to induce blindness. I consider it my duty to make the following notices: Doctor Manlone, formerly a celebrated physician of Dinwidie county, of Virginia, sinee dead, left on record in the margin of one of

Prideaux's works, the following note:—"The gaul of an Eel, laid on with a soft brush, and with great care, and occasionally repeated, has successfully removed a film from the eye. The writer of this, leaves it on record in this place, with the intention that it may be useful to some fellow creature, when the writer is no longer an inhabitant of this world. I most solemnly declare, that I have experienced the good effects of the application, in the course of my practice; but it should be used when the disorder is recent.

C. MANLONE."

Thus we see, notwithstanding the sneers and ridicule of modern infidels, that the story in the apocrypha, of Tobit's blindness being cured by the gall of a fish, is neither ridiculous nor improbable:—Doctor Manlone has been dead about forty years. For the satisfaction of the reader, I will record a case in which I myself was successful in the cure of blindness. Mis Hudson, of Knox county, who resides with her father on the waters of Holston, in this state, came to me afflicted with blindess in one of her eyes, from a *film* which I speedily and easily removed, by introducing upon the surface of the eye-ball, clean hog's lard; it was introduced into the eye with a fine Camel-hair pencil, and with much care.

WHITLOW.

There is an inflammation at the end of the finger or thumb. The pain gradually increases, attended with a throbbing sensation, and always produces in its progress, the most excruciating torment. In whitlow, the finger or thumb affected, always puts on a glossy or shining appearance. After six or eight days, matter forms under the nail or at the side of it, which, on being opened gives immediate relief.

REMEDIES.

The old plan of treatment in whitlow has been entirely laid aside—it consisted merely of poultices and warm applications. The method of cure now adopted in the European Hospitals, which may be said to be an infallible one, is simply as follows. The moment the whitlow is discovered, press the part gently and gradually with your fore-finger and thumb. Then, with a piece of tape or narrow binding bind or wind the sore finger or thumb tightly, from the point upward toward the body of the hand. This bandage must be permitted to remain on, the object being merely *to stop the circulation,* until a cure is effected. You may unwind it once a day to examine the whitlow, but it must immediately be put on again. If the bandage give much pain, so that you cannot bear it, it must be gradually loosened until you can bear the pressure. By this simple method, whitlow may be easily cured, if matter has not formed in it. Were I not convinced that many wise men and old women will laugh at this simple cure, I would not put myself to the trouble of proving its efficacy. Doctor William Balfour of Edinburgh, relates more than *fifty cases* of whitlow being cured, some of them with matter formed and highly inflamed, by this simple method. I will give two cases of success, selected from the London Medical and Physical Journal. "James Briddet," says the writer, "who was a tanner, aged twenty-five years, applied to me on the 25th of August, with a whitlow on one of his thumbs. He knew no cause for the complaint, which had existed for about a week, and prevented him from following his occupation. When I had pressed the parts firmly, and applied a bandage, I desired him to call the next day. He looked at me, as if he would have said—'*Is this all that you are to do for me!*'—I found this fellow, says the doctor, quite doubtful with regard to my cure, and again desired him to call the next day. In the morning he accordingly returned—when I found the inflammation and swelling considerably abated. On the third day the pain was entirely gone, and the man had the free use of his thumb. I now asked him, if he was not *at first,* quite distrustful of the mode of cure I had adopted. He laughed and admitted that he was, expressed his surprise at the quick result, made his acknowledgements, and went about his business.—Peter Fraser received an injury on the 26th of December last, by having his thumb bent forcibly backward in lifting a heavy stone. When he applied to me on the 29th, he complained of having passed three days in great agony, and three sleepless nights. The pain was confined to the first joint, but the swelling extended a considerable way upward. I never handled a more excruciatingly painful case, and believed it must soon terminate in *suppuration*," (breaking and running.) "Such was also the opinion of Doctor Anderson of New York, who happened to be with me when the patient presented himself. I told the gentleman that exquisitely painful as was the complaint, I had no doubt of curing it in a week, without any other application than my own fingers, and a simple bandage of narrow tape. The cure was completed in six days, exclusive of that on which the patient applied to me."—I have thus given two cases, in which whitlow has been cured by the mere application of a bandage: and, I will adventure another suggestion, which is this—that even in cases where suppuration has taken place, and the lancet has been used; the use of an easy bandage would be greatly benficial, applied to every part of the finger or thumb, except immediately over the small point of the discharge.

COW POY

OR

VACCINATION.

This valuable discovery made several years ago by the celebrated Doctor Jenner, is now resorted to as a remedy against the infectious and dreadful inroads of the Small Pox, in almost every portion of the civilized world. Vaccination is merely the introduction or insertion into the arm, by means of the lancet, of the matter by which the *cow pox* is produced in the human system. There is a contention among physicians, and those too of the higher orders, whether the cow pox is, in all cases, a preventive of that dreadful scourge of mankind, the *small pox:* for myself, I am induced to believe, that with very few exceptions, it may be considered an antidote against small pox, especially when vaccination has been effectual on the system. In Prussia, out of 584.000 children, born in the year 1821—40,000 of them were vaccinated for the cow pox. During the above period, there died of small pox, in all the provinces belonging to Prussia, 1190 persons:-and before the introduction of vaccination, from thirty to forty thousand died annually of small pox. Although persons who have been vaccinated may be liable to take the small pox afterwards, yet the latter disease always terminates very mildly. Of many hundred thousand persons vaccinated in London, not a single case of death has taken place from small pox, where the matter of the cow pox had before taken proper effect. The report of the college of physicians in London, for 1807, expressly states, that small pox in any shape, rarely proves fatal, when it attacks those who have been successfully vaccinated. The success attending this operation in the United Stats, has entitled it to the highest confidence of our most distinguished physicians. I have before remarked in substance, and I think the opinion a correct one, that many who have taken the small pox after vaccination, took it from bad management in inserting the cow pock matter: when the proper effect is not produced on the system, by the introduction of the cow pock matter, it is to be expected that persons will still be liable to the contagion of small pox.

To every man of common prudence, and proper sentiments of self-preservation, advice of the necessity of vaccination, as the preventative of the dangers attendant on small pox, would be superfluous; to those who seem to slumber in security, respecting the future ravages of small pox in the western country, I have only to remark—that the facilities of commerce with other countries are daily increasing, from the universal introduction of steam boats, and the rapid improvement of our internal navigation; and that in a few years, through these mediums, the most remote and secluded portions of our country, will stand as much exposed to the mortal inroads of small pox, as our large cities and maratime towns. The great object in vaccination, is the certainty that the matter of vaccination takes full effect on the system; and it is needless to remark, that unless the matter be genuine, no beneficial effects can possibly result from vaccination. Vaccination is an innocent and valuable preventive remedy against *small pox*, in which little if any medicine is required; in children it passes over in a few days. In grown persons, it may produce slight fever and pain under the arm, which usually go off in a few hours. If the person vaccinated be of a gross habit of body, a moderate dose of salts will be of much service on the seventh or eighth day. If the inflammation of the arm becomes very painful, moisten the place frequently with a little weak sugar of lead water, until the sore is dried up; this however is seldom necessary. The great point in vaccination, is certainly to know, that the matter introduced into the system has taken full and sufficient effect. If there is only a slight redness in the arm, where the matter has been inserter, and no other effect is produced on the system, you may certainly conclude that the vaccination has failed of effect. But if, on the contrary, a pustule or pimple arises, of a full and oval form, with an indentation or dent in the centre, not unlike a button mole, about the sixth day containing matter, vaccination has had the desired effect. Great attention should be paid to these circumstances by the operator, or he will probably be the cause of future exposure of the person to the ravages of the small pox, and not improbably to the iminent hazard of death. The influence of the kine or cow pox, over affections of the skin, in many cases in which medical remedies have failed, has lately produced considerable attention and interest in the Hospitals of Europe. The matter of cow pox, can always be obtained pure, by addressing a letter to the Vaccine Institution of New York, Philadelphia, or Baltimore; from either of which, on application, you will receive it by letter. If the matter be received from a distance, it is best to hold the point of the lancent, on which is the matter you intend to insert into the arm, until it softens a little:—then, hold the lancet in such a position, that the matter can gradually go off the point. Next, scratch the skin frequently, but not too deeply, with the point of the lancet on which is the matter, until a little blood may be seen:—this is the whole secret of vaccination. Sometimes the matter of cow pox is sent on thread; when this is the case, make a slight incision in the arm, and lay the threads in it, which must be covered with court plaster to keep it in its place until the disorder has been communicated. If a physician be convenient, it will always be advisable to employ him to perform the operation, because much depends on the exercise of judgment, respecting the future security of the person against that most dreadful of scourges the small pox.

SMALL POX.

How imperfect are the conceptions which are formed by the fortunate few, of the sufferings to which millions of the human race are subject, when afflicted by this dreadful and fatal disorder. How important, then, is the great remedy of *vaccination*, which I have before described, that from some inexplicable principle, renders harmless this potent enemy of human life.

Small Pox is known by the following symptoms:—A few days before its appearance, you feel restless and uneasy, and a great dislike to motion of any kind. Cold chills steal over you, followed by flushings of heat, and accompanied by a slight fever, all of which end as the disease gradually increase. You have a pain in the head, a dull heavy pain in the small of the back, great thirst, increase of stupor—until about the third day, when the eruptions or spots on the skin, something like flee-bites, their appearance on the face, neck, breast and arms, and gradually extend over the whole body. These spots gradually increase in size, until about the fifth or sixth day, when they begin to turn white at the tops, and feel painful. Your voice then becomes hoarse, as if you had a sever cold; your face becomes much swelled; and your features appear much changed.—Your eye-lids, particularly, swell to a considerable extent, so as frequently to close the eyes entirely, and a spitting takes place as if you were salivated. On the eleventh day, these pustules or pimples have increased to about the size of a common pin, and instead of white, contain a yellow matter, on the tops of which pustules or pimples, you will discover a small black spot, whilst all the rest is filled with this yellow matter. About the twelfth day they burst, and discharge their contents, with a horrible stench which is almost insupportable; nor dare you attempt to wash off this matter—the slightest touch giving the most excruciating pain. It is this matter which leaves the scares on the faces of persons disfigured with the disorder. If the matter dries quickly, it leaves no marks; but if from any unhealthy constitutional defect, it lingers for some time on the body, it generally leaves those marks behind it, which disfigure the countenance for life. This disease sometimes, but not frequently, comes on with great violence, with all the symptoms of *typhus* or *nervous fever:*—refer to the head Nervous Fever, where you will see the form of treatment which must be observed in small pox, should it come with symptoms of typhus or nervous fever. When these unfavorable appearances take place in the commencement of the disease, it is called by physicians, *confluent small pox.*

The eruptions appear much earlier in this form of the complaint; they run in patches, and instead of rising, remain flat; and are of a dark livid color. They secrete a dark brown unhealthy matter; the fever, which in the first form of small pox, abates when the pimples become full, in this form of the disease continues constantly throughout the disease, ending in great debility or weakness. In this last form or stage of small pox, which I have described as of the *nervous* or *typhus* kind, it may be considered as very highly dangerous, and as generally terminating, without judicious and skilful treatment, *fatally.*

REMEDIES.

In the treatment of this complaint, you are to avoid every thing, as you value the life of your patient, of a *heating nature*, either as *drink* or *food* or *clothing*. The room is to be kept as quiet and cool as possible. Cover the patient with nothing but a very thin sheet; even the weight and heat of a common linen sheet is painful and oppressive; and unless he complains of feeling cold, you cannot commit an error in keeping him too cool. Let all of his drinks be of the most cooling nature. As a general drink, cold water sweetened with sugar, in which is put a little acid, so as to make it pleasantly sour, is the best drink that can be given. In fevers of every description, and particularly in the one which attends on small pox, acid drinks abate the fever, lessen the thirst, and cool the whole system. The heat and pain of the eruptions will always be lessened by keeping them well moistened with equal quantities of milk and water, or with cold water alone. Cold water, as a remedy used in sponging the body, in the first stage of this complaint, will greatly tend to lessen the heat, and the pain in the head and back. In fact, as I have told you before, there is no danger of cooling remedies, unless the patient complains of being chilly and cold, which is not frequently the case; but if he should do so, moderate the quantity of cooling drinks to the feelings of the patient—*nature usually tells the truth.* If, by any accident, the complaint should strike in, which is not the case once in a hundred instances, the warm bath made pleasantly warm should be used; and a little warm wine whey, or warm wine, given internally at the same time. These measures will again bring out the disorder on the skin. For the proper treatment of this disease, when it puts on the appearance of nervous or typhus fever, and is called *confluent small pox*, I refer you to the head nervous fever, where you will find it at length. When the eruptions burst and discharge their matter, an *ointment* made of cream and common garden parsley, and constantly applied by means of a soft swab, or rag rolled round a small stick, to keep the sores soft, and to prevent their hardening, will entirely prevent any marks or scares from being left on the face. I have omitted to state, that if the bowels are costive, epsom salts should be given in a little cold water:—see table for dose: or you may keep them gently open, by cooling clysters, for clystering, look under the head clysters. The loss of some blood from the arm, is sometimes necessary in the first stage of this disease, if the inflammatory symptoms run high, and the pain in the head is very distressing. This, with the use of cold water as before mentioned, if the inflammatory action is very great, will produce a beneficial effect in relieving the pain in the head and back.

VENEREAL DISEASE.

The prevalence of this dreadful disease among mankind, is another, *proof* among the many others that might be adduced, that it is, the interest of man to be *virtuous* if he wishes to be *happy*, and that a decree of the *Almighty* has announced to him, in language not to be mistaken, "*the penalty of a misdeed* shall always *tread upon the heels of the transgression;* if you violate my laws, which were formed for your *happiness*, I will convince you of that violation, by plunging you into *sufferings* and *misery*,'.

That there are moments of licentious conduct in early life, affording but a short and transitory enjoyment, to which memory in after periods looks back with sorrow and remorse, no man possessed of common sense will deny; but when to the bitter pangs of remorse for a misdeed, are added the pains and sufferings of *bodily disease*, as is always the case in venereal complaints, language has no powers to describe the real condition of the sufferer. What dreadful sacrifices are frequently made by mankind, of *health, wealth, fame, happiness and character*, for a momentary gratification of sensual pleasure, which often ends in shame, and remorse, and the misery of a whole life, inflicted by the *venereal disease*. If the transgressor himself alone suffered, this disease would not present so horrible a spectacle to the eye of humanity; but how often do we see an innocent and spotless wife, in moments of endearing confidence and love, receiving this infectious disorder, and communicating it to her children—I will not say from a husband, it would be a misuse of the word, but from a bruit, who has violated every principle of honor, and the most sacred ties of humanity. But this is not all: how often do we see an innocent, virtuous, unsuspicious wife—her constitution destroyed, her health deeply impaired, and all her hopes of happiness blasted forever, from having received from the man she calls her husband, this loathsome and filthy disorder; and having to submit to an examination of those parts which common decency forbids me to name, in order that she may be cured of a disease, which *always ends in death*, of a most terrible character unless medical means can be used.

This complaint is produced, in most cases, by a healthy person having sexual intercourse or connection with another who has this infectious disorder in the genitals or privates. It took its name from a Greek word, which in our language means *filthy*. The Old testament informs us, that the ancient inhabitants of the Eastern countries, were much subject to diseases of the genitals or privates; and that for the preservation of the Jewish nation, *circumcision* was enforced in the Mosaic laws, and made also a religious rite or ceremony. Circumcision means the cutting off the foreskin or prepuce of the private member, which prevents any poisonous and infectious matter from producing disease, by being lodged under the folds and coverings of this skin. Although no direct mention is made of *venereal disease* among those people, yet the description of some of the disenses of the genitals to which they were subject, leads us directly to the belief, that they were well acquainted with the venereal complaints. Be this however as it may, about the close of the fifteenth century, I think about the year 1494, the venereal disease appeared in Europe, from which it was communicated with great rapidity to every known part of the world, and became such a desolating scourge to the human race, as to become an object of great medical attention. I have neither time nor space, for pursuing the subject of its history any further—indeed it would be both useless and unnecessary.

After you have taken this disorder in the manner I have described, it will depend very much on the state of your system, and other peculiarities of that system not distinctly known, at what particular time the disease will make its appearance. In some persons, whose systems are very irritable, it will show itself on the third or fourth day after you have had sexual intercourse with a person infected with the disease; in other persons, it will be eight or ten days before it makes its appearance—and I have known it to remain a month or more in the system, before it would show itself in any form. In fact, cases are mentioned by good medical writers, in which several men have had connection with a woman known to have the venereal disease, some of whom took it, while others escaped uninjured. This singular circumstance, which we are bound to credit from the goodness of the authorities, must have been owing to the fact of the infected woman making water, immediately before having connection with those who escaped without injury. I am inclined to believe that it has never been fully ascertained, how long the venereal matter will remain, as it were *a sleep* in the system, without making its appearance—some writers say three months, some six months, some a year, and so on. I suspect the fact to be, in those cases in which the disease is supposed to appear after a considerable time, that the persons have not been entirely cured—in other words, that the disease has merely been driven back by quackery, and afterwards shown itself under the following forms:—in the *nose*, in the *throat*, in the *eyes*, on the legs, in swelling the groins, in splotches or sores on the body, &c. This last stage of the venereal disease is called constitutional, because it is firmly seated in the whole body, by the venereal virus or poison having been absorbed, and carried into the whole circulation. The venereal disease may be communicated, by wounding or pricking any part of the body with a lancet, having on its point any particle of this venereal poison. I recollect a student of medicine, who came very near death, from cutting his finger slightly, when dissecting a person who had died of the venereal disease: the poisonous matter was communicated to the slight cut; in twelve hours afterward he labored under violent fever, which continued ten or twelve days before the inflammation could be subdued. This disease may also take place, from an application of the matter to a scratch, to a common sore, or to a wound. Several instances are mentioned, of venereal or pock sores being formed in the nostrils, eye-lids, and lips, from the slight circumstance of persons having the disease, touching their nostrils, eyes, or lips, with their fingers immediately after handling the venereal sores on their own privates. These remarks are made, with the intention of showing how easily this loathsome disease, with all its impure and life corrupting taints, may be communicated—and to place physicians and midwives on their guard against infection.

Venereal disease has two distinct forms: I might say three forms—but the third is nothing more than the one I have just described as *constitutional*, which always arises from one of the other two, or from both in combination. This first is POX, properly so called:—and the other **clap**, called by physicians, *Gonorrhœa*, which is so simple in its nature, that with proper treatment it may be cured, in from three to five or six days.

The *pox* is a most corrupting, dangerous, and destructive disease; and if suffered to progress in its ravages on the human body, never fails in desolating the human constitution, and destroying life at its very core. When it is foolishly concealed, and suffered to run on, or badly treated in attempting its cure, it always ends in distressing, and irreparably fatal consequences. In ten cases out of eleven, if application were immediately made with the proper remedies, the complaint, dreadful as it is, might be cured in a very short time, without affecting the system, for I do know from *actual experience*, having paid much attention to the general practice in venereal cases, that thousands have been *salivated*, and their constitutions destroyed by *mercury*, when more simple and less dangerous practice, combined with adequate and proper attentions, would entirely have removed the disease. Medically speaking, pox is at first a local, and not a general disease of the system—by which I mean that it is more a disease of the part first affected, than of the whole body; and I have no manner of doubt, that many a poor unfortunate fellow, has been pushed and draged through a tedious and destructive mercurial course of medicine, and perhaps for a disease which was not actual pox, who might have been cured by a little *lunar caustic*, a wash made of blue stone, a little red precipitate, or even by sprinkling on the *chancre*, or first venereal ulcer, a small portion of *calomel*. I have frequently observed in the United States, many cases which professional honor forbids me to name, in which patients have suffered infinitely more from the imprudent, and to coin a new word, the *quacknichal* use of *mercury*, than could possibly have resulted from the first insignificant venereal sore itself, with strict attention to *cleanliness*, had the disease been permitted to run on its course. That mercury holds a distinguished, powerful, and perhaps, perfect dominion over venereal disease, in most, if not all cases, I freely admit to be true:—but I as firmly believe, that thousands might have been cured of this horrible complaint, under very mild administrations of this powerful medicine, this Sampson of the Drug-Shops. I have witnessed the progress of this disease, in both Europe and the U. States, from its mildest forms to its most destructive ravages on the human system; and feel perfectly assured that the disease, which is the same in all countries, assumes either a milder or severer form according to the peculiarities of the human constitution, the irritable state of the system at the time this disease is taken, the habits of the persons, the character of the climate, and so on. Very few cases of pox in France, in proportion to the immense population, terminate in injuries to the bones of the face, disfigurement of the nose, loss of the palate of the mouth, &c. This is altogether owing to their proper management of the complaint; with them the pox produces very little alarm, probably not more than the itch does in this country. They are perfect masters of the disease; and there are few cases that do not terminate speedily and successfully, under their strict and judicious treatment. An individual may travel through France, and have promiscuous intercourse of a sexualcharacter for years, without receiving the least injury. On the contrary, in this country, from causes which need not be particularly named, the least deviation from moral propriety, involves the participant in disease and suffering. As my object is the development of truth, regardless of petty objections and servile prejudices, I assert that we use infinitely too much mercury in the cure of pox in the United States: in fact, we very frequently communicate a serious disease by the imprudent use of *mercury*, instead of removing one; yet I trust in God, the day will arrive, and that too at no very distant period, when diseases themselves will be prescribed for, and not their mere *technical names*. There are generally in the venereal Hospital at Paris in France, from five to seven hundred venereal or pox patients. Included in this number there are usually about three hundred women of the town, in other words common prostitutes. "The patients of all the French Hospitals," says Doctor F. J. Didier, honorary member of the Medical society of Baltimore, "are carefully nursed by the *sisters of charity*, a class of nuns whose lives are consecrated to the relief of wretchedness and the calming of pain. With what eloquence does Voltair write, in favor of these charming and admirable women!—'Perhaps, says he, there is nothing on earth so truly great, as the sacrifice made by the softer sex, of beauty, youth, and often the highest worldly expectations, to relieve that mass of every human suffering, the sight of which is so revolting to delicacy.'—I myself have observed one of these angelic women, administering consolation and relief to a man tortured by the agonies of disease and wretchedness. She appeared to take the greatest interest in the poor sufferer. The sweetness, the captivating voice, the winning kindness of these *sisters of charity*, soon dry the tear which flows down the care-worn cheek, and infuse the gleam of hope into the soul depressed by misfortune." It is rather singular to an American, that the French government should license common prostitutes, and exact a tribute from their debaucheries; but such are the facts. The probability is, however, that these measures originate in sound policy on the part of the government, and in sentiments of actual charity, to those who under any circumstances would lead a life of whoredom and prostitution. Several objects are attained by this policy; the *license*, subjects these women monthly, to a medical examination touching their diseases, and tends to check and prevent the spread of venereal infection through their immense population; it furnishes the police offices of their large cities with monthly registers of their names and places of abode, and exacts from them a fund, while in youth and health, for their care and support in sickness and old age, which they themselves would never think of laying up. I think these considerations worthy of the attention of our own governments, general and state, and particularly of the *Medical Board*, lately established by the Legislature of Tennessee. The fact is, that if the Legislature of Tennessee, would compel the loose characters in all our cities and towns, who practice prostitution on a *petty* and *filthy* scale, to take out *license* and *submit to medical examination monthly*, or abandon their commerce in low and corrupt debauchery, we would soon have fewer cases of venereal in our commercial towns, or be rid of the fraternity of prostitutes altogether. I have, in the foregoing remarks, perhaps, strayed a little from the precise track of my subject; but, as the digression will probably not be wholly interesting, I shall make no elaborate apology for it. I will first describe *pox* and *clap*, separately—and next give their *remedies* separately.

POX.

When you suppose you have taken this disease, no foolish or childish delicacy, should prevent you for a moment, from ascertaining the fact. The disease generally makes its appearance by what physicians call *chancres*. These are small inflamed pimples, which show themselves on the head of the penis or yard, or on the side of the penis near the end. In a very few days these pimples enlarge themselves; and become what are called venereal sores or ulcers. In women, these pimples show themselves first, immediately inside of what are called the lips of the privates; and unless arrested in their course of enlargement, extend themselves to the fundament in a short time. The *pox*, also, sometimes makes its appearance, in what are called *buboes*. These are hard lump-like kernels or swellings, which rise in one or both groins. These swellings gradually increase in size, until they become about the size of an egg, and have an angry red color; and unless driven away by the application of medicine, eventually come to a head, and discharge the poisonous matter. These *buboes* generally produce great pain, some fever, and prevent the person afflicted with them, from walking without considerable difficulty. *Buboes* sometimes make their appearance under the *arm-pits*, and sometimes in the glands of the throat: these appearances of *bubo*, however, are not very frequent, and are much oftener the effects of mercury improperly administered in the pox, than arising from the disease itself. The fact is, that I think them produced, generally, from the neglect of many, in not speedily effecting a cure by the proper and efficient use of medicine—in other words, by half way dilatory measures, which neither cure the disease nor suffer it to run its course. When the constitution is very irritable, the disease will sometimes attack the nose, the throat, the tongue, the eyes, the shin bone, and so on, and fill the whole system with the venereal poison in no great length of time; and unless efficient, combined with well judged measures be resorted to, the human system will become a mass of putrifying sores, and the sufferer become an object of compassion and disgust. By this short, and comprisive description, you will be at no loss to know what is the *Pox*, if you should ever have it.

CLAP.

Clap is a simple disease, and may be very easily cured, if timely attention be paid to it. The first symptoms of the disease are, burning and scalding sensations or feelings, in the urethra or canal of the penis, whenever you urinate or make water. There will be a discharge of matter from the penis, first, of nearly a white color, next, of a yellowish color which will stain your shirt, and lastly of a greenish color. After having the disease sometime, or perhaps from the irritable state of your system, you will experience what is called *chordee;* this is a spasmodic contraction of the penis, which gives considerable pain in erections of the yard, as if it were wound with a small cord. In women, this disease called clap, is still more simple; in its *first stage*, merely resembling the whites in their worst stage.—There is, however, this specific difference between *clap* and *whites* in women: in clap, there is always a scalding and burning sensation in making water, and a continual uneasiness and itching about the parts, neither of which sensations are experienced in mere whites.

REMEDIES FOR POX.

As soon as the first symptoms of Pox is discovered, which will in all common cases be known by the appearance of *chancres* or *buboes*, both of which I have described to you sufficiently, take an active purge of calomel and jalap. The object of this purge, is to clear the bowels of all irritating obstructions, and to remove as far as possible, every species of irritation from the system: See table for dose.) If this dose of calomel and jalap does not operate in proper time, take a tea spoonful of epsom salts to assist the operation, and make it fully effective. If you should have dark stools, let the medicine run on its whole coures; but, if the stools become yellow and watery, and you feel much weakened by the operation, take from ten to twenty drops of laudanum, or a tea spoonful of paregoric, to prevent the medicine from working you too severely. Next, obtain from any doctor's shop, a small quantity of *lunar caustic;* cut the end of a quill, and set the caustic into it, which will afford you an opportunity of using it more conveniently, and without handling it with your fingers: Wet the end of this caustic in water, and touch the *chancres* or sores with it lightly, twice a day, until you have killed the poison: always taking care to wash and cleanse the sores well with soap and water, immediately before this operation is performed. The caustic will sting you a little; but never mind this; you are now on the stool of repentance; and are only learning the moral salutary lesson, that "the penalty always treads upon the heels of the transgression," and that the sacred laws of nature and her God, can never be violated without punishment to reform the offender! After using the caustic, as just directed, apply a little dry lint to the sores. If caustic cannot be had, *red precipitate* will answer nearly the same purpose; this must be used by sprinkling a little on the chancre, after cleansing them with soap and water as before mentioned: or you may, if you have neither *caustic* or *precipitate*, use a little *calomel*, in the way that I have directed the precipitate to be used. The better way however, will be where all these articles can be obtained to use the three alternately, or in rotation, until you can ascertain which of them seems best to heal the ulcers—and then to adopt the one which you prefer, from the exercise of your best judgment. I, myself have always found the *lunar caustic* the best remedy. If you are difficultly situated, as to procuring the articles above named, dissolve some blue vitriol generally called *blue stone*, in water, and wash the chancres, or ulcers with the solution *repeatedly*, taking particular care to keep the sores very clean, and entirely free from matter.

If the disease appears under the form of *buboes*, which are such swellings of the groins as I have described to you, and which if left to themselves will rise and break like *boils*, you are to put *blisters* of Spanish flies on them, which extend one or two inches over the *buboes;* and I suppose I need not tell you, that these said blisters, are to be renewed, until the buboes or swellings are what physicians call "*discussed*," in other words driven away, or back entirely. If you cannot get blisters, lie quietly on your back, and apply linen rags to the buboes, kept constantly wet with clear strong ley, which we vulgarly pronounce lye. For this remedy, which is a valuable one, we are indebted to the French Physicians; (I learned it in France.) And now mind me particulary; if these buboes, notwithstanding the application of blisters, or the application of ley or lye, rise to a head, burst, and discharge their offensive and poisonous matter, which they will certainly do if not driven back, you are to take the greatest possible precautions to keep them clean, while discharging their loathsome contents. If you do not, the matter will be very apt to produce other venereal ulcers, especially if it happens to lodge on any sores on other parts of the body. Therefore wash them gently but well. two or three times a day, in strong soap and water; and after drying them well, wash the sores again with a little of the weak solution of *corrosive sublimate.* If you cannot procure this preparation, sprinkle a little red precipitate or calomel on the sores, and dress them with some simple ointment, such as *Turner's cerate,* see under that head —but mind me, these dressings, or either of them, are never to be put on, unless after washing the sores well with soap and water.—During all this treatment, and from the very commencement of the disorder, you are to drink freely of a strong decoction or tea, made of *low-ground sarsaparilla,*—to every quart of which tea, after you have strained it clear, you are to add *sixty* drops of *nitric acid,* vulgarly called aquafortis. Take this tea thus prepared freely, say from a pint to a quart a day; and avoid particularly every kind of strong food, and all kinds of spirituous liquors. These measures, carefully restricted and pursued, combined with time, patience, and the requisite rest, are all that are required to cure this dreadful scourge of debauchery and licentiousness; under any form in which it may appear in the human system, This has been my uniform practice, both in Virginia and Tennessee; and it is well known that I have succeeded in many cases of the most desperate and hopeless character, and where other modes of practice had been resorted to in vain. By these means, which have never before been made known by me, I succeeded in curing a gentleman in Virginia, several years ago, whose case I will dare aver, was as bad a one as can well be imagined.—He had been attended and prescribed for by several of the most distinguished physicians in the United States, and was brought to me twenty miles in a carriage to Montgomery Court-house, where I then resided, in so helpless and dreadful a condition, that he had fainted several times on the short journey, and was but the shadow of a human being. Yet, in the lapse of six weeks, by the practice I have just described, he became a well man. He is now married, and I am happy to add, from late accounts, is a healthy and virtuous husband—and an excellent citizen. I am constrained, however to add, that the real danger of his situation, was as much owing to the effects of mercury he had taken, as to the *actual presence* in his system, of the venereal virus or poison. That his disease was both *venereal* and *mercurial*, I have never entertained the least doubt—in other words, it came under the *constitutional* disease I have before described, as being characterized by sores on the body, blotches, &c. &c.—The venereal disease, in this constitutional stage, has been called by some medical writer, and I perfectly coincide with him in opinion, the *mercurial pox*—which I certainly consider, not only more dangerous, but greatly more difficult to cure, than the real disease itself, if no means other than mercury be relied on. I am perfectly aware, that the idea of abandoning the use of mercury in the cure of pox, will be considered a novelty by many of the Faculty of this country; but I am fully as well a ware, that sarsaparilla, as I have prescribed the use of it here, combined with the *nitric acid* or aquafortis, as before mentioned, will remove the pox from the human system in its worst forms and stages. For the powerful and salutary influence of the *nitric acid* or aquafortis on the human system, the sceptical reader will please to refer to the head "Remedies," in Diseases of the Liver. The practice of treating venereal cases without mercury, has now become general, both in the Hospitals of England and France; and I predict that the day is not far distant, when mercury will cease to be used in this complaint, throughout the United States. The belief, that pox can only be cured with safety and certainty by the use of mercury, is so deeply seated in the minds of physicians at this time, that I am persuaded it will require much time to remove their confidence in its favor. That mercury is, as I have before said, a cure for the venereal disease, is well known;

but, that the effects produced by it are frequently mistaken for the pox itself, I have no more doubt than I have of my own existence.

The French method of curing pox, is by the use or administration of Van Sweeten's liquor, as they call it—or *Antisyphilitic Robb;* for this medicine and the manner of preparing it, (look under the head.) The Robb was used in the London Hospitals, until it was superceded or thrown out of use, by *Swaim's Penacea;* (for the method of preparing which, see under that head.) Both these medical preparations are used with great advantage in *secondary symptoms,* by which I mean what I have said before, in cases where the disease has become *constitutional,,* and is attended with ulcers, sores, blotches, &c. The *Sulphur bath,* or *sulphurious fumigation,* is much used in France. After the fourth bath, the ulcers and venereal blotches begin to heal, and generally in ten or twelve baths, are entirely cured. This last remedy, which is an excellent one, is entirely neglected in the U. States; and I can account for the neglect, if I must speak out, upon no other principles than laziness and inattention on the part of practitioners, and ignorance in their patients. This bath is nothing more than the fumes of sulphur—or sometimes the fumes of sulphuric acid, which is nothing but *oil of vitriol.* For a full description of this valuable remedy, I may add this astonishing one, read under the head *sulphuric fumigation.*

With the foregoing exposition of my own mode of curing Pox, and the material remedies used in other countries, I will now proceed to give the common and general practice in this disease, leaving it optional with the patient to adopt that which suits his opinion or convenience best. Were I to advise, however, on the subject of a choice, I would recommend the *mild method* in the first instance, and the *mercurial* one only when the aggravation of the symptoms seemed to call for it; which I must confess, I think would be but seldom, where the plan of treatment I have laid down had been faithfully adhered to and persisted in. Doct. Rousseau of Philadelphia, a gentleman of distinguished ability, and great practice in this disease, expressly says, "I have never found any benefit to be derived from a *salivation;* on the contrary, those patients who have undergone this dirty, filthy torturing process, have to my knowledge, and to their own sorrow, felt the deleterious effects of it for years, and very many for life." For a full description of this complaint, in its secondary or constitutional symptoms, and the *dreadful effects of mercury,* I refer to this very valuable, intelligent, and honest writer; Medical Recorder, Vol. 3d. "sketches on venereal complaints."

The practice throughout the United States has been, and now generally is, to introduce into the whole system, as much mercury as will produce a soreness of the gums, or *salivation,* by giving small doses of calomel alone, or combined with a small portion of opium, if the calomel alone would run off by the bowels; and by rubbing on the bubo, to disperse it, mercurial ointment known by the country people as *oil of baz,* of which a piece about the size of the end of your finger is to be rubbed in and about the bubo, night and morning, until a salivation is produced, or until the lump in the groin is dispersed.—When the mouth has a copperish taste, or a slight soreness is felt, stop taking the calomel, and omit rubbing in the mercurial ointment; as the whole system is then considered to be under *mercurial influence.* The *blue pill* is now used very extensively in the United States, instead of *calomel;* being a much milder preparation of mercury:—for a description of this pill, and the manner of preparing it, read under that head. The dose is one pill in the morning, and one at night, until they produce the effects on the gums and mouth, required to be produced by calomel; when they are to be continued, only so far as to keep up the effect on the gums and mouth, until the disease is removed. The chancres or buboes, are to be treated as before described in a preceding page. Doctor Cartright, who is among the greatest medical men now living in this, or any other county, recommends the following practice, and relates many cases treated by himself with unbounded success. "I never," says he "prescribe calomel with a view to produce salivation; but to guard against it, I order a clyster or some mild purgative to be taken, in twelve or sixteen hours after the calomel, if it does not operate: and in the event of its operating too much, I direct a little laudanum to check it, so as to limit it to two or three stools—unless the stools are of a dark or green color, when the purging should be permitted to go on, until they change their appearance. As it respects this disorder, when taken in time, I have found by an experience of two years practice, that *pox* is as easily cured by giving twenty or thirty grains of calomel every day, or every other day, as a common cold. In good constitutions, *pox* yields to the native powers of the system. As soon as a *copperish taste* is perceived in the mouth, or the least *tenderness* of the *gums*, or *soreness* of the *teeth*, I order an immediate suspension of calomel, until these symptoms have disappeared —when it should be resumed with caution. The preparation I generally use, says the doctor, is twenty grains of calomel and four of rhubarb, given at bed time. Generally, by the time three or four doses have been taken, the breath will begin to have a mercurial odour, a copperish taste will be perceived in the mouth, or the gums will feel tender. About this time, or even before it, the venereal symptoms begin to disappear, and in a few days more the *chancres* entirely heal. I generally recommend, after the healing of the chancres, a dose or two more to complete the cure of the disease. I have rarely found more than twelve or fifteen pills, each *ten grains* of calomel and *two* of rhubarb, necessary for the cure of a recent infection, or in other words of one that is not of long standing." I have now given a full description of the various methods of treating this loathsome disease called *pox*, in the best manner, leaving the reader to make his own selection among them. Much of my information has been derived from experiment and observation; and I regret to say that I have witnessed the disease in as severe forms, since I have been in Knoxville, as I ever did in the Hospitals of Europe or the United States. The disease was brought from New Orleans, and was of the most virulent or poisonous character. I omitted to remark, that buboes are always to be poulticed with light bread and milk, or slippery elm bark, *if they* are likely to come to a head.

REMEDIES FOR CLAP.

The moment you discover that you have contracted this complaint, the symptoms of which I have plainly described to you, take at bed time an active dose of calomel; see table for dose:—and if necessary, which is usually the case, assist the operation of the calomel in the morning, with a dose of epsom salts; see table, &c. Take care to live on cooling and simple diet, say corn or rye mush and milk, and avoid every thing of a heating and irritating nature, such as salted provisions, high seasonings, and spirituous liquors. When the medicine I have directed has done operating, use the following prescription, and use it with much accuracy too.—Take one ounce. which is about four table spoonfuls of Balsam copaiva; (commonly called *capivi,*) and add thereto one tea spoonful of spirits of turpentine. Mix them well together by shaking, and take sixty drops of the mixture, three times a day on some sugar—and drink freely of flax seed tea, mad by pouring a quart of boiling water on any quantity of flax seed convenient. This tea must be taken cold and used freely as a common drink. If you ride on horse back, or walk much, or take active exercise, clap is difficult to cure, and requires much longer time, than if you remain, quiet and stationary while using the above remedy. I generally cure it in three days, and frequently in less time. A dose of salts should be taken every other morning. Sometimes this balsam operates on the bowels, without producing the proper effect on the urinary organs:—if so, reduce the dose to *thirty-five drops,* twice or three times a day, which is to be taken as usual on sugar. *Cleanliness,* and I wish you to mind this matter particularly, is very important in the cure of this disease; by which I mean frequently washing the parts well, three or four times a day, with soap and water, so as to remove this poisonous matter. Clap is generally more mild, and much more easily cured in women than in men, unless women permit it to remain and run on them for *some length of time;* in this case, the disease becomes painful, and requires the remedies prescribed in the cases of men, only in smaller doses:—say from twenty to thirty drops, of the balsam and turpentine, three times a day. If any attention be paid, nothing more will be necessary than keeping the parts clean by washing with soap and water, and injecting up the birth place with a small *syringe or leaden squirt,* the following mixture: put 15 grains sugar of lead, and 15 grains white vitriol, in a quart of cold water, and let them fully dissolve. Then, of this water, inject or throw up the birth-place, a syringe, full five or six times a day, and drink freely of flax seed tea, using the balsam and turpentine as before directed, *if necessary.*

Doctor Chapman, one of the Professors of the University of Philadelphia, recommends the following valuable remedy, which is admirably suited to weakly persons, and those whose stomachs are much debilitated. It is perhaps better calculated for the summer season, being a much milder preparation than any other. I have used it frequently in my practice; but the first remedy is always *certain* to put a stop to the disease.

Chapman's remedy. Take two table spoonfuls of *balsam copaiva,* the same quantity of sweet spirits of nitre, some of the white of an egg, and mix them together. Add then, one tea spoonful of laudanum, and ten table spoonfuls of cold water. Shake the whole well together, and the mixture will be ready for use; remembering always, to shake the medicine up before taking it. Morning, noon, and night, take a table spoonful of this mixture. You may take it with any thing that will render it pleasant to the taste. It is an excellent, certain, and mild remedy, either for males or females; and I now again admonish you, that if you wish a speedy cure, you are to avoid every heating article of food or drink, and to repose much on the bed.

When clap is permitted by neglect to go on, or when you ride much on horse-back, you will be apt to have what is called *chordee,* which I have fully described under the head clap, and which it is needless to repeat: in these cases of chordee, take a dose of laudanum on going to bed—see table; and when the *spasm* comes on, which it will with a partial erection, pour cold water over the parts which pain you.—Should a discharge of blood take place, which is sometimes the case, apply cooling poultices of light bread and cold milk, to the *affected member*, or a poultice of slippery elm bark.

The old plan of curing clap, which is scarcely worth-while to mention, was by weak injections of sugar of lead and white vitriol; equal quantities mixed in water and thrown up the canal with a syringe. This old and imprudent practice, which in many instances occasioned swelled testicles, gleet, and what is called running of the reins, has entirely ceased. The methods of cure I have laid down, are infinitely superior in every respect, and are attended with none of the dangers of the old manner of cure.

GLEET.

This disease sometimes called running of the reins. It is a discharge which resembles in consistence, the white of an egg. Men who have frequently had the clap, also, those who have been old soldiers in the wars of Venus, are very liable to have the *gleet*. It is also produced, by too frequent intercourse with women, in those enjoyments which ought always to be bounded by virtue and moderation. The disease is also produced, by that horrible practice of self-pollution, called onanism; and also by the use of strong diuretic medicines, or such as cause a great flow of urine. This complaint sometimes resists the powers of medicine for years; and operates as a constant drain on the strength of the system, by which the constitution and the vital energies are sometimes prostrated, it is a disease that ought never to be neglected.

REMEDIES.

You are to bathe the parts three or four times a day in cold water; this cold bathing will act so as to give tone and strength to the parts. Obtain a phial of muriated tincture of iron, and take thirty drops of it, three times a day, in a wine glass of strong tea, made of the dog wood bark; it must be taken cold. By persevering steadily in this remedy; and in cold bathing for a month or two, you will probably be relieved of gleet. You may at the same time, use an injection of red-oak bark, made by boiling a little of the bark in water, and straining it clear. A little of this tea, can occasionally be thrown in the canal, by the aid of a *small syringe*, which you can obtain at any Doctor's shop; it must be thrown up cold, four or six times a day. In throwing up this injection, you are to press your left fore finger pretty hard on the lower side of the penis near the root, to prevent any part of the injection from getting into the bladder.

After a fair trial of the above remedies, and are baffled of success, commence with taking *ten* drops of tincture of cantharides or Spanish flies, instead of the iron, in the tea three times a day, gradually increasing the dose to thirty drops and no more. This is generally a certain remedy. Women may use the iron as directed; but not the least tincture, unless in very small doses of eight, ten, or fifteen drops, three times a day—bathing frequently with cold water, and with a female syringe throwing the bark water up the birth place, five or six times a day. Cold water thrown up will also answer a good purpose. As the western country abounds with chalybeate springs, they ought to be resorted to, and used freely of, by all persons laboring under gleet. I suppose I need not tell you, that chalybeate water is such as is impregnated with *iron*. The gum called turpentine, of our common pine tree, taken in common sized pills, one three times a day, is a valuable remedy in gleet, and has been known to cure it when all other remedies have failed.

POISONS.

Any substance, which, taken into the stomach, or into any other part of the body, or applied externally to the body, so as to produce disease or death, may be called a *poison*.

The most active and powerful remedies we use in medicine, if given in large doses, operate as poisons. But when given in small ones, are not only innocent but valuable. There are, also, many medicines, which, when taken into the stomach are quite harmless, indeed very valuable in the cure of diseases; but, when taken into the lungs by breathing or respiration, are dangerous and destructive in the extreme. The poison of the *Rattle-snake*, when taken into the stomach, is entirely harmless; but the same poison, when inserted into the flesh so as to reach the circulation, immediately produces disorder and death, unless relief can be obtained. I make these introductory remarks on *poisons*, to throw as much light on their operations as possible, in the fewest number of words.

When *Mineral poisons*, such as *copper*, *arsenic*, *corrosive sublimate*, *lead*, *lunar caustic*, *&c.* &c. are taken into the stomach, in too large quantities, you will feel a burning and prickling sensation in the stomach, and great pain in the bowels, accompanied with a constant puking, and a thirst which cannot be satisfied. Your mouth and throat will become rough and dry, as if you had chewed and swallowed unripe parsimmon—and the pain will gradually increase, until it becomes almost insupportable. In this stage, unless speedy relief is had, inflammation will take place, and terminate in *mortification* and *death*. Should the dose of poison taken, not be sufficient to destroy life, a fever will take place, which will last for some time, attended with a constant trembling of the nerves.

When *vegetable poison*, such as *James-town weed*, *hemlock*, *opium*, *hen-bane*, *deadly night-shade*, *fox-glove*, *wolf's-bane*, *laurel*, &c. &c. are taken into the stomach in too great portions, they produce *stupor* and a constant *desire to sleep*. The James-town weed, usually produces effects peculiar to itself:—for which, and a description of the plant, read under that head.

When the *poison of animals* is introduced into the human system, it is communicated by the bites or stings of *serpents*, *spiders*, &c. &c. requiring prompt and immediate attention to the following remedies, which, together with those applicable to other species of poisons, mineral and vegetable, are arranged under the proper heads.

REMEDIES.

When any poison has been swallowed, whether *vegetable* or *mineral,* the first thing to be done is to empty the stomach, by an emetic or puke of the most active kind. *White vitriol,* from five to ten, and even twenty grains, should be given in a little warm water, and repeated every fifteen or twenty minutes if necessary, until free and copious puking is produced, which you must encourage and keep up by large draughts of warm water. The white vitriol is an innocent puke, and acts almost instantaneously: and if the emetic should require assistance, apply tobacco leaves, steeped in warm vinegar or water, to the stomach; they will materially assist the operation of the vitriol. If the patient cannot be made to puke, you must immediately give repeated clysters, made of strong flax-seed tea and sweet milk—let your patient drink freely of vinegar and water, sweetened with sugar. If the poison taken into the stomach is of the mineral kind, beat up the whites of fifteen eggs with a quart of cold water, and give half a tea-cupful every three or four minutes—this will greatly assist the puking. From taking large doses of opium or laudanum, your patient will sometimes sink into a stupor, or deep and insensible sleep. When this is the case, stimulants must be given, of sufficient power to rouse him if possible. In these cases, I have sometimes resorted to scalding the soles of the feet with boiling water—and in one instance, saw the life of a young man saved, by whipping him to keep him in motion. There is one simple and certain remedy, however, to be found in almost every house:—take two tea-spoonfuls of made mustard, or in other words common mustard seed, pounded fine and mixed as if for eating; put them into some warm water, and give the whole as an emetic, and copious puking will almost be immediately produced. This simple and effective remedy, has been the means of saving hundreds, who have accidently or intentionally swallowed poison.

I have mentioned, that poisons might be taken into the

lungs, by breathing or respiration. Doctor Paris, in his book on diet, speaks decidedly against the introduction of *gass lights* into the interior of dwellings, and says, "that carburetted hydrogen is a deadly poison, which, even in a state of great dilution, is capable of exerting a baneful effect on the nervous system. I have been consulted," says the Doctor, "on several occasions, for pains in the head, and distressing languor, which had evidently been produced by the persons inhaling the unburnt gass in the boxes of play-houses." Sir Humphrey Davy, the celebrated chemist, made an experiment on himself, by inhaling pure carburetted hydrogen: and the result was, that after three inspirations, his vital powers were so completely suspended, that he did not recover them until the next day. Many instances have occurred, of persons sleeping in close rooms during the night, where small charcoal fires have been kept up for warmth, who have been found dead in the morning;—I mention this as a caution; and will also, notice some other facts respecting poisons, which ought to be attended to by those who value their safety.

Medicines should always be strictly examined, especially if to be given by inexperienced persons, and those who are not well acquainted with their appearance and qualities: even those who make a practice of selling medicines, sometimes make dangerous mistakes in them. I have now in my office, three pounds of *emetic tartar*, which I received for *cream of tartar*; and, had I administered this medicine without detecting the mistake, the results must have been fatal to many. A merchant of Knoxville, of the first respectability, received from a young man who attended a drug-store in Baltimore, emetic tartar, for cream of tartar, and was in the very act of giving it to a friend who was indisposed, when the master of the shop arrived in great alarm, having discovered the blunder, just in time to prevent the fatal consequences. I will give one case more, by way of caution respecting mistakes in medicine.

During the summer of 1825, a gentleman from South Carolina, stopped at the house of Mrs. H——, of Patrick county, Virginia; he felt somewhat indisposed, and desired to have a dose of salts: through mistake he received and took saltpetre. Nothing saved him but the early arrival of the son of Mrs. H. a gentleman of superior intelligence, who immediately administered a powerful emetic and relieved him.

Poisons, communicated by the bites of snakes, spiders, and other insects, are immediately to be attended to. The moment you are bitten by a snake, you are to tye a tight and strong bandage immediately above the bite. This will prevent the circulation of the blood, and give you time to apply the remedies needful for relief. As soon as possible, dissolve six grains of lunar caustic in six table-spoonfuls of water, and wet the bitten part with it constantly. Every man in the country, ought to keep a small piece of lunar caustic in his house: it is sometimes called nitrate of silver, and is made of pure silver, nitric acid, and pure water. If the caustic cannot be obtained, make a poultice of quick lime and soap, and apply it to the part affected; and give the patient as much red pepper tea as the stomach will bear; and also every hour, give him a table-spoonful of the juice of the plantain. In all cases where a physician can be had, the best remedy is to cut out the bitten part. The Indians, when bitten by a poisonous snake, always extract the poison by sucking the wound. There is no danger in this operation:—I have told you before, that the venom of a snake if even taken into the stomach, is attended with no danger: The blood should be encouraged to flow from the wound, by scarifying the parts immediately about it, and applying the cupping instruments. When you are bitten by a spider, or injured by any other insect, apply a linen rag constantly moistened with laudanum, spirits of hartshorn or strong ley.

I shall record a few cases, in which it will be evident, that the bite of the rattle-snake may be very easily cured by extremely simple and always practicable remedies. The cases may be found in detail, on pages 619, 620 and 621, of the sixth volume of the *Medical Recorder*. I shall abridge them. 1st. One evening, at my residence, on the hills of

Santee, says Wm. Mayrant Esq. (formerly a member of Congress,) I heard a violent scream at no great distance. In a few minutes I was called out and informed that a negro had been bitten by a rattle-snake, and was dead or dying. I found him motionless and speechless, his jaws locked, and his pulse fluttering and scarcely perceptible. I had heard of the successful use of *spirits* in such cases; both among the Whites and Indians. I therefore took a glass of whiskey; put into it a table-spoonful of pounded red pepper; and poured it down his throat. In a few minutes it was puked up; as were also three or four succeeding doses. After the fourth glass it remained on his stomach. His pulse improved greatly in a short time: and after getting five or six glasses to remain, I ceased giving him any more, until the pulse fell very fast, and nearly ceased beating. I again commenced giving him the whiskey and pepper, and soon discovered that on ceasing the stimulants, his pulse would again sink to nothing. After taking more than one quart of this liquor, a copious stool followed:—the spirit was again administered, until his pulse became steady. During the night he took three quarts of whiskey: in the morning he was much better, but very weak—he finally recovered.

3d. About a year afterward, I was called to another slave who had been bitten by a rattle-snake; he was in great pain about the chest, and was puking a green fluid. I gave him repeated doses of whiskey and pepper, until his pulse returned, which had nearly ceased to beat: in twelve hours, by the use of about a quart of this liquor, he was a well man.

3d. I related the above cases to a friend, who had lately arrived from Rio Janeiro, after a residence of thirteen years. He told me that the serpents of that country were so extremely venomous, as in many instances to produce death in fifteen minutes; and that the natives effected their cures, by giving large doses of spirits, in which herbs had been stewed. He related an instance in which a man was found with one of these most poisonous snakes on him and biting him repeatedly. The snake was killed, and the man taken to the house, to all appearance dead. In a short time he came to himself, and was unhurt by the poison. The fact was, that he had been very drunk, and had fallen on the snake: the stimulons of the liquor had no doubt, counteracted the influence of the poison; this was the solution of the difficulty.—These three cases coincide strongly, with a case, published several years since, in the National Intelligencer, by the celebrated Doctor Ramsey; in which large doses of brandy and opium were given with complete success, in the bite of a rattle-snake.

The tincture of *cantharides*, which is nothing more than the Spanish or blistering flies, or our common potatoe fly, steeped for a few days in whiskey or spirits of any kind. Of this tincture, apply a few drops to the wound until it occasions a redness. By this application, the poison is rendered harmless; and the stings of insects or reptiles are entirely removed as soon as the blister raises. This is a late discovery, and truly a valuable remedy.

I cannot quit this interesting subject, without noticing particularly, that a most excellent remedy in the bites of both venomous snakes and spiders, is the immediate application of the soft black mud from spring branches, or such mud as is used for the daubing of houses. I have never had occasion to try the experiment myself, but fully believe from the best authority; that it is an efficient and powerful application.

PAINFUL AFFECTION OF THE FACE

This disease is called by physicians, *tic douloureux*, and happily for mankind, is of very unfrequent occurrence. It is an acutely painful affection of the nerves of the face, particularly over the cheek bone; in which the pain shoots with great quickness and suddenness, and is almost insupportable for a few seconds, when it as suddenly becomes easy. The slightest touch will cause it to dart instantly, and sometimes by opening the mouth quickly, it will return with a jurking and spasmodic affection of the muscles of the face. There is in this complaint, neither swelling of the cheek nor any species of inflammations, nor does the pain seem deeply seated.

REMEDIES.

Remedies for curing this complaint, have long been objects of retentive research, with the most distinguished and able physicians. The remedies usually resorted to, but I confess with very little success, are sulphat of ten, which is white vitriol; Peruvian bark; opium; and carbonate of iron, given in doses of twenty grains every fourth hour. As I have just remarked, these are remedies attended with very little success; the carbonate of iron was for some time considered efficient and beneficial; but at length, like the other remedies it fell into disrepute. We are now indebted to a common weed for the cure of this complaint, a weed which infests our gardens, high-ways, and barn-yards;—it is the common Jamestown weed, usually called the stink-weed and thorn-apple: read under the head Jamestown weed. A physician of much distinction, Doctor John Eberle of New York, speaks thus in substance of this weed—In July last, I was called to see a lady aged about twenty years, who was suffering very much from this complaint in the right side of her face. The paroxysms of fits of pain, were sometimes, so very violent as to produce temporary *loss of reason!* She had been treated by other physicians with the usual remedies; all of which had been found incompetent to afford relief in the slightest degree. I prescribed for her the extract of stramonium or Jamestown weed, and gave her a grain of this extract every four hours. She commenced with this in the evening; and toward morning had intervals of ease, and slept some. She continued this medicine during the succeeding day, and experienced much less pain than she had done for eight days previously. After the fourth dose, she felt some vertigo or dizziness of the head, and was directed to take the

AA

medicine only every six hours; in which she persisted until entirely relieved and fully cured, which was in a few days. "The Jamestown Weed, says this eminent physician, is undoubtedly a medicine of great and valuable powers. In *chronic rheumatism*, I have employed it in several instances with the most unequivocal advantage. In *sciatica*, (by which the doctor means *hip gout.*) also, I prescribed it with complete success in three cases. We are chiefly indebted to Doct. Marcet for our knowledge of its efficacy, in affections of this kind," &c. "If I were called upon says this writer, to express in a few words the general opinion which I feel inclined to form from the opportunities I have had of studying the properties of *stramonium*, (Jamestown Weed,) I should say, that when given with due caution, and in proper doses, in all cases of chronie disease, attended with acute pain, it will invariably lessen the sensibility to pain and suffering." I fully accord with the Doctor in his opinions, and refer the reader to the head Jamestown Weed, where he will find an interesting development of the medicinal powers of this plant.

The following remedy is taken from the New York Medical Inquirer:—Mr. Abernethy has administered the *nitrate of silver* in this disease, [which means *lunar caustic*] in the dose of one grain twice a day, made into pills, with conserve of roses," [which is nothing more than a syrup made of rose leaves and sugar, or honey.]

"A Mr. Thomas also recommends this preparation in this most distressing disease. The following is a copy of Mr. Thomas's prescription. Take nitrate of silver, one scruple; nitric acid, fifteen drops; [which is commonly called *aquafortis*] pure water three ounces. From forty to sixty drops to be taken twice a day, in two table spoonfuls of camphorated julep." For a description of the method of preparing the camphorated julep, read under that head.

LOCKED JAW.

This disease is called by physicians, *tetanus;* which means *spasm* with *rigidity*—it is from the Greek word which means to *stretch*. It may be considered an involuntary contraction of all the muscles of the body, while the patient remains perfectly in his senses. It generally arises from wounds; and I have even known it to originate from the slight puncture or prick of a needle, in which case it terminated in the death of and amiable lady. It comes on with a dull stiffness of the neck and head; in a short time the head and neck becomes difficult to move; the tongue also becomes stiff and difficult to be moved about or put out; the swallowing becomes painful; there is a tightness across the breast, sometimes attended with pain in the small of the back: the jaws gradually become stiff, and the *teeth clenched;* this is *locked jaw.*

REMEDIES.

You are immediately to open the wound, if that be the cause, with a lancet or other sharp instrument, and remove any matter that may be in the wound. Then apply spirits of *turpentine* to the wound, and if the person is strong, hearty and in full habit, you are to draw blood freely from the arm. Then put your patient in the warm bath; I mean here, that the whole body is to be immersed in warm water for some time and give two grains of *opium*. During the time these operations are making, a skilful physician must be sought for; because the immense quantities of opium which must now be given, will make even the best physician dread his own practice. Yet such are the fatal consequences of delay and timidity in locked jaw, that unless bold remedies are used, particularly the use of opium in heavy doses, death must certainly take place. Opium has to be given in this complaint, according to the situation of the patient, and the violence of the disease, almost without regarding the quantity. That it is the proper remedy in spasm there can be no doubt; and that the quantities sometimes given in locked jaw are almost incredible, is a fact well known to practitioners of medicine. Tobacco is highly spoken of in this distressing spasm, given in the form of clysters. Doctor Thomas tells us, "that many cases are on record, where the astonishing quantity of an ounce of opium has been given in twenty-four hours." To proportion the quantity of opium to be given, combined with the administration of clysters of tobacco, must always require the judgment of a skilful physician, and I therefore, recommend that one always be procured where practicable. In desperate cases, where, by reason of the clenching of the teeth, the patient cannot receive any thing in the mouth, it is necessary to remove a front tooth, and sometimes more than one. I have never heard of nor seen the practice; but should a case of desperate *locked jaw* occur in my practice, I would try the effect of a strong bath made of *warm ley* or lye, in which the body of the patient should be entirely immersed, at the same time, that I would give a clyster containing fifteen grains of tarter emetic—in addition to which I would stimulate the patient freely with warm toddy.

CANCER.

Cancer generally makes its appearance about the lips, the nose, and about the breasts of females. It sometimes, also, but the instances I am happy to say are not very frequent, makes its appearance in the womb, in which the cure is very doubtful. Those who are advanced in life, are much more subject to cancerous affections than young persons: particularly, if they have scrofulous constitutions, which have descended to them from their ancestors. A *cancer* commences with a small inflamed pimple, of a bluish color, which becomes a sore with hard rising edges of a ragged and uneven appearance. On a close examination of the sore, you will discover two whitish lines, crossing from the centre to the edge of the sore. At first, a burning sensation is felt in the sore, which is accompanied as the disease increases with sharp shooting pains. After sometime, these pains subside, and the cancer discharges a highly offensive matter; this discharge increases gradually, and the matter communicating to the adjoining parts, finally ends in a large offensive sore or ulcer, of a most dreadful and exhausting nature, always terminating, unless a cure is effected, in a lingering, painful, and horrible death.

REMEDIES.

The moment cancer is discovered, dissolve ten grains of *corrosive sublimate* in a gill of whiskey, or a gill of strong spirits of any kind. Apply cautiously this mixture to the affected part: it may be done by making a small rag swab, wetting it with the solution just named, and touching the affected or sore part with it gently. This operation is to be performed once a day, until the cancer is destroyed. This is a powerful medicine, and the pain produced by it's application is very severe; but by an early application of this remedy, and bearing the pain of its application fifteen or twenty minutes for a few days, it will kill the cancer. It should never be used on large ulcers or cancerous sores, the pain it inflicts being as severe as if a red hot iron were applied. In many cases, when applied at an early stage of cancer, I have known this remedy successful. The sores should be washed with salt and water, and dressed with charcoal plasters. To kill the pain give opium or laudanum: see table. But notwithstanding, what has been said of the foregoing remedy, in order to ensure a successful cure, I think the parts ought to be removed or cut out at an early period of the disease. I have performed the operation fifteen or sixteen times with success; the last operation was performed on Mr. H——, of Monroe county Verginia, during my residence in Botetourt county, of the same state, assisted by my medical friends Doctors, M'Dowel and Foot, two gentlemen of distinction in the medical profession. The gentleman on whom the operation was performed, was about 48 years of age. The *cancer* was seated in the lower lip, and was of such size as to require the removal of the lower lip entirely. By the suggestion of Doctor M'Dowel, but with great caution, I cut well down the chin, and secured the edges of the incision together, after taking out the cancer. Singular as it may appear, a new lip was formed.

The wound healed with the first intentions; and when it was entirely well, the mouth was so extremely small, as scarcely to admit the end of the fore finger. The mouth, however, gradually distended itself by the exertions of nature, and is now both useful and beautiful. Before the operation, the mouth was large and the lips coarse and fleshy. On my way out to Tennessee, I presented to Doctor Powell of the *Boat yard*, the old lip, and I doubt not he has it now in his possession. A remedy for cancer, appeared in the public journals some years since, which, from its marks of authenticity of statement, and success in the case of Thomas Tyrrel, I think proper to place on a more durable record. It is simply the use of "a strong potash;" made of the ley of the ashes of redoak bark, boiled down to the consistence of molasses. With this substance, the cancer must be first covered, and in about an hour afterwards, the whole is to be covered with a plaster of tar. This must be removed after a few days, and if there are any protruberances or lumps in the sore, the applications are to be renewed. As far as an opinion can be relied on, without actual experiment, I think the remedy a good one.

SCALDS AND BURNS.

Because we all know well what scalds and burns are, and because the saving of space for matters of high interest, is important to both, the subscribers to this work, and myself, I shall not attempt to describe them.

REMEDIES.

In these accidents, which sometime unfortunately arise from negligence, the important point is to use such remedies as are immediately at hand, or are easily obtained for affording direct relief from excruciating pain. Nature always a tender parent, bountifully affords the best and most soothing remedy, *cold water:* in which the parts affected are to be immediately plunged. If ice can be obtained which is but water under another character, its application will be as good, if not better than mere water, which sometimes cannot be had of sufficient coldness. If the body is severely scalded or burned, apply cloths kept continually wet with the coldest water. Where the scald or burn takes place in children, and to no great extent, the application of common tar immediately to the injury, is a valuable remedy not often resorted to, but which I earnestly recommend.

The application of carded cotton to a scald or burn, is also an excellent remedy, and one which is nearly always convenient. The old method of applying sweet or olive oil *immediately* to a scald or burn is a bad plan; and ought never to be resorted to, until cold water or ice has been applied for reducing the inflammation; then olive or sweet oil will answer a valuable purpose. If oil is not convenient, which is often the case, the application of poultices made of raw Irish potatoes, carrots, or turnips, will be proper; the oil however, if possible to be obtained is preferable. When the patient has been in the greatest pain, and every remedy I had applied give but little relief, I have always been able to give instant ease, if I had or could procure it, by the application of *Turner's cerate*. For the method of making this very valuable salve, look under that head. It must be applied by spreading it on linen rags, and covering the burned or scalded parts with them; and I suppose I need not tell you, that these cerate plasters are to be supplied by new ones, every day laid on fresh. This cooling and soothing remedy seems to act like magic, in giving relief from the most horrible suffering. On my arrival in Montgomery county, Virginia, I was called in consultation with Doctor Joseph Miller, who was a physician by nature, and a man of the highest native genius; a man who must have stood at the head of his profession, had his great intellectual power been aided by adequate opportunities of education. With this gentleman I attended on Maj.——. He had been taken with a fit, and fallen into a large fire by which he was sitting, after his family had retired to bed. Before he was discovered by his family and taken out, he was litterally roasted; his ribs were perfectly exposed on the right side, and the motion of the abdominal viscera, (the intestines or guts,) could easily be distinguished through the thin membrane. His situation was as truly horrible as can well be imagined; and his sufferings were so very great, as frequently to induce him to pray to us, that something might be given him to end the miseries of his existence. Those sufferings indeed must be unspeakable, which destroy in man the deep seated love of life. By the application of Turner's cerate, which was spread on a sheet and applied to him, and slippery elm tea given internally, this gentleman recovered and is now living in Montgomery county, Virginia, near Christianburgh. I mention this case in all its horrors, to induce every family into whose hands this book my fall, always to have in their possession, Turner's cerate for immediate application.

CORNS.

We all know what corns are, and it is useless to consume time in describing them.—

Remedies.—To get rid of them in the shortest possible time, bathe the foot or feet in warm water, about half an hour before going to bed. Wen the corns have become soft from bathing, shave down the horny parts smooth, but not so close as to produce blood. Then moisten the tops of them with spittle, and rub over them a little lunar caustic, which you can easily procure. This caustic must be gently rubbed on, until a sufficiency of it sticks on the corns, to change them first to a dark grey color, and next to a deep black. Put a little cotton over them to prevent the stocking from rubbing them, and in a few days they will come out by the roots:—This is the remedy of doctor Brown of Philadelphia, and it is a good one.

WARTS.

We all know what warts are, and it is also useless to describe them.

Remedies.—Put on each wart, a small blister of Spanish flies, which can easily be confined by adhesive plaster, of any kind. In a few days the warts will come out, when you may use the lunar caustic, as in the case of corns: or you may wet the warts with a little sulphuric acid or oil of vitriol, which will soon bring them off; or with nitric acid or aquafortis, which will produce the same effect.

THE

DISEASES

OF

WOMEN

AND

CHILDREN.

DISEASES OF WOMEN.

When we consider the important relation, in which woman stands to man in every department of life; when we consider, that in one relation, she is the wife of his bosom, the chosen companion of his heart, the voluntary sharer of his prospeirty and misfortunes, the *mother of that offspring*, in whose life and prosperity, man even in the decline of life and the decay of health, lives over again the youthful vigor and tender passions of his early years: when we consider that in another relation, as the sincere lover of his virtues, and the admirer of his heroic and noble achievements, she urges man to perseverance in the performance of his moral duties and to those sentiments of patriotism which gave to the ancient *Republics* their statesmen and heroes—to Ireland her Emmets, to england her Sidneys, and to America her Washingtons: and, when we consider, that in another and important relatian, the minute and apparently ignoble cares of a family devolve on her, where there are no witnesses to support her under endless sufferings and trials, and where no civic crowns or public honors await her victories over *domestic miseries*, and *ignoble sufferings and misfortunes*, we cannot but be astonished at the fortitude, the courage, the devotedness, the fidelity to her duties, and the heroic virtues of woman! Place man in her situation, and compel him to perform the duties of woman, and he would soon either degenerate into a savage, or sink into perfect insignificance. Placed in the limited sphere of the employments of woman, and man would soon feel himself an obscure and lonely slave: doomed like her, to a life of obscurity and domestic cares, where the anticipation of no honors would await the performance of his duties, his boasted magnanimity and fortitude would expire like meteors of night, and leave him a monument of powerless and fallen ambition

And, how soon would his boasted philanthropy and love of mankind expire, were there no historians to record his deeds of benevolence, and patriotism, and transmit them to future ages, and especially, were there no honors to be gathered but such as grew on the brows of obscure and suffering humanity, and such as would fade in the grasp and be remembered no more.

Woman! when we reflect on thy blameless life, thy artless tenderness, thy pious simplicity, thy confiding love, and the meek and lowly resignation of thy heart and feelings, under the pressure of miseries and misfortunes of almost every possible character, it seems difficult for the most humane of mankind, duly to appreciate either thy *sufferings* or thy *worth!* But, when to these considerations are added the multiplicity of diseases entailed on thee by nature and sexuality, as well as by the *ignorance* of the *Midwives* of this country, thy lot and condition of present existence seem hard indeed! Most of the midwives of this country, and indeed of most other countries, are those who take up the employment from too great laziness to exert themselves in other walks of life; from utter ignorance of the great responsibilities attached to such a calling; and from a heartless destitution of feeling and humanity, which permit their ignorance and officiousness, to entail diseases originating in mismanagement, on thousands of women for life. These people are always seen wishing to officiate in something which had better be let alone; in fact, if I must speak in plain terms, in attempting to force nature into premature and exhausting exertions, who, if let alone so far as not to be retarded in her operations, would finish her own work without injury to the sufferer. I do not mention this to cast censures on all midwives; I am acquainted with several of excellent qualifications; who are kind, feeling, and experienced; and who possess the excellent good sense, never to hazard or exceed the due bounds of prudence; and, who, in all cases where there is lingering and difficulty, always so far distrust their own judgment, as to require the aid of a *skilful physician.* Women should never dread the time of child-birth; but always reflect on the innumerable millions of cases, in which women have passed safely through the trial, for one perhaps which has been unfortunate. When a physician is called in, which in many cases is absolutely essential to the preservation of life, and the safety of the child, his whole solicitude should concentrate in feelings and sentiments of humanity; in such cases, therefore, no woman however delecate or fastedious in her feelings or sentiments, ought to feel any hesitation in permitting the assistance of a physician:—life is always to be preserved, and the safety of human beings ensured, by much greater sacrifices than those which appertain to feelings of mere bashfulness, or even sentiments of modesty. When I speak of calling in a physician, with permission to render the essential assistance to nature and child-birth, I mean a man of delicacy of sentiment and feeling, tried and well known discretion, and dignified elevation of character; I do not mean a beardless boy, who has dosed over a medical book for year or even two, without understanding its contents, and who is as proud of the name *Doctor*, as is a child of a new pair of morocco shoes; such a physician would be worse than an ignorant and officious *midwife*, who always wishes to be doing something *right* or *wrong*. When young in my professiou, I always thought it necessary to be giving some little article in all cases; in other words, something that would do neither good nor harm: this kind of conduct will do well enough, so far as it has a tendency to keep up and animate the spirits of the patient, but here it ought to stop: —my good old preceptor or master, who had for more than forty years officiated successfully as a man midwife, gave me the following advice, which I recommend most sincerely to the attention of all my readers: "neither hurry nor retard nature; give her time to perform her own operations, and when she fails *assist her*."

BB

OUTWARD PATS
OF
FEMALE GENERATION.

I would omit a description of these parts altogether, were not a slight delineation of them essential to understanding the medical doctrines and diseases relating to them. The front exhibits what is called the *mons veneris* which is shielded by nature with a coat of *hair*, as if she aimed at the concealment of these parts, intended for the procreation of the human species. The labia or lips as they are called, shaded by this covering of hair, extend downward on each side of what is called the *cleft;* they unite and form a thin skin or membrane called the *perineum,* which divides these parts from the fundament.

On opening the labia or lips, you will observe a small part which appears more full, and rises higher than the rest: this by physicians is called the *clitoris,* and is the chief seat of pleasureable sensation, in the intercourse or connexion of the sexes. It may as well be remarked here as any where else, that cleanliness, by frequent bathing these parts with soap and water, has a powerful tendency to remove or quell those venereal desires which frequently arise from the irritability of the parts, and lay the foundation of many evils for life:—read, in addition to these remarks, under the head warm or tepid bath. Immediately under the *clitoris,* you will find on close examination, a small orifice or hole; this is the end of the canal which leads to the bladder, and it is through this orifice or hole that the urine or water passes off. My object in explaining these parts so plainly, is to enable any woman of common sense, by the use of the *catheter,* to draw off her urine or water herself, whenever it may be necessary, instead of being exposed to a physician on every trifling occasion. [For a description of the catheter, and the use of it, see the head *catheter.*]

Immediately under the part out which the urine passes, is the mouth or entrance into the birth-place, called by physicians the *vagina,* at the further end of which is situated the *womb*, at the distance of three or four inches. The mouth of the vagina, or entrance of the birth-place, is usually, but not always defended by a thin tough membrane resembling a fish scale, called the *hymen;* which was once supposed to be the test of virginity, and which is always destroyed on a first connection with a male. Some females have this membrane so strongly formed by nature, as to prevent their *menses* or *courses* from flowing; when this is the case, they collect in the womb in such a manner as to resemble pregnancy. I have seen several cases of this kind; and I recollect one particular instance, in which a lady of great respectability had to undergo an operation, before her husband could have sexual intercourse with her. When the *menses* do not flow at the usual period, and the proper means have been used to bring them on, it is always proper for the female parent to examine particularly into this matter, or the consequences of neglect may be fatal. The method of relief, when the hymen is *imperforated*, or in other words, has no hole in it through which the menses may flow, is simply to puncture or open the hymen with a lancet, or any other instrument that will answer. In some females, this hymen does not exist; but this is no evidence of the want of virginity, for the membrane is very often destroyed by jumping, romping, running, &c. at an early period of life.

About the age that females usually marry, the vagina or entrance of the birth-place, is from two to three inches in length, and capable of some distention. At the upper end of the birth-place or vagina, is the mouth of the womb, which can be felt with the finger. Midwives should be very particular in becoming acquainted with these parts, and particularly with the mouth of the womb, because it is from the peculiarities of its feeling, that we become confident of the presence of *actual labor:* Labor means nothing more nor less, than the efforts of the womb itself, to expel the child. at the period fixed by nature for its entrance into life. Labor is considered *natural*, if the head of the child presents itself *fairly*. If the time of *labor* is longer than twenty-four hours, it may be called a lingering or difficult labor. If any part of the child other than the head, presents itself. the labor is called *pretenatural;* and every other case requiring assistance, is called *complex.*

The *bones*, necessary to be described, are those which form, or appertain to the pelvis or basin. The pelvis resembles in form, a wash basin with the bottom out. In women, it is very shallow and very wide; and it is by these marks, that the skeleton of the female can be distinguished from that of the male: in women, the bones of the pelvis are very slender, and the opening at the bottom so wide as easily to permit the child to pass. In some instances, this opening suddenly becomes so wide, that the head of the child presses with violence on the soft and fleshy parts, and tears the *perineum*, which is the membrane between the birth-place and the fundament. This pelvis or basin, is formed by four bones; the ossacrum behind, the ossa innominta on either side, and the os coccygis below—the vulgar sometimes call this the *crupper bone.* This last bone is so formed as to move back when the woman is in labor; and frequently makes a grating noise in women who have been married late in life. I have now explained to you the external parts, and also the hard or bony parts which it will be well for you to remember.

The bladder is very near the front bones; so near indeed, that for want of an instrument called a catheter, when in the country, I have frequently drawn the water off by a common goose-quill. The *womb* lies next the bladder; in shape it resembles a pear, is of an oblong form like a pear, and in its natural position has its largest end turned upward toward the stomach, and the vagina neck downward toward the external parts. The womb is supported by small membranes or little strings, interwoven together and to the sides of the pelvis or basin, which I have already described to you: it is so commodiously and admirably arranged, as to float about occasionally. On each side of the womb, and coming out from its sides, are two fleshy tubes which are called fallopian tubes, from the name of a physician who discovered them in 1547. These tubes are about three inches in length, and the ends look as if they had been cut off with a dull knife. On each side of the pelvis or basin, is found a lump about the size of the end of the thumb: these are the female *testicles*, which supply the seed at the time the female conceives the child. These ovaria or testicles, have small cells in them, which burst like small blisters, in the act which gets a woman with child. The tubes which I have mentioned are constantly floating about, and the moment the seed of the male comes in contact or touch with them, it stimulates them to take up the contents of one or two of the small cells I have mentioned; and to convey their contents through the tubes of the womb; by what is called by medical men *peristaltic motion*. The seed being now deposited, the child commences its formation and growth; this commencement of growth takes place, as is supposed, about three weeks after the sexual commerce has taken place; because about that time the ovaria or egg passes through the fallopian tube into the womb. About the fourth month, the woman feels a peculiar sensation about the womb; this is called *quickening:* and is caused by the womb suddenly rising above the brim of the pelvis or basin, and as suddenly pressing on the inside of the belly. The womb is much thicker at the sides than any where else; it is a hollow fibrous mass, which means that it is composed of fibres or threads, interwoven with each other. It has the power of contracting or drawing up, and of expelling its contents whatever they may be. These fibres secrete and hold the discharge called the menses or courses. I have now given you a full and plain description, of the female organs of generation; of what is believed to be the manner of *conceiving;* of the formation of the womb; and of the different presentations of labor: and I have been thus particular, in order that you may the better understand the information I have to communicate on the diseases of women.

MENSES OR COURSES.

The early or late discharge of the menses or courses, depends very much on the climate; the constitution of the woman, as to strength or weakness; on the emotions and passions of the mind, or in plain terms on the *lasciviousness* or *chastity* of her venereal desires. In all cold climates, this discharge is later in making its appearance than in warm ones! Fruit ripens sooner in warm latitudes than in cold ones: and it is the same with females. In the genial climate of Italy, girls have their courses at nine years old: but in the colder regions of Russia, this discharge does not come on until women are from twenty to twenty-five years of age, and then not unfrequently in very small quantities. In all warm climates, says a distinguished writer, women exhibit all the splendor of their charms, when they are mere children in understanding; but, when their minds have arrived at maturity they cease to be objects of love.

In the western country, although the climate is mild, it is much subject to sudden changes, particularly in East Tennessee. These changes produce powerful effects on the health of women, and also on their constitutions. The western country is damp and wet during the winter season; in sonsequence of which, women from being exposed to wet feet, are subject to more irregularities in this discharge called the menses or courses, than in any other part of the U. States. When the usual period for this discharge comes on a little attention on the part of the parent will be sufficient to discover the symptoms: Many girls have their discharges without inconvenience, while others suffer considerably when the period is about to come on—such as a great restlessness, slight fever, head-ache, heavy dull pain in the small of the back and bottom of the belly, swelled and hardened breasts, and so on The appetite becomes delicate, the limbs tremble and feel weak, the face becomes pale, and there is a peculiar dark streak or shade under the eyes. When these symptoms and feelings occur, every thing should be done to assist nature in bringing forward this discharge. This is a critical period of life, and much depends on the result. The greatest possible precaution should be used, to prevent the girl from taking cold at this time; because by very slight exposures, *nature* may be prevented from performing this very important office, by the failure of which some of the most fatal female diseases are produced. Exercise should be taken on horse-back at this time, or indeed any exercise that will give free circulation to the blood: the emotions and passions of the mind, ought also to be particularly attended to; a cheerful disposition should be produced and kept up, at the same time that every effort should be made to banish grief, despondency, or any of the depressing passions, which I need not tell you have a powerful effect in preventing the due discharge of the menses or courses. The discharges, in their first appearance, are in small quantities, and rather irregular as to time; but they gradually, in healthy women, become regular and flow monthly, While in a state of pregnancy, or when suckling children, women do not have these menses or courses; nor do they ever become pregnant, or in plain terms get with child, until this menstrual discharge make its appearance on them. Women also cease to breed, when this menstrual discharge leaves them, in advanced life. The period when this discharge commences on women, and the period when it leaves them, are critical and dangerous periods of time, to the health and constitutions of women. As I shall describe the remedies more fully, in cases where the menses have been established, and have suddenly stopped, from cold or other causes, I shall merely remark here; that in all cases where the first symptoms of menses make their appearance in young girls, they should use all mild and gentle methods of courting nature to the performance of her office, by sitting over the steam of warm herbs, bathing, their feet and legs at the same time in warm water, as high as the knees, or what is preferable, use the warm or tepid bath: [see that head,] and drink freely, of warm pennyroyal tea. These remedies should be used a short time before going to bed, so that a gentle moisture or sweat may be produced on the skin, which generally causes the menses or courses to flow. This discharge is usually at first very small; but, by attending to this simple course, which I have laid down, when the proper or expected time has arrived for their appearance, *nature* will gradually become regular, and the menses or courses be produced. The quantity, as I have observed, will at first be quite small, perhaps just sufficient to stain the linen or shift—which will in quantity increase at every period or monthly return. As this discharge depends very much on climate, constitution, manner of living, and exercise, you will easily account for its differing in quantity, not only in different women, but even in the same woman, increasing or diminishing as to the state of the system. In all southern or warm climates, the quantity discharged is from eighteen to twenty ounces; but, in colder climates, it diminishes accordingly even to one or two ounces. The length of time the menses or courses remain on and the time of their monthly return, differ very much in women: in some it will remain but a few hours or a day—in others from two to four days—and I have even known it to remain ten days. The common or usual time, however, is from three to six days. In the western country, the menses generally cease at about the forty fifth year. This however depends very much on the period they make their appearance—if at an early age, they go off earlier, and if at a later period, they sometimes continue to fifty years. About the expected time that the menses or courses should flow. which will be easily known from the description I have given you of the symptoms, you are to avoid every thing that may injure the digestive powers, and particularly costiveness or being bound in the bowels, loss of sleep, exposures of any kind, such as damp feet, or sudden changes from warm to thin clothing. Girls in the country should be prevented, about this time, from wading in the water, or walking bare-foot through the dew, as it often stops this discharge. Getting cold, from any imprudence or unnecessary exposure, must also be avoided. On the subject of medicines, you are particularly requested, as you value the health of your child, to give no strong medicines in the first stage of the menstrual discharge, called vulgarly forcing medicines. This indeed is a proper name, for you are truly forcing nature, which is contrary to every principle of common sense: for this discharge, unless stooped from some one of the causes I have mentioned, will assuredly yield to patience and simple remedies; after a full trial, and sufficient time allowed, and you are disappointed at bringing them on, you will try cautiously and mildly, the following remedies under the following head—"obstruction of the menses," where you will find the valuable remedy "Seneka Snake-root"—for a full description of which important root in the stoppage of the menses or courses, read under the head Seneka Snake root.

OBSTRUCTED MENSES.

When the menses or courses have been once regular, and have been stopped from any accidental cause, such as cold and so on, they are said to be obstructed. This is sometimes attended with pain. When this is the case, it is called obstructed or painful menstruation, and is attended with greater or less misery, according to the state of the system at the time this obstruction takes place particularly, if any other part of the body is laboring under disease; for the womb, from whence the menses or courses flow, is subject to great varieties of diseased action, and it is utterly imppossible for me to describe the close sympathy and connexion, which is immediately and sensibly felt, between the womb, the stomach, the head, and the influence or power it has on the pulse. In six cases out of ten, where hysterics, despondency of mind, sickness at the stomach, pains in the head, coldness of the hands and feet, flushings of heat over the whole body, and not unfrequently fever, arise from *obstructed menses* or *courses*, or some disordered state of the womb. I have had in my practice, many females who became greatly alarmed from the spitting of blood. This is frequently the case, where the obstruction has been for any length of time, accompanied by frequent bleeding at the nose, dry short cough, pains in the bottom of the belly, and in the small of the back, pulse hard and quick, skin hot, and burning sensations in the palms of the hands and feet. When these last symptoms take place, immediate attention should be paid or consumption will take place. A skilful physician must be sought for, if the remedies after a fair and steady trial, should not produce the discharge. In some instances, this obstruction of the menses or courses, arises from debility or weakness of the constitution. This will be known by the *whites* making their appearance. When this is the case, you must not force nature, but give tonic or strengthening medicines to restore the system. First, then, the remedies that follow; beginning with those that are the most simple, until the menses or courses are produced.

REMEDIES.

If the woman is of a robust or full habit of body, the loss of some blood from the foot will be proper. A short time before the return of the menses or courses, warm cloths wrung out of hot water must be applied to the bottom of the belly: this is to be done a few nights before the expected time; or you may sit over the steam of common pine tops, on which boiling water has been poured; or you may sit in a tub of warm water for fifteen or twenty minutes before you go to bed—and while sitting in warm water have your feet bathed in another tub or vessel, in which the water should be as warm as you can conveniently bear it: or plunge your feet and legs in and out frequently, as you may be able to bear the heat of the water. While you are bathing or steaming over the pine tops, use the following remedy, which must be prepared and kept ready for use when you are going to bathe. One ounce of Seneka snake-root is to be bruised with a hammer; then put it into a quart of boiling water, and stew it over a slow fire to half a pint. Of this tea, take a table-spoonful every ten minutes while bathing; or while over the steam. For a full description of this valuable root, see the head *Seneka snake-root.* When you have used these remedies for a quarter half an hour, retire to bed, and have the bottom of your belly well rubbed with a coarse warm towel, or a soft brush; this is called friction, the intention of which is to rouse the circulation, excite the womb to action, and cause the menses or courses to discharge or flow. You will find the following medicine to be a valuable assistant in producing this discharge: and it should be taken for one, two, and even three nights before the expected time:—Five grains of aloes; five grains of rhubarb; and five grains of calomel; and must be finely powdered and mixed together well; and should the dose produce a stool or two by morning, you are to take a small dose of epsom salts to assist the operation. If the dose should purge you too severely, the next dose should be less: say three grains of each instead of five; or even two grains of each will answer. Your own judgment will easily regulate the dose to the costitution of the person. Or you may apply a small blister a day or two before the time, between the fundament and birth-place called by physicians the *perineum;* giving at the same time, a purgative twice or even three times a day of aloes; each dose five grains. Should these remedies all fail, inject or throw with a syringe or squirt, into the vagina, a mixture of strong whiskey and water,so as to irritate or excite an action in the womb. As I have remarked in the first instance, the loss of some blood will generally be found beneficial, unless the constitution or the health of the woman will not admit of the loss of blood, which is not very frequently the case. The loss of blood, always attends to assist the womb to return to its natural action. Madder, which is known to every person in the country as a dye, and may be purchased at any of the stores; is highly recommended by the late Doct. Barton of Philadelphia, late professor of the medical school in that city, in doses of twenty or thirty grains. The tincture of gum guaiacum, in doses of a table spoonful in half a cup of new milk may be given. This tincture is made in the following manner; obtain one ounce of the gum guaiacum, which is worth about ninepence; mash or pound it fine with a hammer, and put it in a pint of spirits of any kind. Let it steep for ten days, shaking it daily, and you have the tincture of gum guaiacum, it being then fit for use. Doctor Dowees, professor of midwifery, in the medical school of Philadelphia, asserts, that in the experience of thirty-tow years, it has never failed him in producing the menses or courses. Of this spirit, put a table spoonful in the milk and gently pour off the spirit, so as not to shake it at the time you are about to use it. I have now given you the different and important remedies, out of which you may select which you please for use: they are all valuable. You will however bear in mind, that the efforts to be made to bring on the menses or courses, should take place about the expected time, or a little time before it. The constitution of the woman, must be fully and properly examined, so as not to force, but to assist nature in her operations.

GREEN SICKNESS.

When the menses or courses have been retained or stopped for any length of time, and the whole system becomes diseased from a want of discharge, so necessary to the health of every female, it terminates or ends frequently in what is called chlorosis or green sickness. When this is the case, the skin turns of a pale yellow or greenish hue; the lips become of a pale or purple color; the eyes have a dark or purple tinge around them; on making the least exertion, the heart palpitates or beats; the knees tremble, and there is a frequent sighing without knowing the cause. The mind is very ficle, and the woman dislikes, or seems to want the power to attend to her domestic concerns. The cheeks are frequently flushed, similar to consumption; the feet swell; and the whole system seems to sink under debility or great weakness. I have now described to you the symptoms which I alluded to, when I directed you to examine the constitution, and not to force nature, especially when tonic or strengthening medicines are required to restore the whole system, before any attempt ought to be made to bring on the menses or courses. The treatment in this last stage called green sickness, should be as follows:—as little medicine as possible should be given: in fact, nothing but simple medicine, such as will prevent costiveness by keeping the bowels open, such for instance as a tea spoonful of epsom salts, and a tea spoonful of magnesia, ground finely and well mixed together, to be taken in a cup full of cold water when necessary for this purpose; travelling on horse-back or moderate exercise. Good Maderia wine, taken frequently and in small quantities; bitters made of equal quantities of wild cherry tree bark, and poplar bark, usually called swamp poplar, steeped in wine for several days, and taken in moderate doses; or tea made of the flowers of garden chamomile, and taken cold, the dose a wine glass full, three or four times a day. The chalybeate water should be used very freely. The western country abounds with these waters; for they are to be found on almost every branch or creek. Chalybeate waters, are those springs which are impregnated with iron. By these remedies, the whole system will be restored, and in due time the menses or courses will again appear; at which time, mild and gentle remedies are to be used, to court nature to the proper performance of this necessary and important discharge.

THE GREAT DISCHARGE

OF THE MENSES OR COURSES.

When the menses or courses come on suddenly or irregularly, and the discharges for several days are greater than usual, by which the woman is greatly reduced and weakened—this is called excessive menstruation. The causes are too great a determination of blood to the womb; or in other words too great an action in its vessels. This over quantity, or large discharge, generally take place in delecate women, particularly those who takes but little exercise, or those who sit a great deal; such as milliners or seamstresses, and in fact all who lead sedentary lives, and are addicted to such unhealthy habits.

REMEDIES.

Draw blood from the arm immediately; and regulate the quantity taken, by the constitution, the habits, and the strength of the woman: there are few cases that do not admit of a little blood being drawn. Give a purge of epsom salts or castor oil, and let your patient go to bed and there remain: she must be kept as cool as possible, with her hips a little raised. The room also must be made and kept as cool as possible. If the discharge of blood is considerable, apply cloths wet with cold water to the birth-place, and even push them up it; at the same time injecting cold water up with a female syring or pewter squirt. There is no danger whatever in these cold applications; therefore do not hesitate to use them if necessary. I have always used *ice* in my practice in Virginia, by putting it in a towel or piece of flannel, and applying it to the belly. If the blood flows rapidly, make a plug with cloth, and push it well up the birth-place; so as to prevent the blood from flowing, or that it may congeal and stop. Should these remedies fail, you must resort to the following remedy, which should only be used in extreme danger:—Mix two grains of sugar of lead with a quarter of a grain of opium; give a pill of this mixture every two hours, made with a little honey, until the discharge of blood is lessened. If the patient is very much exhausted, give laudanum in the dose of fifteen drops, occasionally—or administer opium, see table for the dose: administering either laudanum or opium, according to the urgency of her situation—pains *&c.*, as both these medicines will give strength, and allay the great irritation of the nervous system. Or if there is great pain in the womb, administer a clyster–look under that head. The clyster must be made of the bark of slippery elm, by pouring boiling water on the inside part of the bark. It is to be perfectly cold, and in it put a tea spoonful of laudanum. Throw this clyster up the fundament, out of which passes the stool. These clysters are to be given every hour, until relief is obtained. Every thing used at this time as a drink, should be perfectly cold. Nothing heating of any description ought to be given, either as food or drink, during this great flow of the menses or courses.

To prevent a return of this discharge when once relieved, take moderate exercise: bathe the back and belly frequently in cold water, and take the salt bath—see the head cold bath. Take moderately, the best old Maderia wine; and a short time before the expected discharge, lose some blood from the arm. At all times you are to pay partienlar attention to your bowels: that is not to permit them to become costive or bound. Morning, and night, when you rise or retire to bed, use *friction;* which means rubbing the whole body, for twenty or thirty minutes with a brush or coarse towel—this should be done by a servant or assistant. This last remedy is truly worthy of strict attention.

CESSATION OF THE MENSES OR COURSES.

A cessation of the menses or courses, means an entire stoppage of these discharges, or a change of nature in this respect, at an advanced period of life. This revolution or change takes place, generally speaking, from the forty second to the forty seventh year: it is a critical and extremely dangerous period of a woman's life, and although thousands pass through it without experiencing any great inconvenience, it is a period which requires particular attention and care.

All exposures to cold and damp must be scrupulously avoided; and particularly *wet feet,* and remaining any length of time on the damp ground. Sudden changes of dress are also extremely hazardous at this period; in fact, every thing that produces sudden revolutions in the bodily system, from extremes of heat, cold and dampness. By not attending to what I have laid down, you will be sure to lay the foundation of diseases of a multiplied and stubborn character, which will be sure to embitter and distress the remainder of your life, be it long or short.

The courses about this time of life, begin to lessen in quantity, and to become more or less irregular in their discharges. When you are likely to suffer some inconvenience in this change of *nature*, you will have *warning* by the occurrence of the following symptoms:—You will have pains in the head and small of the back, trembling of the knees, flushing and burning of the face, choaking sensations in the throat, sickness of the stomach, dizziness or swimming in the head, and frequently mists before your eyes. You must now live on spare diet, and as I have just told you, avoid all kinds of cold, damp, and wet.

REMEDIES.

Very few medicines are to be taken in this state of the system, and those that are taken must be of the most simple, mild, and innocent kind. For the purpose of keeping your bowels open, and removing all causes of irritation, use all purges of epsom salts, or castor oil when necessary: they will always cool the system, and allay any dangerous irritations. If you are of a robust and full habit of body, and have dizziness and have pains in the head, *cupping* on the temples, so as to draw some blood will give relief. For the method of *cupping*, which is very simple, look under that head. Or, if you should not like the plan of cupping, or if it be inconvenient, you may occasionally draw a little blood from the arm, when those unpleasant feelings I have described make their appearance. *Temperance*, or in other words, abstaining from strong food, and living on very spare and simple diet, is greatly more important than any medicines that can be taken; nor will any medicines be necessary in most cases, other than such as will keep the bowels in a gentle laxative state, as mentioned before, with cupping if considered necessary. You should take moderate exercise in good weather on horse-back, and above all other remedies, use regularly *friction:* which means rubbing the whole body, twice a day with a brush or coarse towel—*morning* and *evening*. This friction you are not to neglect, because it is very important at this period. You are also, to keep the birth-place perfectly clean, by washing daily those parts, in milk-warm water and soap. Unless these parts are kept perfectly clean, they retain a secretion which I need not name, which *irritates* and *excites diseased action in the womb.* Whenever you feel pain in your *back, belly, &c. &c.*, take the warm or tepid bath, which you are to make sufficiently warm to be pleasant. For a description of this bath, see the head warm or tepid bath. If pain is felt in the *head, stomach* or *breast*, a blister must be applied between the shoulders, which will give relief. You may take off the blister after it has been on two or three hours if the pain has been removed by its application; as is sometimes the case, after the skin has become red from the blister. But the warm bath, moderate bleeding, and keeping the bowels open with the mild medicines I have described, will afford you the necessary ease and relief in your situation, provided you keep yourself in a perfect state of rest, on your bed.

If the pain in the womb be considerable, and you have any fears of an inflammation, in those parts, apply a large blister over the belly—which blister is to be dressed with sweet oil. You are, also to give clysters frequently, which are to be thrown well up the bowels, three or four times a day. They are to be made of slippery elm bark, by pouring boiling water on the inside bark, and letting the water stand until about milk warm; this water is to be thrown up, as directed under the head clystering. If the inflammation is great in the womb, throw up the birth-place, with the clyster-pipe, the slippery elm water, five or six times a day: but remember it is to be perfectly cold, when you throw it up the birth-place: when thrown up the fundament into the bowels, it is to be milk-warm. There is an excellent preparation, which can easily be made, to throw up the *birth-place*, which is perhaps better than the slippery elm water. Take two tea spoonfuls of sugar of lead, and put them in a quart of the coldest water. After the lead is dissolved, it will be fit for use. Of this lead water, throw up about a gill, mixed with a about a gill of slippery elm water. Do this occasionally.

Should an ulcer or sore break out on the legs, or any part of your body, be very careful not to heal it up immediately or very suddenly: it is an effort of *nature* to relieve herself of the discharge. It may be necessary for me to remark, that if the womb is painful, and there is no danger of inflammation, apply over the belly, and to the small of the back, warm herbs, or warm salt; or bladders filled with warm water—and take a dose of laudanum or opium; see table of doses. By attending closely to these instructions, which I have laid down plainly, you will pass through this change of nature with safety, and no doubt, enjoy through the winter of old age, an exemption from those complaints which are too apt to occur, from neglect of this important change of the female constitution.

THE WHITES.

This disease is called by physicians *Fluor Albus*. It is an unnatural and white colored discharge from the birth-place, and is produced from various causes: such for instance, as the power of the womb being impaired, by severe labours, repeated miscarriages, getting out of bed too soon after child-birth; or by taking cold at this time, or any other time when the menses or courses are about coming on; or by over fatigue or weakness, produced by general bad health; or when the general secretions and excretions have been deranged by disease; as the womb always more or less sympathises with the whole system. Women who are of weakly or delecate constitutions, and take but little active exercise, and such as have had many children, are much subject to *fluor albus* or whites. I have known many instances, in which the *whites* make their appearance *monthly*, instead of the natural menses or courses. This is generally the case, where the woman is laboring under the suppression of the menstrual discharge, or some weakness or derangement of the whole system. I shall now describe the means of knowing the *whites* from the *clap*.

In the *clap*, there is a swelling of the parts, an itching and uneasy feeling, and much *heat* in making water. In a little time, both the inside and outside of the parts become inflamed, and give much *heat* and *scalding* in evacuating the urine: if these symptoms occur, you may be tolerably certain you have taken the clap, in which case you will find the means of relief distinctly laid down under the head *clap*.

The whites are called by this name, because the discharges resemble the white of an egg, or the mucus or slime, which runs from the nose when you have a cold. There are three or four stages of this complaint, between its mildest and its severest forms: and if permitted to run on, it will entirely destroy the constitution of the woman, by reducing her flesh and muscular strength. Her complexion will change to a sickly pale color; she will become very weak; and her heart will palpitate or beat, with the slightest personal exertion. As this disorder seldom stops without medical assistance, means ought always to be immediatly used, or it will commit great ravages on the female constitution. The whites come on very irregularly, sometimes the discharge is in lumps, but more frequently, it is of a white, slimy, or ropy consistence. If the disease is of the mildest form, the discharges resemble the white of an egg, having no smell, and no color but that just mentioned. In the second stage, the discharges are of a light yellow or straw color, and something offensive to the smell. In the third stage, the discharges are of a greenish color, of a tough and gluy consistence, and quite offensive in smell. In the *worst stage* of the disease, or when the complaint has been permitted through ignorance or negligence to run on, the discharges are very offensive, and mixed with blood; the face becomes of a sickly greenish hue; under the eyes there is an unnatural color; the lips become purple; the feet and legs swell; the face becomes subject to flushes of heat; there is a dry cough and great difficulty of breathing, particularly on the slightest exertion: and unless relief is obtained, the disease will, *after this stage*, terminate either in *Consumption* or *Dropsy*.

I shall now proceed to describe the effects which the disease produces, in the different stages of its advancement. When it is slight, or in its mildest form, and the general health of the woman is not much impaired, there is a pain in the back, the menses are not regular, and, on the slightest exertion, the woman feels a *shooting*, and afterwards a *heavy pain in the back*. In the second stage, the above symptoms are felt more constantly and severely; the stomach becomes disordered; the head aches; the bowels are costive or bound up; there is a dizziness or swimming in the head; and there seems a heavy pain in the bottom of the belly, and at the upper part of the thighs. In the severest form of the disease, the symptoms of which I have already described, all the indications or marks of dyspepsia or indigestion take place: for a description of which complaint, refer to that head. The whole system becomes disordeied and unhealthy; the menstrual discharge entirely stops; and the woman, from general debility and weakness, sinks rapidly into a decline, and ends either in *Consumption* or *Dropsy*, as I have said before.

REMEDIES.

There is no remedy in the first stage of this complaint equal to scrupulous cleanliness; or bathing well those parts in cold water,, three or four times a day: and injecting up the birth-place, frequently, the same thing, *cold water*. Sleep on a matrass instead of a feather-bed, or in other words, a hard bed of any kind. Rise early, and take proper exercise; and if convenient to a chalybeate spring, or one whose waters are impregnated with iron, drink freely of those waters. The western country abounds with waters of this description; and they are a most valuable remedy for women laboring under this disease, or any irregularity of the menses or courses. The bowels are to be kept open, with mild laxative medicines, such as epsom salts or castor oil. From fifteen to twenty-five drops of *balsam copaiva*, are to be given on sugar, three times a day; which if necessary, are to be continued eight or ten days, or even more if found essential. I have relieved this complaint, when all the different remedies had been tried, by simply using the *turpentine* from the common pine tree.

It must be made into pills with honey, and one of the pills given two or three times a day: using at the same time the following injection, which is to be thrown up the birth-place three or four times a day. A tea spoonful of sugar of lead, is to be put into a pint of spring water, and permitted to remain until dissolved. Obtain at any doctor,s shop, a female syringe, which is a *pewter squirt* with holes in the end of it. With this instrument you are to throw up the lead water, three or four times a day. You will find this a valuable remedy. If it be inconven ent to get the sugar of lead, make a decoction of white oak bark, by boiling it in water—and of this water when perfectly *cold*, throw up the birth-place as often, and about the same quantity that you would of the lead water.

If the discharge is very offensive from the parts, you should introduce up the birth-place every morning and night, about a common tea spoonful of *charcoal*, pounded as fine as possible. This will entirely remove the offensive smell.

If the directions I have given, do not restrain the discharge, you will apply a large *blister* to the small of the back, at the same time using the injections freely as directed. Should the constitution be much injured, and the woman greatly reduced by the discharge, obtain from any doctor's shop, a phial of tincture of martis, which is a preparation of *iron* dissolved in *muriatic acid*. Obtain also a box of *soda powders*. On these boxes you will find directions how to use them; if not look under the head soda powders. When you have mixed your paper of soda powders with water in two tumblers, and before you have poured them together, drop into the tumbler in which you have put the contents of the *blue paper*, eight or ten drops of the medicine in the phial. Being now ready, pour it all into one tumbler, and drink it down immediately while it is foaming or effervessing. This drink should be taken three times a day. I have merely to remark, that this is a preparation of one of the most valuable *mineral waters* known in Europe, and is admirably adapted to debility or indigestion of the stomach, affections of the womb, and indeed debility of any kind. After all these remedies have failed, *polypus* of the womb may exist, which always requires the call of an able physician.

PREGNANCY.

When the sexual connection between a male and female. has been favorable to the increase of our species, the seed of the man and that of the woman are conveyed, as already described, through the *fallopian tubes* into the womb, and there deposited. Here the growth of the *fœtus* or *child* commences, whilst at the same time there is formed, a bag or covering for the whole, (called the membranes,) which lines the womb. At the same time there is a fleshy substance formed, which very much resembles the liver: this substance is called the after-birth, and by physicians the *placenta.* This fleshy substance, called the after-birth, receives and prepares the blood, which is supplied by the womb for tne child. From the after-birth to the navel of the child, there is a small cord or tube called the navel cord, or umbilical cord. This tube admits the circulation of the blood, between the mother and the child. There is also a fluid, known by the name of the waters, in which the fœtus or child moves and increases in growth.

You will now readily perceive, that the womb contains when pregnant, the *child,* the *waters* in which it moves, the *membranes* which support it, the *navel cord,* and the *after-birth.* From eight to ten days after the woman has *conceived,* the first formations of the child may be distinguished; it is however so extremely delecate, as to require the most minute attention to discover it with the naked eye. The face and form of the large features, are as yet not sufficiently plain to be distinguished; you can merely discover the formation of the head and trunk; the trunk being the longest and most delecate: the whole resembling a bit of jelly of an oblong figure. You will perceive, by close examination, the resemblance of a small feather, which comes from the navel, and ends in the membrane by which the whole is enclosed. This fine feathery fibre afterwards the navel cord, connects the young with the after birth.

In about three weeks after conception, the formation of the infant may be plainly distinguished: because by this time, the head and features of the face begin to assume something of a strong outline; in other words they begin to show the realities of what they are. The arms and legs are next seen to project from the body; two black specks represent the eyes—and two extremely small holes make the places of the ear. The ribs on each side are about the size of common threads; and the fingers and toes about the same size or magnitude. The arms are something longer than the legs, in consequence of their growth being more rapid.

In about one month after conception, the fœtus or child is about *one inch* in length: and it now takes a bending posture, in the middle of the water or liquor, I have before described to you. About this time, the *membranes*, sometimes called the bag or covering, become enlarged, and get thicker and stronger, and the whole mass together, is about an inch in length, and nearly the shape of an egg.

In about six weeks, the motion of the heart of the child may be perceived. In fact, in surgical operations which I have seen performed, when the child was taken from the womb, the heart was seen to beat for a considerable length of time.

In three months, the child is three inches in length, and its weight from two to three ounces. Women assert, that they have felt the motion of the child about this time, but I would suppose it doubtful at this early period. In about fourteen weeks, the head of the child is bent forward, and the chin rests on the breast; the knees are lifted up; the legs bent back on the thighs; and both the hands lifted up towards the face.

In the lapse of time, the child acquires more strength, and is constantly changing its posture; but the head most commonly inclines downward. Near the fifth month, the mother can distinctly feel the motion of the child, which is called *quickening*, and which is often accompanied with *sickness* at the stomach, and *vomiting*, particularly in the morning. When this quickening is felt, it is a very certain proof of pregnancy. About the time of this quickening, the womb seems as if it were loose in the lower part of the belly. As long as the womb is detained in the pelvis or basin, you can, by introducing the finger up the birth-place, the woman being in a standing position, distinctly feel the mouth of the womb, which is lower down than in the natural and *unimpregnated* state. This is occasioned, by the weight of the womb and its contents, continually and gradually bearing downward. Thus, the mouth of the womb can be felt, after the woman has become with child, for several weeks, and affords another evidence of pregnancy.

After this time, the womb begins considerably to increase in size, and ascends gradually up into the abdomen or belly, growing at last so large that it remains mostly above the bones of the pelvis or basin, and partially rests on them.

In the beginning of the fifth month, the belly becomes hard, and the navel of the mother is perfectly even and smooth. From this onward, the woman increases in size: pregnancy being now evident, a further description of its progess would be unnecessary. In *nine months*, or in *about forty two weeks* from the stoppag of the menses or courses, the child is prepared for its entrance into life; and *nature* prepares herself for a delivery of her burthen, by a contraction of the fibres of the womb, which are no longer able to bear the irritation. Here commences the pains of labor; in other words, restless and uneasy sensations, pain in the small of the back, frequent desire to make water, accompanied with *bearing downwards*, particularly at the bottom of the belly; constant desire to go to stool, perhaps without being able to pass any thing; costiveness, with a small discharge of mucus or slime from the birth-place, &c. &c.

I have mentioned to you, the waters in which the child moves, and changes its position. As to the quantity of these waters at the birth of the child, it varies very much in different women. In some I have seen not more than a gill; in others not more than half a pint; and in others, I have known nearly two quarts. Those who have written on the subject before me, state that these waters resemble the white of an egg, and have very little smell. This is however, not always the case: the waters are sometimes very offensive. The fact is that their color and consistency depend on the peculiar state of the system.

The *after-birth* prepares the blood in a proper state, which is then conveyed by the navel cord to the child for its support and growth: you will therefore, understand, that the growth is produced through and by the *after-birth.* This after-birth or fleshy substance, which resembles the *liver,* is generally in weight from a pound to a pound and a half; and depends both for weight and size, not on the appearance of the women, but on the health or diseased state of the womb and its secretions. For I have very often seen in my practice, very large women produce quite small after-births, whilst on the contrary, I have seen very delecate women produce astonishingly large ones.

The *navel cord* called by physicians the *umbilical cord,* is formed of *two veins* which come from the *after-birth,* and an *artery* which comes from the child; these being *twisted* nicely together, is the reason why it is called the *navel cord.* The blood which passes through the veins of this cord, enters at the navel of the child; and by the proper vessels is conveyed to its heart: it is then conveyed again back from the heart, to the various parts of the child's body for its growth and support, as I told you before. After returning again, the heart forces it back through the *artery,* which I have mentioned as a part of the *cord,* to the *after-birth,* which prepares it for the fœtus or child.

I have now given you a plain explantion of pregnancy, and the means by which the child is sustained in the womb, and the parts connected with the womb, necessary to be known and understood. This explanation will enable you, with a little attention, to understand something of the astonishing powers possessed and employed by nature, for the procreation, increase, and preservation of the human species,

SIGNS OF PREGNANCY.

Sickness in the morning, often attended with vomiting or puking: heart-burn and sourness of the stomach; loss of appetite, and dislike of the sight of food; craving for things which before you were indifferent to, or even disliked; and *stoppage* of the menses or courses: this last symptom, however, is sometimes occasioned from cold &c. Pregnancy is also known by palpitations, or flutterings of the heart: faintness accompanied with a desire to vomit: these last symptoms are generally felt by young married women in their first pregnancy. The breasts become more full, the nipples more firm and hard, and the rings around them assume a darker color. The rising of the navel so as to become flat and smooth with the belly, may be considered an almost certain evidence of pregnancy. I omitted to mention that tooth-ache is frequently an indication of pregnancy. The pulse of a woman with child is considerably quicker than common: there is also frequently, a dizziness or swimming in the head; the complexion of the face generally changes, either by becoming much improved, or by exhibiting a more sallow, pale, and sickly color. There are few women who do not undergo some peculiar change of countenance in pregnancy, so as to indicate to those well acquainted with them, their real situation. There is, however, no certain sign of pregnancy, but the motions of the child felt by the mother; and all the symptoms I have mentioned, although sufficient to induce the belief of pregnancy, may be deceptive. For instance, the menses or courses may stop, and it may be produced by cold, or some cause other than pregnancy; therefore, until about the third or fourth month, doubts may exist as to the actual situation of the woman.

I have mentioned, that after conception, and before the womb began to rise above the pelvis or basin, by introducing the finger up the birth-place, the mouth of the womb might be plainly felt. This is the fact and the reasons are obvious. The increasing weight of the womb at this period, lowers its mouth in the vagina or birth-place, so that it can be easily touched with the finger; and an experienced physician or midwife, by such an examination could easily tell whether the woman is with child or not. The indications, however. are more plainly felt in young married women, than in one who has borne children. In making this examination, the woman should always be in a standing posture, leaning on the shoulder of the operator, so as to relax the parts as much as possible. In women who have borne children, or suffered injuries from child-birth, the mouth of the womb is very apt to protrude downward through the birth-place, and is called falling down of the womb. This is caused by the ignorance and stupidity of common midwives, from pulling the alter-birth away, and producing this descent of the mouth of the womb. You will be made fully acquainted with this *falling down of the womb* in the proper place.

CAUTIONS

DURING

PREGNANCY.

When the woman discovers her change of situation, or in other words that she is with child, she is to attend to her bowels particularly, so that they may not become costive or bound up. She must steadily bear in mind, that more than half the diseases which arise during pregnancy, are more or less occasioned by neglect to keep the bowels regular. If you cannot have a stool daily, take a clyster of simple milk and water.. There is no indelicacy in this matter. There are instruments called self-pipes, which you can use yourself, and there ought to be one of these in every family. For a description how to prepare and administer clysters, read under that head. I have known many women, who by neglecting their bowels during pregnancy, were compelled to submit to having the hard excrement removed from the fundament, before a passage could be obtained. This is certainly more indelecate than using a clyster-pipe, and merely throwing up a clyster of milk and water; and I do assert. that if these clyster-pipes were more used in the United States; both by women and men, there would be many constitutions saved, and very many diseases and sufferings avoided. Is it not reasonable to presume, that more danger is done to the stomach, by eternally keeping it loaded with drastic purgative medicines, than would be done to the system by the simple use of the clyster-pipe.

Women, during pregnancy, may be said to labor under constant irritation, however delecate their constitutions; and therefore, clysters, not only afford an easy and pleasant passage or stool, but cool the bowels and allay the irritation of the whole system. The tepid bath for directions see that head—ought to be used during pregnancy. It will entirely soothe, not only the bodily irritation, but also tranquilize the mind and feelings. You will recollect, that the water of this bath is to be but pleasantly warm, because hot water has been known to produce *abortion*; which means losing the child. The bathing I recommend, will have an effect to preserve and equalize the healthy action of the womb, and all the parts connected with it. Particular attention should be paid to your diet or food. Let it be simple and plain, and of such a quality as agrees with you. If you will but attend to these instructions, I may assure you that you will pass through this period, not only with safety, but with great comfort, and produce in due time, not only a healthy, but a vigorous offspring.

By all means banish gloomy and depressing fears: nor listen for a moment, to the *idle tales* of misfortunes which are said to have happened to others. All these tales are without a shadow of truth. Think of the countless and innumerable millions, who have passed through these feelings and trials, without the slightest accident. Therefore, place full and implicit confidence in the benevolence, wisdom, and mercy, of that GOD *the Great Father* of the Universe, who rules and governs all human destinies!—Be cheerful, collected, and serene, for in multiplying and replenishing the earth, you are fulfilling an imperious command of an Almighty power, in which he will never desert you,

---

DISEASES

OF

PREGNANCY.

The many diseases to which women are generally liable during pregnancy, mostly arise from the causes I have already enumerated; such as costiveness, improper diet, and so on. The womb at this period is extremely irritable, and always sympathises with the other parts of the system, and particularly with the stomach and head. Some women suffer a great deal during pregnancy, and others very slightly. The fact is, that the mind. the passions, and even the feelings of women, sometimes participate strongly with the physical system *during pregnancy;* not only leaving powerful impressions on the fœtus or child itself, but exercising a strong influence on the very conduct of the woman herself. I hardly need instance such matters as *longings* for particular articles of food, or the vast and countless variety of whims, caprices, sympathies. antipathies, and so on which beset some pregnant women; nor need I point out to the reader, the abortive proportions of birth, and the varieties of injury sometimes sustained by the child, through the mind, imagination, and feelings of the mother.—Pregnancy also, and not unfrequently, exercise a moral influence. I recollect a lady in New York, of the very first respectability, whose husband was long an associate of the legislative coucils of the nation, who never visited or left her house, after she had felt the *quickening sensation* of pregnancy, in other words the *motion of the child,* without experiencing an irresistable propensity to *steal;* nor could she ever combat successfully, or restrain the unaccountable desire to pilfer. This, however, is only one case among a million which might be adduced, to prove the existence of *influences* in pregnancy, which baffle the whole powers of genius and human reasoning.

Doctor Rush, or some other physician of equal celebrity relates the ease of a medical man in some part of Europe, in whose *natural disposition* the propensity to steal was so strong, that he never was known to visit a sick chamber, without stealing some articles of value, if they were not put out of his reach. His practice was very extensive, he was wealthy, and his propensity to theft so well known to society, that after a few years had been passed, in *stealing the same article over and over again,* nothing was said about the matter. The fact is, that he had *stolen* the same artcles só often, shat it became the business of his wife, on his return home every night, to search his pockets, assort out, and send home the articles he had so often stolen. If this delineation of native character be correct, which we are not even permitted to doubt, why need we be surprised at the few instances of a *natural propensity to petty roguery* and *hook-fingered avarice,* which our own country presents? Or why need we be in the least surprised, to find men whose *native* and *irresistable* propensities to swindling, petty fraud, and diminutive rascality, will lead them to cheat in *weight,* and *measures* on all paacticable occasions.

This subject, however, presents itself in another, and a much stronger point of view. It bears strongly on the criminal laws and jurisprudence of our country and must at some future period arrest the attention of our legislative bodies. If there is such an influence in nature, as leads to the commission of crime, and that too in defiance of *moral restraints,* and *fears of punishment,* are there not cases in which *moral justice* would revolt at the punishment of *involuntary* and *irresistable* criminality? I have not space in this work to give this subject such an investigation as it really and intrinsickally merits; but should it be in my power, as I now intend to publish a second volume of this work, when time and circumstances will permit, this subject will be one which shall be particularly embraced. To speak plainly, I have long entertained doubts, whether, under circumstances in which it is practicable to *banish a man from society, deprive him of his liberty, and prevent his committing future crimes*, it can ever appertain to *justice* and the *security of society*, to shed *human blood!*

It is very true, that the scripture thus denounces the murderer:—"whoso shedeth man's blood, by man shall his blood be shed;" but, ought we, not to take into serious consideration, the simple fact, that at the period this penalty of murder was announced to the Jews, *solitary confinement* for life, was unknown to the policy of human laws.

That a diseased state of the mind may exist, on one particular point, and that the same mind may be sound, and sane in all other respects, no medical man in his senses will deny. The daughter of a wealthy merchant of Philadelphia, was in the habit of stealing from the different stores in which she purchased goods. Being extremely wealthy, and her propensity known, *private accounts* of the articles stolen were always kept, and always *duly paid* by her father. She married, and was never known *during her pregnancies* to steal the smallest article: and candidly confessed, that during these periods, she had not the smallest propensity to steal or pilfer; and, what was equally extraordinary, so soon as her deliveries were over, the old and natural propensity to theft returned. How are we to account, on any thing like known principles, for the above facts and delineations of character? Medical philosophers, I propound the interrogatory to you! The value of the articles, this woman often repeated, had nothing to do with the natural impulse to theft: was it a disease of the mind, derived through the physical system, from impressions made on the fœtus or child in the womb, from the mind, and passions, and feelings of the *mother?*

SICKNESS

OF

THE STOMACH.

This is common in the commencement of pregnancy, particularly with the first child; it generally lasts until the quickening sensation is felt, and no longer. If the vomiting or puking is not severe, it will do no injury; but if it should continue or become severe, which is sometimes the case, you will find relief in the following remedies.

REMEDIES.

If the habit of the body be full, that is strong and fleshy, the loss of some blood from the arm will be proper. But if the woman should be weakly and delecate, omit the bleeding, and use the following remedies. Of columbo root and chamomile flowers make a strong tea, in which you may add a little ginger. Let this tea get perfectly cold, and give three or four table-spoonfuls occasionally. Or you may obtain the columbo root in powder, and give fifteen or twenty grains, mixed with a few drops of peppermint, and a little good old spirits of any kind. Or take an ounce of columbo root, and bruise it with a hammer; then pour a pint of boiling water on it, and let it get cold. Take a wine glass of this decoction, with a few drops of peppermint in it, three or four times a day, or when you feel this sickness of the stomach. This bitter is very serviceable in weak stomachs, and laxative bowels. Where the vomiting or puking is very severe, apply the stewed leaves of the garden mint to the pit of the stomach; the application must be warm, and it will stop the vomiting or puking without fail. Or purchase a box of soda powders, on which you will find directions: or if there are no directions, see the head soda powders. Give these powders three or four times a day. Ginger tea, and mint tea are also good remedies. Or use elixir vitriol, in doses of ten or fifteen drops, three or four times a day, in a glass of cold water. Should the vomiting be extremely severe, rub a little laudanum over the pit of the stomach; if this does not stop it, give ten or fifteen drops of laudanum occasionally in a little mint or ginger tea. In very stubborn cases of vomiting, the following will always give relief. Mix in a phial, equal quantities of *compound spirit of lavender, laudanum,* and *spirits of harts horn.* Of this mixture, give a tea spoonful in a little cold water, three or four times a day, or as the sickness and vomiting may take place.

COLIC.

This is a common complaint during pregnancy; and this is the reason why I have cautioned you so particularly, respecting your diet or food, and by all means to avoid costiveness, or in other words, by permitting yourself to be too long a time without a stool. The bowels during the time you are with child, will always be much subject to flatulence or wind, which is called in the country *windy colic.*

REMEDIES.

Bathe the belly with warm water: or sit in a tub in which there is warm water, and take a table spoonful of castor oil. Or you may apply to your belly warm salt. Or you may apply cloths wrung out of warm water to the belly, and throw up the fundament with the clyster pipe, the following injection. Make a pint or quart of thin gruel: strain it clean, and put into it a table spoonful of hog's lard or less: let it stand until it becomes milk warm, and take it as a clyster. See the head clystering.

PAIN IN THE HEAD

AND

DROWSINESS.

When there is pain in the head, or a heavy dull drowsiness is felt, it is apt to arise from the blood vessels being too full. This is generally the case, with fleshy, strong, healthy young women. In delecate and weakly women, pain in the head and drowsiness are sometimes felt; but they generally arise from an opposite cause, from a want of due circulation of the blood, which induces debility or weakness.

REMEDIES.

If the woman is fleshy and strong, and is thus afflicted, draw blood from the arm; and give a dose of laxative medicine, such as epsom salts, castor oil, &c. But if, on the contrary, she be delecate and weakly, bleeding in any way would be highly improper. She is to take moderate exercise on horse-back: attend to the state of her stomach, and also to her food; use freely the tepid bath, see that head; take very gentle medicines, or a clyster to keep her bowels regular if bound; bathe her forehead and temples frequently with spirits, in which camphor has been dissolved: and take occasionally through the day, a glass of real good wine, or some toddy, made with any kind of spirits. If this pain, or heaviness of the head still remains, after the above means have been resorted to, it may arise from the stomach: if so, the columbo root, as already described, will be found of great benefit.

HEART BURN.

This complaint generally arises from *acid* in the stomach, and very few women escape it during pregnancy. If the heart burn is attended with a constant hawking up of a tough phlegm, the stomach should be cleansed with a gentle emetic or puke, of fifteen or twenty grains of *ipecacuanha.* But if the heart burn is accompanied with a sour taste in the mouth, or a belching up of sour water, it will be relieved by the use of very weak lime water, or a tea spoonful of *magnesia* in a cup of cold water. This last, or either of them, may be taken whenever these acid tastes take place. The magnesia is generally preferred in lumps, and may be eaten in moderate quantities, being perfectly innocent. When a considerable lump is used, it will act as a mild purgative. By adding a little rhubarb to the magnesia, it is an excellent purge for women in a pregnant state. As both articles are quite innocent, they may always be used, when found necessary for opening the bowels.

SWELLED LEGS.

This swelling is produced by the womb, which is enlarged during pregnancy: the weight of the womb presses on the vessels which return the fluid from the lower parts on the body. When the woman is far advanced, these swellings frequently give much pain: there is however, no danger: nor should they give any distress to the afflicted woman. These swellings are very apt to go off if she will take rest on a bed, bathe her feet at night in strong salt and water, or steam herself over mullen on which boiling water has been poured. As rest in a recumbent or lying posture, lessens very much these swellings, it would be advisable for the woman to remain as quiet as possible, and lose a little blood from the arm occasionally. Attention to these things, with a little cooling medicine, such as epsom salts, or a little cream of tartar, will nearly always allay these swellings of the legs.

CRAMP.

Cramp generally comes on about the fourth month after pregnancy, and is often very troublesome at night, while the woman is in bed. Its attacks are generally in the legs and thighs, but sometimes in the bottom of the belly and hips. Those women who have never before been subject to cramp, are very apt to have attacks of it, during the last stages of pregnancy.

REMEDIES.

When the cramp is frequent and severe, the loss of a little blood will be proper. Cramp sometimes arises from costiveness or constipation of the bowels: when this is the case, you may give a clyster, or a cooling purge, such as epsom salts.—Standing a few minutes on a *cold hearth* with the *feet bare*, as a simple remedy, and will always give relief. I have known a small garter or belt, in which was confined some pounded brimstone or flour of sulphur, relieve several ladies who were much subject to cramp.

CONSTANT DESIRE

TO

MAKE WATER.

The constant desire to make water, or pass off the urine, is occasioned by the weight of the womb constantly pressing on the neck of the bladder. Whenever this desire becomes troublesome, rest quietly on your bed as much as possible, taking at the same time a cooling purge. If convenient, and whether so or not, the use of the warm or tepid bath will be very beneficial: by which I mean that the whole body is to be placed in water a bout *milk warm* if this be impracticable, for a want of a vessel large enough, you may sit once a day in a tub of water of this warmth. The fact is, that by bathing occasionally in water milk warm, during any stage of pregnancy, much benefit will always be derived.

STOPPAGE OF URINE.

This is called suppression of urine by physicians, and means when the water is stopped from flowing from the bladder, at those periods when nature requires the evacuation. When this stoppage takes place, the bladder becomes distended or swelled with the water, and is also severely painful. Relief must immediately be had, by applying to the lowest part of the belly, cloths wrung out of warm water, and taking a clyster of warm milk and water: see the head clystering. Clystering is extremely beneficial, in this and all similar cases, and women should be early taught to know, not only that there is no indelecacy in the operation, but that in all warm climates it is absolutely essential to most women in a state of pregnancy. All the *lying in* hospitals of Europe, are furnished amply with the apparatus for clystering; but in the western country of America, where there is certainly as much general intelligence as in any part of the world, seems that you might as well desire a lady to swallow an elephant, as to take a clyster instead of a purgative medicine. This is all *false modesty;* the women of all countries ought to know, that the more simply the diseases are treated, and the more according to nature, the better will their health and safety be ensured. After the remedies just mentioned, have been used without affording relief, you are to send for a physician, who will draw off the water with a *catheter:* for a description of which, and the mode of using it, look under the head *catheter.*

WANT OF SLEEP.

On or about the last stage of pregnancy, most women become restless and uneasy, and their sleep very much disturbed. They are also troubled with a choaking sensation, and a difficulty of getting their breath. This last affliction is sometimes so great, that they are sometimes obliged to get out of bed, and throw up a window to get fresh air, which generally relieves them.

If the woman who is subject to these unpleasant feelings, be of a robust and unpleasant habit of body, the loss of a little blood from the arm will be proper; in addition to which, some mildly laxative medicine ought to be taken to open the bowels. If the woman is of a delecate constitution, and much debilitated or weakened, bathe her feet and legs in strong *salt* and *water*, made pleasantly warm, before she retires to bed; and give her fifteen or twenty drops of laudanum; or if laudanum cannot be had, give her a glass of toddy, made with any kind of spirits.

PILES.

This is an uneasy and troublesome complaint, which frequently attends on pregnancy, and generally afflicts fat stout women. The fact is, however, that most women are subject to *piles*, after the fifth or sixth month. In addition to the remedies I shall mention here, for further information refer to the head *Piles*, where you will find a full description given of piles.

Women who have never before been troubled with this disorder, are apt to be afflicted with it, as I have just mentioned, during the last months of pregnancy. It is almost invariably produced from costiveness or constipation of the bowels. The common oak-ball pounded fine, and stewed down in butter without salt, is an excellent remedy. The parts are occasionally to be rubbed with this ointment; whilst at the same time you are to take a gentle purge.

You may also, occasionally bathe the parts in cold water. Or you may put a tea spoonful of sugar of lead, into a pint of cold spring water, and frequently bathe the parts with it during the day. As much rest as possible is to be taken; in other words, walk or ride about as little as possible.

FALSE PAINS.

These pains resemble the pains of labor very much, and are frequently the cause of alarm, and much inconvenience to all concerned. False pains are always produced from some deranged state of the system; or from the improper conduct of the woman herself, by excessive and sometimes slight fatigue. Anxiety of mind; sudden exposure to cold or heat; want of attention to the bowels; indigestion, or eating such articles of food as produce wind in the bowels, will frequently produce these pains. Dysentary accompanied with severe griping, will also produce these pains.

When these pains occur frequently, it will be proper to employ an experienced physician, because their too frequent presence may produce miscarriage, or in other language, the loss of the child. On discovering the pains to be false, which must be ascertained by the physician or midwife, either of whom should be well acquainted with the mode of conducting an *examination*, they are to be removed as speedily and easily as possible. If there is much pressure on the mouth of the womb from above, and if it is perceived to dilate or open during the continuance of the pains—they are not false, and the woman may be considered in labor: but, if neither pressure nor dilation or opening can be felt, *the pains* are *false*, and are to be removed.

When these false pains are caused by fatigue, the patient should be kept as quiet as possible, and take the necessary rest to remove the fatigue. If she be of a feverish disposition, she must lose a little blood; and generally, it will be proper to give a gentle dose of laxative medicine, or some mild and opening clyster.

FLOODING.

Flooding is a disease incidental to pregnancy, often of a dangerous and fatal character, in which there is a loss of blood from the womb: It is, fortunately, of not very frequent occurrence; but when it does come on, you are to lose no time in obtaining a skilful and experienced physician. It is a case in which merely common skill and experience will seldom answer; because it is frequently attended with abortion, and often with the loss of life. Flooding is usually produced by a sudden fall, by over exertion, by fright and alarm, and not unfrequently, by the *gloomy* and *depressing passions of the mind.* It is also produced, by weakness of the womb, originating in miscarriage, or other injuries derived from severe labor in child-birth. It also, sometimes arises, from the *after-birth* separating from the *womb*, and the large blood vessels entering into it, discharging their contents through the mouth of the womb. This complaint is very alarming to persons well acquainted with its dangers; because death frequently comes on suddenly, and with very little warning of its approach.

No discharges of blood ever take place from the womb in a natural and sound state of pregnancy; the idea of regular discharges in pregnancy, is entirely erroneous, and perfectly farcical; and whenever they do take place, they always prove to the man of skill and judgment, that there is something *wrong*. They are always either produced from the passage of the womb, or from the womb itself.— When they merely come from the passage to the womb, they are seldom if ever attended with danger; but when they proceed from the womb itself, there is considerable danger that disagreeable consequences may be the result. When but a little blood comes away from much walking or riding, or from standing in an upright posture, and there is only a trifling pain in the lower part of the belly, attended with no symptoms of fever, and no increased or inflammatory action of the blood vessels, the blood may always be presumed to come from the passage to the womb. This can always be removed, and that very easily, by lying a short time in a recumbent or horizontal position, and afterwards avoiding much walking and riding, and long continuation of standing in an upright posture. But, mind me particularly, when the discharge of blood is preceded, or accompanied with flushings of the face, considerable heat in the palms of the hands, and *great thirst;* or when there are great pains in the lower part of the abdomen or belly, in the loins, or in the back, it is evident that the discharge of blood is from the womb itself, and also that there is much danger.

REMEDIES.

The first step to be taken, when the flooding proceeds from the womb itself, and may therefore be considered dangerons, is to place the woman in bed. and to keep her as cool as possible, by removing the bed clothes, admitting the cool and fresh air; and, as you value the life of your patient, give her nothing to eat or drink of an inflammatory or heating nature; in other words, nothing that will *increase the action of the blood vessels:* I have told you before, that in this case, which is a dangerous one, a skilful physician must be obtained if possible. The women should be immediately bled from the arm, freely, copiously, and *rapidly,* so as to produce *fainting:* because this is the moment if ever, when those clots of blood are formed and congealed, which put a stop to the great discharge of the blood vessels. Apply at the same time, to the belly, cloths wet with the coldest water, or even ice wrapped in very thin cloths, if it can possibly be procured. If the blood should still continue to flow in any considerable quantity, a soft piece of cloth ought to be introduced up the birth-place, also wet with cold water. These cold applications, however, ought not to be continued so long as to produce a *chill;* but, while they are continued, they ought to be occasionally and often renewed. A clyster of cold water occasionally thrown up the fundament, will also be very effective in stopping this flooding.

If the above remedies should fail, which is sometimes the case, you are to give the patient *two grains* of sugar of lead *every hour*, for five, six, or even seven hours. This is a powerful remedy, and most generally an effective one. You may, also, put twenty or twenty-five grains of sugar of lead in a quart of water: and when it is dissolved, you may throw about one fourth of it up the bowels, and with the residue occasionally wash the birth-place—these measures will greatly assist the cure; and if necessary they may be repeated two or three times. The last remedies mentioned, are generally attended with relief; but there is always considerable danger of the return of the flooding. Therefore, it is very immaterial, how well the patient may feel after relief, she must continue in bed three or four weeks, and be kept cool and quiet, and always ready for the application of cold wet cloths to the belly, and also up the birth-place: her situation will still be dangerous for that length of time, and without this cautious and circumspect conduct, she may still be lost without three hours warning of her fate. If, however, all these remedies should fail to stop the flooding, and to prevent its reaching the stage in which the woman must inevitably perish, an *abortion* must be resorted to, as the only possible means of saving her life.

ABORTION,

AND THE MEANS TO BE OBSERVED IN PREVENTING OR PROCURING IT.

I intend by *abortion*, the expulsion of the fœtus or child, at such an early period of pregnancy, that the child is either dead when it is brought forth, or dies soon afterwards. Whilst speaking of *flooding*, many of the symptoms and circumstances attending miscarriage or abortion are named; but, there are several others which precede and cause abortion, which must be particularly mentioned. They are the following; and are always to be guarded against or removed by pregnant women, if they wish to preserve their burthens, until the expiration of the period fixed by nature. Severe and oppressive exercise; violent and sudden exertions of strength; sudden and agitating frights; fits of excessive and violent passion; excess of venery, by which I mean too frequent sexual communication with the male; a morbid or diseased state of the womb; external injuries of all descriptions which affect the generative organs; and general and excessive debility or weakness of the whole system. I say nothing of those means of procuring abortions, which are sometimes used by pregnant women, with the *intention* of relieving themselves of their charge: these are matters to be referred to the lofty and unerring tribunal of God himself; they are accounts between such woman and their Maker!

Generally speaking, before abortion comes on, there will be felt some slight pains about the lower part of the belly, and also in and about the loins: there will be a looseness and flabbiness about the breasts, and some general sensations of shuddering and boldness; and in women of full, strong, and muscular habits of body, there will nearly always be some considerable degree of fever. Next to these symptoms, slight discharges of blood will take place from the womb; and these discharges will continue to increase, perhaps occasionally stopping a short time until they amount to absolute *flooding*, which I have already particularly described. When these discharges return, after they have become copious and debilitating, they are always attended with a sense of *dead weight*, and a heavy *bearing down* about the womb, great *sickness of the stomach*, and sometimes *frequent faintings*. These are self evident indications, of immediate miscarriage or abortion, which soon takes place; and is always followed by profuse bleeding, which however soon subsides. After the expulsion of the contents of the womb, and the bleeding has gone off, there is a serous or watery discharge mixed with a little blood; but this is a matter of no consequence.

This is an abortion, according to the dictates and operations of nature herself. It may sometimes, however, be avoided, by observing the following simple treatment:—On the occurrence of the first symptoms of abortion, the woman must be placed in bed, and kept cool and quiet until the matter be decided. If she is of a full and strong habit of body, she must be bled. Every thing of a heating, irritating, and stimulating nature, either as food or drink, must be entirely avoided. Nothing but cold water or very weak tea is to be drunk by the patient. The bowels may be opened, if costive, and kept open, by merely injecting up them some milk warm water. The *irritation* of the *womb* is to be lessened immediately, and much as possible: to effect the lessening or reduction of this irritation, the woman ought to be placed in a tub of warm water; and when taken out, to have large quantities of sweet oil rubbed about her back, loins, belly, and breasts. If these means fail in preventing the abortion, nature will effectuate the expulsion of the child, in the manner I have just described. She may, however, be assisted in her exertions, by the following means. The woman is to be kept quiet, and treated as in common labor; after which, cloths wet with cold water must be applied to the belly, to aid in the contraction of the womb, after the expulsion of its contents.

When abortion is to be brought on, in order to stop profuse and dangerous *flooding*, it is to be done in the following simple and easy manner. I will here adopt the language of Doctor Bard with some abreviations. The woman is to be brought down to the edge of the bed, either lying on her side, with a pillow or two between her thighs, which are to be drawn up—or lying on her back, with her hips a litte raised, and her feet on the lap of an assistant *on each side*. The operator must sit on a *low seat* immediately before her: whilst a double sheet, thrown over her body and that of the physician or mi wife, must protect her from cold, and form a decent covering. The hand of the operator, well rubbed with good oil or hog's lard, with the fingers collected into a point, must then be slowly introduced through the birth-place into the mouth of the womb; which will sometimes make considerable resistance against attempts to open it. This resistance must be overcome by cautious, gentle, and patient efforts. When the mouth of the womb begins to dilate or widen with the efforts of the operator, one of the fingers must be introduced into it, then another and so on, until by patience and gentle attempts it admits the hand. The efforts to dilate or widen the mouth of the womb, and you must remember this particularly, is always to be *suspended* or *stopped*, whenever the *pains come on*, and whilst they are *on*. In other words, whenever the *pains cease*, you are to proceed, in your efforts to widen gently the mouth of the womb. When the hand passes into the womb, it is to be opened and laid flat; this will prevent a contraction on the knuckles, which might rupture the neck of the womb, and do much injury. The mouth of the womb being sufficiently widened; if the hand can then be easily passed over the parts of the contents, called by physicians the placenta or after-birth, which are *separated* from the womb until the fingers reach the membranes, this is to be done; and breaking the membranes, it is to be immediately passed into the womb.—But if you cannot readily pass the separated portion of the *placenta*, and the *flooding be great*, you are to pass through it: which is less dangerous than to separate the *larger portion*, by passing the hand between it and the womb. The hand being now in the womb, the neck will generally cling so close to the wrist, as to prevent the escape of much water, and you will find room to act with freedom. Here you are to deliberate, and to refresh the woman with some proper drink. You ought now to get at the *feet* of the child, by all practicable and gentle means. You are to recollect, that the most *natural presentation* is the most common; and that in that case, the child's head is at the brim of the pelvis or basin with the *face* and *belly* to the back of the mother, the knees bent to its breast, and the *feet* towards the *upper part* of the womb. As therefore, the child must ultimately be *turned*, this is the best time to *push the head and shoulders* up towards the fundus, and to turn the face of the child to the back of the mother; which is most easily done *within the membranes*: by this movement the feet of the child will be brought within reach of the hand; and having secured them, they may easily be brought, by a waving motion into the vagina or birth-place. You are always to remember, that you are to pause, whenever a pain comes on. Next, you are to bring down the hips and body of the child; and take care, if it be necessary, to turn the child gently, so that when it is delivered to the arm-pits, the belly of the child shall be to the back of the mother, which is the position in which the arms and head can be most easily delivered. Now or before this time, examine the navel string, and occasionally pull it down a little, so as to prevent its being stretched. If the pulsation has ceased in the cord, or if the woman floods freely, either the child or the mother may be lost by delay; and you are to finish the delivery as soon as you prudently can, in doing which, you are, always to remember, that *gentleness*, *caution* and *dexterity*, are always to be used in preference to *force*.

There are few conditions more truly dangerous and alarming, than flooding to any excess, toward the expiration of the natural term of pregnancy; and I therefore strongly, and most emphatically advise, that in all such cases, where an experienced and skilful physician can possibly be had, he be immediately sent for—and especially where a forced abortion is essential to the preservation of the life of the woman. Such cases always require the skill, judgment, promptness of conduct, and decision of resolution; he must therefore, be a man who can decide coolly, and act with firmness and caution. After the delivery, or rather the *abortion* has been produced, the womb may be assisted in its contraction, and the flooding retarded and stopped, by the means I have already noticed so plainly: in addition to which, the rest of the woman will be promoted, and her recovery much hastened, by small or weak anodynes, in some cordial julep, such as spirituous cinnamon water, or a little good weak toddy with nutmeg. These are the remedies first called for: and they are to be succeeded by small portions of nourishing diet, repeated with caution whenever called for, and by strengthening articles, such as tonics in which peruvian bark has been infused and Port Wine in which cinnamon bark has been infused.

LABOR.

The commencement of labor means, the time the woman begins to be delivered of her child. She is always warned of the approach of her time, by pains which are called *labor pains.* They are produced by contraction or drawing up of the womb, which at the *commencement* expells or forces out a *slimy matter*, generally colored with blood, which is called the *shew.* As soon as this matter is discharged, the mouth of the womb, at each pain, begins to open and widen itself; so as to permit the contents of the womb to pass. You will recollect, that I have before informed you, what the womb in pregnancy contains. These pains increase gradually, the belly diminishes in size, and the womb seems to sink, or approach nearer to the birth-place. The pains at first are quite short, and only come on after considerable intervals: the woman is now restles, first hot, then cold, and not unfrequently sick at the stomach. She is also, often griped, and frequently belches wind, or passes it off backward, which should never be restrained from false delicacy. These pains now fly quickly to the back, and then again to the bottom of the belly. The woman has now a great desire to *urinate*, or make water frequently, and to go to *stool.* These inclinations are always to be attended to; because emptying the bladder, and evacuating the bowels frequently before actual child-birth comes on, are highly important and ought never to be neglected. The pains having been sharp, and some-time between them, she then begins to be uneasy and fretful, and requests something to be given her, to bring the pains on more rapidly.

This is the precise point of time in which so many injuries are done, by ignorance and officiousness, in attempting to force nature in to premature exertions; who if let alone a little while, would in almost all cases perform her office, according to the dictates of *divine wisdom*, and with safety both to the mother and child. for you may be assured, that what you so much dread, is intended for your eventual benefit, by permitting the womb, *gradually* to distend or open, with perfect safety to the parts and in order that you may be blessed with an *easy birth*, and a living and uninjured offspring. You will always know the pains I now speak of, by an irresistable desire to catch hold of every thing within your reach, such as the bed-stead, a chair, and so on. These pains, as I have already told you, arise from the constant efforts of *nature* to open the mouth of the womb; and they must and will continue, until she accomplishes her end,

When this is the case, and the mouth of the womb is sufficiently widened, *nature* will immediately commence her efficient and powerful operations, to press down the infant so as to empty the womb. You will immediately know this change, by a *pressing down pain*, if I may be allowed the expression, which gradually increases to a strong sensation of *bearing down*. Although these forcing pains are powerful and strong, yet the woman will bear them with more apparent ease and forti ude, than those which were felt in the first stage of *labor* At this time, the membranous bag which contains the *child* and the *waters* which surround it, and which I have before described to you, is pushed out of the womb *by degrees* at every pain. The distance which this bag extends out, varies in size in different women; sometimes it is very small, and sometimes of considerably larg dimensions. It continues gradually to force open, and to widen the mouth of the womb, until it opens the parts sufficiently to permit the *head of the child to pass*. You will now perceive, that by these gradual exertions of *nature*, to arrange and prepare all things properly, those delecate parts, which by sudden and powerful exertions would have been torn and seriously injured, are now sufficiently enlarged to permit the birth of your infant without injury. And you will also discover, by what I have just disclosed to you, that if nature is hurried by an imprudent physician or midwife, by forcing the child away before the parts are sufficiently widened, great and signal injuries *must* be the consequences, both to the woman and child.

As soon as the parts are sufficiently prepared for the birth of the child, this membranous bag bursts open and the waters are discharged: sometimes however, these events take place at an early period of the *labor.* When this is the case, the labor is never so easy as under other circum stances. The quantity and quality of this water, differ in different women, as I have before to told you. When these waters then burst forth in proper time which I have pointed out, the *bearing down* pain continues, and the child gradually enters into the world. As soon as the child's head *passes,* the woman's relief is very great, and a little rest ought to be allowed her; you are by no means to pull the body out by force; for by so doing, you will produce great injury to the soft parts, and at the same time render it very difficult to deliver the woman of the *after-birth.*

I must here remark *emphatically,* that this is another stage of *labor,* at which thousands of women are injured materially and fatally, by the hurry and officiousness of midwives, in hastily forcing the birth. Give time and I will ensure that nature will exercise sufficient power to expell the child in her own time.—The *body of the child* is not to be pulled and forced outward: let it a lone—converse with the sufferer, and cheer her spirits: and tell her that from the time the child's head makes its appearance, she is not to *force* and *bear down.* Tell her that by so doing, she will force the child forward before the parts are ready; and, that the consequence may be the tearing or rupturing the *perineum.* This is the part between the fundament and birth-place. Tell her that such an injury would leave her in a wretched condition for life, and must be avoided by all means. It is the duty of the midwife or physician, as the child's head passes to keep one hand pressed firmly, yet *cautiously* against the perineum which must of course, from distention or stretching, be very thin and easily torn: and at the same time *gently press* so as to incline the head of the child upward toward the *pubes*.

When the woman has rested, and the pains again come on, the hand must again be pressed against the perineum with steadiness and care, until the shoulders and hips of the child pass, at the same time gently supporting the child —and the delivery is over so far.

The child being now *born*, you are to permit it to be still a few minutes without being molested. Give it *fresh air*, and *time to breathe*, and the *pulsation in the navel cord* will begin to diminish. This pulsation by all means should be suffered to subside before you *separate* the child from the mother. You will then, with a waxed thread, or a small string, make a moderately firm tie about the navel cord, about three inches from the navel of the child. Then make another tie, about three inches further from the child on the navel cord, and cut the cord asunder between the two ties, with a scissors or sharp knife.

You are now to hold steadily, but by no means as you value the life of the mother, to pull the navel cord which has been tied and cut off: because this cord is attached to the after-birth, which is till in the body of the mother, and is yet to be delivered. Permit me to caution you, to implore you, to *command* you not to pull away by force the after-birth; for I do now know some of the finest women in the United States, who are suffering daily and hourly, and will continue to suffer during their lives, from officiously and imprudently forcing away from them the after-birth—which *nature* herself would have effected, without risk or pain, had she been left to her own exertions. By pulling away the after-birth, before the proper time, and before nature expells it, by what are called *after-pains*, the consequences will and must always be *flooding* and *great loss of blood;* because you force the separation before you give time for the contraction of the *blood vessels*—in other words, before the *mouths of the blood vessels*—have had time to close. In fact, the exercise of common sense cannot fail to teach you, that where the after-birth is yet connected with, and strongly adheres to the womb, force will always tear the womb from its connexions, and be productive of unspeakable injuries. From this plain statement of facts, and the reasoning I have employed, I am convinced you will exercise due caution, in a matter of such vast importance to the future *health* and *safety* of the mother.

According to the old usage and practice, the child would be immediately washed in warm water, and not unfrequently in spirits. Either of these plans of treating the *infant*, in fact, both of them are highly improper, and have been the means of destroying thousands of children. Warm water or spirits ought never to be used in this manner, unless the infant be born apparently dead; in such a case, warm water merely is to be applied. For a further explanation of this important matter, look under the head, treatment of new-born infants.

The woman having rested for a short time, after her separation from the child in the manner I have described to you, the *after-pains* may be expected to come, for the expulsion of the *after-birth*. These pains are produced by the contraction or drawing up of the womb, to deliver or expell this *after-birth:* they generally come on, in the lapse, of from fifteen minutes, to an hour, after the child has been brought forth. You are now to remember, that none but gentle and simple measures are to be used, in order to produce the expulsion or delivery of the after-birth. You are now to rub the belly of the woman, and gently extend or pull the *cord*, at the same time that she blows with *some force* into the palms of her own hands; the policy of this blowing is obvious: it will cause a gentle and natural *bearing down*, without *straining* which would arise from *holding* and *forcing* the breath. If the woman be healthy and stout, if she has lost no blood, and if she feels able; let her *stand up*, and support herself on the shoulders of the operator or physician, while he is endeavoring by the means just pointed out, to relieve her of the after-birth. I have, however, often succeeded in delivering the after-birth when the womb would not contract, and when the woman was in a lying posture, by introducing the finger up the birth-place, and gently turning it round in the mouth of the womb; in this case, the sensation felt in the mouth of the womb, will generally cause it to contract and expell the contents.

If all these means fail, and an hour pass without the expulsion of the *after-birth*, you are to introduce your hand with great caution, (the parts being very sore,) and open your fingers inside and round the edges of the womb; at the same time that you feel cautiously, and slowly separate, between the edges of the after-birth and the womb, any parts which may adhere as the womb gradually closes. When the *after-birth* is expelled or brought away, and any great discharge of blood takes place, apply to the belly some cloths wet with cold water, and put one up the birth-place as directed in flooding. The woman is then to be wiped or very gently rubbed dry, and suffered to rest quietly for several hours.

DIFFICULT LABOR.

Most cases of tedious labor, arise among women with their first child, with women who have married late in life, and with those who are so healthy, robust, and corpulent, that the parts seem to relax so slowly, as hardly to permit the birth of the child. The loss of some blood from the arm will be proper; and I have frequently after bleeding, put them in warm water—in doing this however, you must be careful as to the child. I have known instances in which women have had their children in the close-stool or pot, while in the act of endeavoring to urinate or have a steel. The warm bath and bleeding will relax the system, sufficiently in all probability for the child to be born: but take care that the child is not injured by the water while the woman is in the bath.

When *convulsions or fits* take place during labor, and the woman has before complained of great pain in the head, and dimness with loss of sight, remember that you are to bleed freely, and to open the bowels with clysters, or some gentle laxative medicine. The most powerful means, and the best known for relieving tedious or difficult labor, is blood letting from the arm; and it should always be done if the woman is strong, healthy, and of a vigorous constitution.

TWINS.

What I have already said on the subject of labors, relates to cases in which nature presents the mother with but one offspring from a pregnancy. You are well aware, however, that she sometimes presents a parent with two children; and, in the western country, if rumor speak the truth, she in more than one instance, has not even stopped at this number. In about ninety nine cases out of a hundred, the directions I have given you, which relate to the birth of one child, will be found sufficiently ample and particular; but I must not omit to instruct you also, as to cases of child birth, in which more than one child is to be born.

It is not easy to ascertain, that there are twins, or more than twins to be born, until after the birth of the first child; and if there are three to be born, not until after the birth of the second. Where twins are to be produced, the membranes of both children may be felt at the birth place, sometimes before the delivery of oue of them, but not often; and sometimes, but very seldom, it may be distinguished on examination, that different parts of both children present themselves. Twins are always considerably smaller than single children, which generally causes their birth to be more easy and rapid: in fact the rapidity of a first birth, generally produces the first suspicion that there are twins. Generally speaking, immediately after the birth of the first child, another may be felt by very accurate pressure on the belly of the mother. But if the womb be very capacious or large, rather than subject yourself to great uncertainty, the hand may be very cautiously and gently introduced, and the child distinguished by the touch. Where there are twins, the second child is brought forth, within about an hour of the first, and in a position directly contrary to the first: so that when the first is presented with the head foremost, the second may always be expected, with the breech or feet foremost.

"The first child being delivered," says Doctor——, "as prescribed in single cases, some time must be allowed to recruit the woman's strength, and to afford nature time for bringing on the next delivery. There are cases, in which it would be necessary to wait even three or four hours. 1st. When artificial aid was used in the first case. 2d. When the child presents unnaturally. 3d. When fits of flooding come on.

When both children present naturally, and the labour of the first ends without aid, and without much fatigue to the patient, I wait for the secondary pains; but should these not come on in a reasonable time, *four hours*, I introduce my hand cautiously, and rupture the membranes; when, commonly, the second child passes readily through the pelvis or basin. If the first labor has been natural, and the second child presents in a wrong direction, I have generally, without delay, extracted it by the feet. If the first labor has been unnatural, with but little delay, the membranes are to be ruptured; and, whether the child should be brought down immediately, and delivered by the feet or not, the operating physician or midwife must decide. The rules applicable to twins, will equally apply to cases where there are three or more children."

Where a woman has brought forth twins, or more, great care and attention are necessary to prevent her from fainting. She should, therefore, not have her head raised or elevated: and even in moving, should have herself rolled over in the bed. A broad bandage round the belly, should never be omitted in the case of twins, to support the belly of the mother. The directions I have already laid down, respecting the *after-birth* of single children, are fully and entirely applicable in the cases of twins, and more children even than two.

DIRECTIONS

FOR

MIDWIVES.

The following remarks are especially intended for the *serious* consideration and benefit of *midwives;* and, indeed of all such as are in the practice of *officiating* in the delivery of pregnant women. Regularly *bred* and *licensed* physicians, are always presumed to *know* their duties, and to *perform* them with skill and judgment, in this highly responsible department of their profession. The practice of *midwifery,* by those who are not regularly taught the medical profession, and who are presumed to know little or nothing about the real organization of the human system, implies the assumption of a most awful and dangerous responsibility; especially when it is considered, that the *fatal consequences,* of *ignorance* and *presumption* if combined with total disregard of moral feelings, duties, and principles, are nearly as chargeable with criminality as if they proceeded from voluntary and intentional violations of the laws of GOD! There is very little difference, in other words, between the disregard of those duties which are enjoined by the laws of justice and humanity, and their palpable and unconditional *violation.*

The directions which I shall lay down for your considerate adoption, will be plain, simple, and natural; they will be obscured by no technical language, and rendered unintelligible to you by none of the mysteries of the medical profession; and if you scrupulously attend to them; they will enable you to be successful in ninety nine cases of midwifery out of a hundred, in which you may be engaged. If you wish to be esteemed great and skilful in your calling, and if you desire to be an instrument in the hands of *Divine Providence*, for affording consolation and relief to your sex in the hour of affliction, treasure up the salutary advice, and never lose sight of it, that you *are never to force nature*; that you are *to give her time to perform her operations*; and, that *if you have any doubt as to the success of the delivery, you are to run no risks*, but to call in the aid of a *skilful* and *experienced physician*. By attending to this course of conduct, you will relieve yourself of dangerous responsibilities, discharge your duties to a fellow creature, and appear in the presence of your *Creator*, with the consciousness of having acted in obedience to the most solemn injunctions of humanity.

1st. Immediately on your being called to deliver a woman, your first inquiry of her should be as to the state of her bowels, whether she has had a stool, and whether she is bound or constipated in her bowels. I need not tell you, that the discharge of the bowels, and also of the urine or water from the bladder, are both *important* and even *necessary*—first, in preventing injuries to the parts, as the child enters the world—and second, to render the labor and birth more easy and safe. You will of course, therefore, strictly attend to these evacuations, and in proper time.

2d. You are now to ascertain and determine, whether *actual labor* has taken place or not; and, the only certain and satisfactory signs of actual labor, are such as I have before minutely described to you. The mouth of the womb is to be felt, by introducing the finger with much tenderness up the birth-place: and if you feel that it dilates or opens, during the time that a pain takes place, the woman is in *actual labor*.

3d. When examining, conduct the operation with caution and tenderness; and at the same time, take care to have your nails closely and smoothly pared—because your finger will feel the membranous bladder or bag containing the waters. If the labor be not much advanced, you will only feel the mouth of the womb, and its dilation or opening at every pain.

4th. Place a pillow between the thighs of the woman, so as to give sufficient room for the child to pass, and for its head to rest upon as it enters into the world, and let the woman draw up her legs.

5th. As the head of the child advances, press your right hand firmly and steadily against the part between the fundament and birth-place, called by physicians the perineum, so as to give it support and prevent its rupturing or tearing; at the same time, that you incline the child's head toward the *pubes*, which are the parts which form the arch in front. If you will recollect, and if you do not read the part over again, I have fully described and enforced the necessity of your being extremely careful to prevent injuries to the *perineum;* for by its being ruptured or torn, which is sometimes the case from incautiousness and imprudence, as well as from *hurrying the birth*, the lower gut or fundament and the birth-place itself, become *one opening* from the tearing or laceration of the perineum. On this point, then, let me again urge you to be extremely careful.

6th. If the child's head advances forward too rapidly resist or stop its passage outward, for *one* or *two pains*, with your hand: by these means, you will increase the powers or energies of *nature* in the *mother*, avoid all of risks of injuring the *perineum* and give ultimate facility or ease in the delivery.

7th. So soon as the head is delivery, the woman will have some respite from her sufferings. You must then converse with her, and encourage her to be *patient* and *firm in her resolutions.* Remember now that the head of the child is to be supported, and that no force or pulling whatever is to be used. You are to wait patiently for the next exertions of nature, who will always perform her operations in *due time;* the woman is by no means to *strain, bear down, or force her pains.* As I told you before, and gave you the reasons, she may blow strongly into the palms of her hands, but exercise impulsion or force no further.

8th. The child being born, you have now nothing to do for a few minutes but to give it *fresh air*, and permit it to *cry*. After it has had sufficient time to breathe freely, and the *navel cord* has in some measure ceased its pulsation, the cord is to be tied about three inches from the navel of the child, and then again about an inch and a half from the first knot—and cut asunder between the two ties, with a scissors or any other sharp instrument. But I have told you this before.

9th. When the child is separated from the mother, you are *not to wash it*, according to the old custom; this is a wrong and highly improper plan, and frequently produces serious injuries to the child, as you will be fully informed by reading under the head *treatment of new-born infants*, which you will find among the *diseases of children*.

10th. Now comes the period in which so many women are injured *for life*, by ignorance and imprudent batse. Let the woman rest a short time, and await patiently the return of the pains which are to expell the *after-birth*, which the womb will do by *contraction*. Your own good sense will teach you, that if you pull or force down the *after-birth*, you will also pull down the womb, or separate the *after-birth* before the womb has contracted, so as to stop the blood vessels from pouring out their contents. Now if you do pull, after all the advice to the contrary I have given you, the consequence will be, that the woman will *bleed to death*. I have told you before, how to excite the womb to action, so as to bring on the pains for expelling the after-birth. You are to rub her belly; and if she is a strong woman, and feels able, you may by *assistants* raise her up by supporting her under the arms. She may then blow in her hands, a long breath, for the reasons I have already given you. As soon as an after pain comes on, the midwife is gently to stretch the cord, but not to pull it or use any force. By the motion of the cord or its gentle extension, the *after birth* is very apt to come away. If you do not think proper to use these measures, you may turn the woman over on her belly, and introduce your finger into the mouth of the *womb*, with much care, the parts being extremely sore: then, by turning the finger gently round the mouth of the womb, as you would round the edge of a cup, the womb *will contract*; now gently stretch the *cord, and* you will extricate the *after birth* generally speaking with safety. An hour, an hour and a half, or two hours, may be allowed for the expulsion of the after birth.

When it cannot thus be delivered, proper means are to be taken for its *expulsion*, in other words for its *discharge*. These means are the following:—Let the midwife introduce into the birth place, her hand with the fingers collected into a point, and made as small as possible. At the mouth or edge of the womb, let her open or extend her fingers, and rub them carefully round the edge. These measures will cause the womb to contract: then, with the fingers gentle introduced between the *after birth* and the *womb itself*, she must slowly separate them from each other, should they adhere or stick together. Recollect distinctly, that all this is to be done, while the contraction of the womb is going on.

11th. If the discharge of blood is great, after this operation, apply cloths wet with cold water to the belly of the woman, as in flooding: and push up the birth place gently, and not too far, a soft cloth also wet with cold water, as directed in flooding.

12th. When the woman is relieved of the *after birth*, let a wide bandage be placed round her, pleasantly tight, and let her also be wiped dry. The cloths which are wet, and those which were placed under her, are now to be removed, and she permitted to remain perfectly quiet, and to take her repose. If she complains of faintness, or seems exhausted, give her some wine and water, or a little toddy on which some nutmeg has been grated. I have now given you a full description of what I intended, and I am persuaded in such plain terms, that any woman of common sense can afford the requisite assistance in common cases of *labor*.

DIRECTIONS AFTER LABOR.

After labor, the more quiet the woman can be kept the better. The fact is, that she is to move or be moved, as little as possible, and to lie principally on her back. Her nipples are to be washed with milk warm water, before the infant is put to the breast, which ought to be done within twelve hours after the birth. If the woman has lost considerable blood during the labor, the milk will be longer in flowing than otherwise. When this is the case, apply bread and milk poultices *warm* over the nipples; these will soon cause the milk to discharge.

You will frequently observe, in women who have had children, that their bellies protrude or stick out, as if they were always in a state of pregnancy.—This is owing to neglect and bad management. To avoid it, on the second day after child birth, you are to apply round the whole belly, moderately tight, a *broad bandage* of cloth or flannel, the last is the best, which is to be worn for at least one month. It is not to be too tight, but merely tight enough to support the parts pleasantly. This will prevent the woman, after having recovered, from having a large and ill-shaped belly.

You are now to bear in mind, and that too particularly, the advice I am about to give you, especially if you value your health, and probably the preservation of your life. On the second day after delivery, you are to take a dose of castor oil or epsom salts. More than two thirds of the women who have been afflicted with, and finally died of child bed fever, have owed their fate to neglecting, after the birth of their infants, to attend to the evacuation of their bowels. If you do not like to take salts or castor oil, evacuate the bowels with clysters: see the head clystering. The fact is, you are not to let twenty four hours pass, after the birth of a child, without a passage or stool. The consequences of this neglect always are, that it is not only an injury to yourself but the child. When you have had such passages as I have told you are necessary, you are not to exert yourself by getting out of bed, but to bave a basin or other handy convenience placed under you; folding a blanket at the same time so as to prevent you from getting wet. In this way without any danger or indelecacy, have these passages, from which you will receive much relief in body and mind, and dorive much benefit in your recovery.

You are every day, without fail to have the birth-place washed with milk warm water and good clear milk. This is to be done by putting under the bed-clothing, a basin of warm water, and having your hips and thighs raised with a pillow or some bed clothes. In this situation a common squirt made of elder or cane may be used, or a female syringe, which can be procured at any doctor's shop in the country. Every day warm water is to be thrown up the birth-place so as to cleanse the parts: and to remove any clots of blood or matter, called by physicians *lochia*, which by remaining would produce irritation and fever. If you wish to escape *child-bed fever*, and the whole train of afflictions incidental thereto, you are particularly to attend to these directions.

In two or three days after delivery, for a short time, you may sit up in the bed, supported with a chair at your back, covered with pillows; this will assist the natural discharge from the birth-place. You are not to stand up before the sixth day; and in making any change, you are to do it very gradually. You are to be kept neither too warm nor too cool; the air of the room is to be kept pleasant and agreeable; and you are never to be exposed to a current of air. Two weeks after delivery, is about the general time of leaving your room; this however will depend on your situation; caution must always be used in the change, so as to bring it on gradually. Sudden changes are always dangerous to women immediately after delivery, and indeed until they are completely restored.

From the moment the woman is delivered of her child, the whole system becomes inclined to fever, and particularly, for three or four days after delivery. Your own good sense will now teach you, that the practice of giving in such cases spirituous liquors, highly seasoned food, heating meats,

GG

and strengthening medicines, is directly contrary to what ought to be done: giving such matters as I have just named, keeping the woman in a constant sweat, and closing the room so as to confine all the foul air around her, are the very means of bringing on the fever which you should endeavor to escape. Therefore let me tell you in as plain and emphatic language as I can find, that whatever adds to the heat of the woman's body, or to the febrile or feverish action of the system, will always encourage the coming on of fevers, or increase it if it has come on. On the contrary, light and cooling dict must be used: the woman must neither be subjected to extremes of heat or cold; her clothing and bedchamber must be so attended to, as neirther to oppress her with coldness nor heat; attention to these things in ten days or two weeks, after she has had her child, will so exempt her from fever, that in a little time her health will be fully established.

LOCHIA.

This word is derived from the Greek. It means *to bring forth*, and also *the cleanings:* by which are intended here, the serous or watery and often green colored discharges, that take place from the womb and birth-place, during the first three or four days after delivery, when they generally subside. During the first three days, these discharges, are apt to change their color, and frequently become offensive, unless due caution and cleanliness have been observed.

If they are profuse or great, and there is considerable weakness, cloths wet with cold water must be applied to the belly. There must also be cold water thrown up the birth-place, and also a clyster of cold water taken, at the same time that some laxative medicine is taken, to open the bowels: as these, however, are necessary discharges, they are not to be suddenly checked, unless they seem to be going on to a dangerous extent.

On the contrary, if they should stop too suddenly, they must be immediately brought on again, by a course of treatment directly opposite to that I have just laid down. Applications of a warm nature must be made to the belly; and clysters of milk warm water, instead of cold ones, must be given: see the head clystering. Should the woman be feverish, or of a full habit of body, the loss of a little blood will be proper.

FAINTINGS.

If the woman should faint after the delivery of her child, ascertain immediately if there is a flooding. Should this be the case, use the coldest applications, as directed under the head flooding. On examination, should there be no flooding, give her wine, or some toddy, or some spirit and water, and draw the bandage tight for an hour or two round the belly. If her feet and legs are cold apply hot bricks, or other warm materials to them.

CHILLS.

When the woman complains of cold after her delivery, or that cold chills are stealing over her, which is sometimes the case, make warm applications to her belly, feet and legs, and give her nothing but warm balm or sage tea to drink. If the shake is very severe, let the persons round the bed, grasp with both hands her thighs and legs, and hold them firmly, but tenderly, until the shivering subsides. Recollect now, that you are to give no heating spirits at this time, or you will certainly produce a fever. Should the chills continue, you are to have recourse to laudanum or opium: [see table of dose.] These last articles are not however to be given, unless the chills continue, or are very severe.

AFTER PAINS.

These pains are brought on by the contraction of the womb, in the exertions of expelling the clots of blood and secretions, which are contained in the womb after the birth. When not very severe you are to let them alone; but if too excruciating and severe, you will generally relieve them, by applying cloths wrung out of warm water to the back and belly. If the pains continue to be severe, throw a clyster up the bowels or fundament, made of thin gruel milk warm, in which put a tea spoonful of laudanum: [see the head clystering.]

INFLAMMATIONS.

From difficult or tedious labor, the parts frequently become inflamed and swelled; and sometimes there are quantities of blood, which from a substance in the mouth of the birth-place, which I believe has no name.. Although there is no danger in this matter, yet it frequently produces great pain and uneasiness.—These inflammations are to be relieved by cold applications, such as cold poultices of light bread and milk; bathing the parts with, and throwing up injections of cold water: or by making use of the following preparation:—In a pint of cold water, put a tea spoonful of sugar of lead, and bathe the parts with the mixture. Or you may rub them well with sweet oil, keep them cool, and daily cleanse them with cold water.

If the belly feels very sore on being pressed, bathe it often with warm water; apply cloths to it wrung out of warm water; and rub the belly well with the following liniment:—Get equal quantities of spirits of hartshorn and sweet oil; and mix them well together, and rub the belly two or three times a day with this mixture. This, with the warm bathing as just directed, will give immediate relief.

INFAMMATION

OF

THE BREASTS.

This disease generally arises from want of care, after delivery; by which want of care I mean, that proper attention has not been paid to your system, in order to prevent *fever*, which is always produced from eating or drinking stimulating articles too freely, and before the milk has had time to secrete freely. This effect is also produced, by permitting the breasts to remain distended too long with milk. In this case, great pain with inflammation comes on; in other words, *fever* is the consequence of this neglect.

If there seems any disposition to inflammation, the best preventive is to apply, a few hours after delivery, warm poultices of light bread and milk to the breasts, for at least three hours. This will assist the natural discharge of the milk. If the child refuse to suck, fill a common black bottle with *warm water*, and apply the nipple to the mouth of the bottle, which will gently draw the milk, as the water becomes cooler. Bathe the breast well with sweet oil or hog's lard, at the same time. If the inflammation continue, put a tea-spoonful af sugar of lead, in a pint of cold water, and keep a cloth wet with this mixture, constantly to the breast; but recollect, you are not to wet the nipple with this mixture, by which means it may get into the child's mouth. When the inflammation is severe, Doctor Physic recommends a blister over the breast. When matter is fully formed, make a small puncture or hole with a lancet, so as to permit it gradually to escape. I have always, however, relieved by poultices and sugar of lead, as above directed, without the painful necessity of using a blister.

MILK FEVER.

This fever is owing to the change of the system, after the delivery of the child, by the swelling and irritation of the breasts, from the milk secreted in them. This always occasions the discharge from the womb to lessen in quantity. You will now recollect the advice I have given you before, as to applying poultices to the breasts for a few hours, anointing the breasts well with sweet oil or lard, taking some laxative medicine and living on low diet. These measures and precautions, will enable you to avoid the following unpleasant feelings: heat, thirst, head-ache and fever. Although this fever is quite common, and may be easily removed, yet the imprudence of neglecting the above advice, may be the cause of other complaints, which I shall in their proper places mention. If the breasts are painful, take a dose of salts to cool the system: and if the fever continue, the loss of a little blood from the arm will be proper. Drink mild balm or sage tea, in which put about twenty drops of antimonial wine. This drink may be given occasionally, so as to produce a gentle moisture or sweat on the skin. Take no heating articles, and live on light cooling diet. In a few days the milk will flow, and the fever go off.

SWELLED LEG.

This disorder takes place after child-birth, and I am happy to say that it seldom occurs, when due caution and cleanliness have been observed. I am of opinion that it arises from some irritating matter being left in the womb, or at its mouth. When you discover this disorder, which is known by a *pain inside of the leg*, extending to the heel and the groin, the limb always begins to swell, so that the slightest motion gives great pain. The pulse becomes quick, the skin hot, the tongue white, the urine thick.

There are, also, slight pains about the womb, and the discharge from the birth-place is dreadfully offensive.

REMEDIES.

On the appearance of this complaint, get a syringe for females, or what will answer the same purpose, make a squirt of elder or cane, and throw up the *birth-place*, several times during the day, some warm water to cleanse it—and in the intervals of time, some good *sweet oil*. Wash the parts well with water made pleasantly warm, and rub the leg or legs with the following ointment. Take a gill of sweet oil, a table-spoonful of laudanum, and to these add a gill of spirits in which camphor has been dissolved. With this mixture, rub or bathe the legs twice a day; and provided the woman has no purging of the bowels, let her take at night, and also in the morning, two grains of *calomel*, mixed with the same quantity of squills, and made into a pill. This is to be repeated until relief is obtained.

CHILD BED FEVER.

This disease is called by physicians puerperal fever. It generally comes on from the fifth to the eighth day after the woman has been delivered: but its being earlier or later, depends very much on the woman's *constitution*, and the particular *state of her system*. I have before mentioned to you, that you are to be very prudent in your conduct, respecting your *food, drink*, and the *state of your bowels:* for on these three things depend, in a very great degree, your uniform health, and exemption from this dangerous disease, puerperal or child bed fever. This fever sometimes arises, from a stoppage of the discharge which I have described to you, called *lochial discharge*, and from the putrid matter which I told you it was composed of, and which I directed you to cleanse: see the head lochia. An undue secretion of milk, a stoppage of the lochial discharge, the absorption of putrid matter from the womb, exposure to too great cold or heat, all these things are capable of producing child bed fever. This fever is extremely dangerous, and requires the immediate attendance of an able physician; but, as you may be so situated as to be unable to obtain one, I shall explain to you clearly the symptoms of this disorder, and also the proper remedies.

CHILD BED FEVER comes on, with a *chill* in the first instance, then a *flushing heat;* next the woman becomes *restless,* and a sweat brakes out. In a short time this sweat dries up, and the skin becomes dry and burning to the touch: there is now great thirst; flushing of the face; whiteness and dryness of the tongue; great pain in the head and back; sickness at the stomach, sometimes attended with puking. In a short time the belly swells, feels full, and becomes very painful: so much so, that the weight of the bed clothes, gives considerable increase of pain. The bowels become quite loose in some cases, and in others, much constipated or bound; so much so that it is difficult to get a passage through them. By these symptoms you are to know this fever.

I must here remark. that if this fever continues for some time, it is very apt to change to a *typhus* fever. When this is the case, the inflammatory symptoms subside, the tongue and teeth are now covered with a dark brown coat; small sores break out in the mouth and throat, similar to those in a child that has the *thrush;* the breath smells very badly; the stools are dark and very offensive; and not unfrequently, small purple spots appear on different parts of the body. When the last symptoms appear, the case is certainly a very doubtful one. In the *typhus* stage of *child bed fever,* for further instructions refer to the head Nervous Fever, and you will find the remedies under that head. The remedies in the first stage I have described, or child bed fever properly so called, are as follows.

REMEDIES.

While the cold stage is passing over, warm applications to the feet and legs are to be made; and, when the inflammatory or hot stage comes on, as before described, the woman is to be bled from the arm, and immediately purged freely with calomel: [see table of doses.] This purge of calomel is to be followed up with a dose of epsom salts: [see table.] If the woman is of a full, stout, and healthy habit of body, and the *pains* and *fever* in eight or ten hours do not begin to give way: and if the pains in the head and back continue severe, generally draw more blood from the arm. During this fever obtain a phial of antimonial wine and one of sweet spirits of nitre; mix as you can, equal quantities of these two articles, and give a tea spoonful of this mixture every half hour in a little water or tea: in other words give it in such a manner as to produce a little sickness of the stomach, attended with a gentle moisture on the skin. If it be inconvenient for you to obtain these articles, put into a pint of milk warm water, ten grains of tartar emetic, and give of this water one or two table-spoonfuls, every one or two hours, so as to produce and keep up a constant sickness of the stomach. This will lessen the fever. Rub the belly well with sweet oil, and by injecting a little up the birth-place occasionally, the irritation will be greatly lessened. The application of flannel cloths, frequently wrung out of warm water, and laid to the belly, will also be highly important in lessening the pains and inflammation.—Should the pain continue in the belly, apply a blister at the upper part of each thigh. I would advise blistering on the belly, that being the proper place, but then you could not apply the warm cloths, which are highly important. It will therefore, be better to apply the blisters as directed. Clysters made of slippery elm, and about milk warm, thrown up the fundament with a proper pipe, three or four times a day, will answer a valuable purpose, and be a cooling and soothing remedy in this complaint. You will recollect particularly, that in this disease, operations must be had by the bowels, during the inflammatory period: and, that when the disease changes its appearance and character to *typhus*, as it will sometimes do, you are to gently keep the bowels open, but not to purge so as to weaken the patient. In this event, the continuance of mild clysters will be found truly a fine remedy. For the method of clystering; &c., see that head.—When purging comes on, so as greatly to weaken the woman, which is not unfrequently the case, you are to check it by giving a clyster, made with *common starch* on which hot water has been poured. This clyster must be about the thickness of gruel, and to be about *milk warm*, in which you are to put twenty-five or thirty drops of *laudanum:* it must be repeated three or four times a day, as the pain and looseness may require.

At the commencement of this *child bed fever*, the diet or food must be very cooling and light; but as the disease advances, and the woman becomes weaker, let the nourishment be increased: and if necessary, from her loss of strength in purging, or from other causes, or if the disease seems to be approaching to the *typhus* or *nervous fever*, the symptoms of which I have fully explained, it will be necessary to support her system, by the assistance of good wine or toddy, and such nourishing food as will support the enfeebled action of the system. In these cases, wine and barks may be given also: or chamomile tea made strong, and taken cold occasionally through the day; or you may give a strong decoction of dog-wood bark, wild cherry tree bark, and swamp poplar bark, made from equal quantities of these barks boiled together and perfectly cooled, in the quantity of about a wine glass full three or four times a day. These remedies are all valuable *tonics*, or strengthening medicines to support the system. Remember particularly, that no tonic or strengthening medicines are to be given, until after the system has been entirely cleansed of its impurities: and also, you are most particularly to bear in mind, that tonics or strengthening medicines are never to be given, when they produce or increase fever.

SPIRITS OF TURPENTINE. I am induced to believe, from testimony not to be questioned, that this valuable medicine, *spirits of turpentine*, has not yet received the attention, or been employed sufficiently in *child bed fever*. So far as my studies and experience will enable me to form and deliver an opinion, I would prefer its use to that of the *lancet* in this fever, in the reduction of febrile and inflammatory symptoms. I have been in the practice for several years past, of using spirits of turpentine as a medical remedy, and feel no hesitation whatever in asserting, that a fair and impartial trial of it, in a great variety of cases would entitle it to rank and appreciation among medical remedies of the very first order. In obstinate costiveness of the bowels, and when every other remedy had failed, I have frequently used it with signal success; nor is there any thing superior to it in colic, and in various inflammatory or spasmodic affections of the abdominal viscera. In *enterities* which means inflammation of the intestines; in *dysentery;* and in *hemorrhage*, which means a discharge of blood, I know from practical experience, that it is a very valuable remedy. With these remarks, which I consider amply due to the subject, I will subjoin such testimonials of the efficacy of spirits of turpentine, as will entitle it to much attention in the treatment of *child bed fever.*

Says Doctor Payne, in substance, pages 98—9, of the 6th vol. Medical Recorder—"Puerperal or child bed fever, within the last fifteen years, has raged with its usual violence in many parts of this kingdom, particularly in the westriding of Yorkshire, when but few of these attacked by it escaped. Before the publication of Doct. Brennan appeared, recommending the oil of turpentine in this fever, blood-letting was usually resorted to; but there was much less success attending it, than appears to have followed the application of the same remedy, in the cases of Doct. Campbell. After reading Brennan's work, I was glad to try a fresh remedy in child bed fever, because I had seen so little good result from blood-letting. It is now nearly eight years since I was called to visit a female who labored under this disease; when the surgeon who had only seen the patient a short time before, proposed giving the oil of turpentine, which was assented to, and given in doses of *half an ounce* every *two hours.* The effect was a very copious discharge from the bowels, appearing to consist of a cerous or *watery fluid tinged with green*, in which were seen floating numerous pieces of *white matters* like coagulated lymph. Soon afterwards, the patient became maniacal or deranged, and continued so for several days, when her intellects were restored, and she gradually recovered.

"Since that period," says the doctor, "I have seen several cases of child bed fever, one of which had been attended by a surgeon who had discontinued his visits. I believe she had not been bled. Her friends seeing I had an unfavorable opinion of the case, called in a more experienced physician, and it was agreed to try the turpentine as a last resource. Two drachms of it were given every two hours, which soon brought on a purging, of a matter of the like nature, as before mentioned. I have stated in the case first mentioned, that mania had taken place from giving the turpentine; and the probability is, that the largeness of the doses produced the effect, by throwing too much blood to the head, in the case I am now speaking of, two drachms only were given at a dose, and the result was, that although the patient seemed to be at the very verge of eternity, she quickly recovered."

I will give but one case. It is one communicated to the Medical Recorder 6 vol. page 615, by Doctor James H. Lucas of the County of Madison, and State of Georgia. It is ably and clearly detailed, and will be highly satisfactory to the reader.

"On the 15th July, I was called to a woman who had been delivered five days before of her child, after a lingering labor of two days and nights. When I saw her, there was a wildness of expression, and great anxiety, with considerable sharpness of the features. Her pulse was from 100 to 110. She had a severe pain above the eyes, a hot and dry skin, and great restlessness; the tongue furred in the middle and a red appearance of the edges. There was much tenderness of the belly; with an appearance like a ball over the pubes. Her bowels are costive; her extremities cold every morning about two o'clock, with a scarcityof the lochial discharge: the restlessness was also much more troublesome, in the afternoon. The child and placenta were both delivered as usual. As a preparatory means, ten grains of calomel were given, to be worked off with castor oil. This brought away several dark green fetid stools, which she said relieved her considerably; particularly her head. The next morning, the 16th. I ordered her to take two tea-spoonfuls of *spirits of turpentine*, in a solution of gum arabic, or beaten up with the white of an egg, with a table-spoonful of castor oil in the evening, to assist the operation of the *turpentine*. On the 17th. the tenderness of the belly had nearly subsided; the pulse was less frequent; and four more stools, of a green and offensive smell from the *oil* and *turpentine*, were voided. She was ordered to continue the medicine. On the 18th. the tenderness was gone, except on pressure, and the pulse was about 90 in a minute. Three stools had been passed of a less offensive smell, and but slightly tinged with green. The skin was much cooler than on the day before. The medicine was still continued. On the 19th. the pulse was natural, with a slight perspiration on the surface; the tenderness of the belly was entirely gone; the lochial discharge of its proper quantity and color; five stools had been voided, the two last of which were of a natural appearance; and her appetite was good. On the 20th. I found her up quite cheerful, and perfectly free from fever or disease, and she has continued so ever since." From these cases which are drawn from high authorities, the value of *spirits of turpentine*, as a most valuable remedy in child bed fever, will probably be acknowledged by every reader of this work.

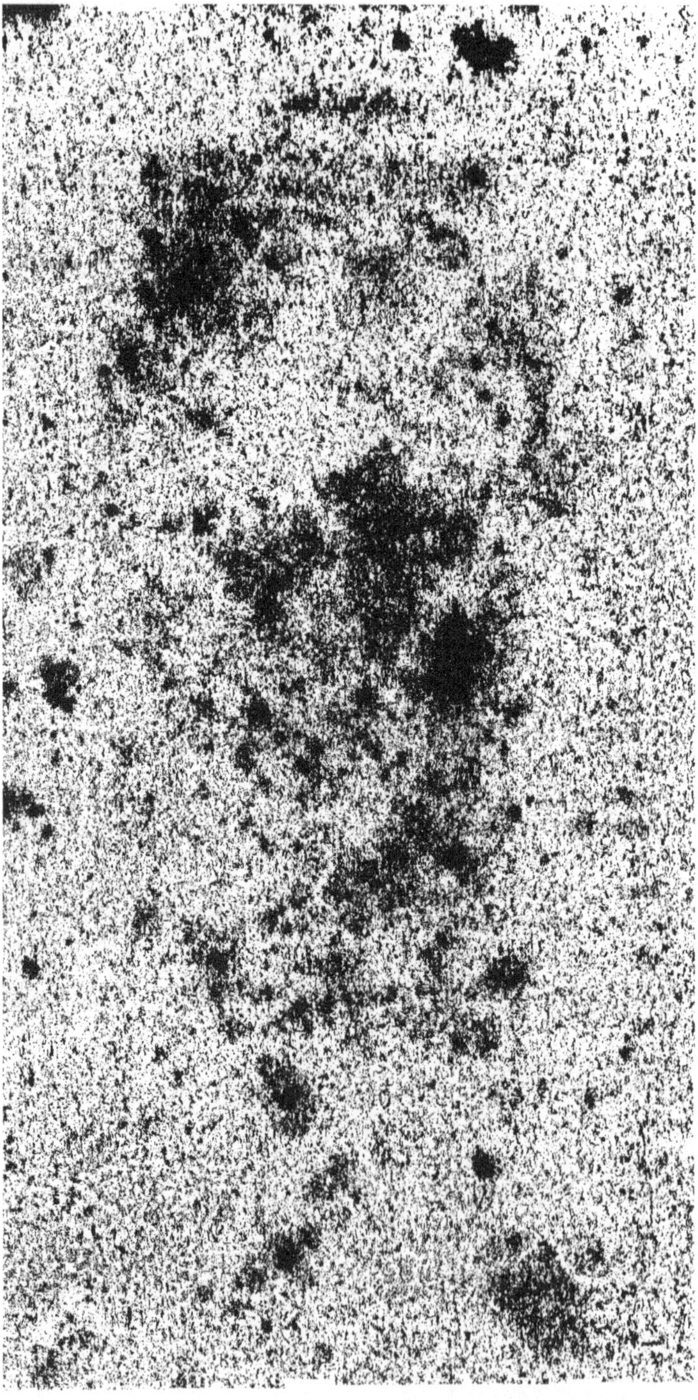

DISEASES

OF

CHILDREN.

Surely there can be nothing more painful and distressing, to a mind of sensibility, than to be compelled to witness, in very many cases without being able to relieve, the various and often fatal diseases to which infants are liable. That most of them are of a morbidly *irritative* character, is probably well known to every physician who has attended to their symptoms; but, what it is that particularly excites this diseased irritability in the intestinal canal, it would probably be difficult for even the most learned and skilful of the profession to determine.

The foolish and dangerous custom, of giving infants medicine the moment they are born, in order to keep them quiet, is a practice which ought always to be discountenanced, as laying the foundations of many disorders, sometimes destroying life itself, or entailing on the constitution maladies which last for life. Various medicines are given to infants, for very foolish and frivolous reasons, which had better be let alone entirely. such, for instance, as Godfrey's cardial, Bateman's drops, &c. &c. all of which contain opium, and do inconceivable injury to infants. I do not mean by these remarks, that these medicines are not sometimes beneficial; but to be constantly administering them on all occasions, and for nearly all possible purposes, must convince any person of common sense, that they are injurious both to the health and constitution. By suckling infants, then feeding or rather stuffing them, and then following up both by medicines, *to keep them quiet*, their tender stomachs are kept constantly loaded; and, if they are not fortunate enough to puke up part of what they have been compelled to swallow, *furmentation* must and will take place, the stomach being unable to master such a mass, followed by colic, and purgings. The above remarks are made in terms thus plain, that they may be distinctly understood by my readers, and that they may profit in the treatment of their infant children, by their true meaning.

STILL BORN.

When an infant is born apparently dead, or giving no signs of life, it is said to be *still born*. This appearance, however, should not prevent the midwife from making every possible exertion for the restoration of the child: by patience and perseverance, thousands of infants have been restored to life. If no pulsation or beating can be felt in the navel cord, and if there be marks of putrification or decay, I need not tell you that all your efforts will be fruitless. The infant, in this case, where there is hope, ought to be separated from the mother as early as possible, and wrapped in a blanket made warm by the fire. As soon as possible, after this, its breast is to be bathed in warm spirits, at the same time that you gently apply to its nostrils spirit of hartshorn. If these remedies fail to restore the circulation, put it in warm water, keeping its head in such a position as to prevent suffocation. You may loosen the string on the navel cord, so as to let it bleed about a table-spoonful, when it must be again tied. While these measures are in operation, you are to prepare a clyster, made of a table-spoonful of spirits of any kind, and three table-spoonfuls of warm water; and if the child does not breathe, you are to give this clyster up the bowels with a proper instrument; look under the head clystering. The lungs are to be *filled with air*, by means of a common syringe, the pipe of which is to be introduced into one nostril, while the other nostril and mouth are to be carefully closed; when you are then by gentle pressure on the breast of the child to empty them; in this way the lungs are to be frequently filled and compressed until natural respiration or breathing takes place. Sometimes the application of a little cold water to the chest will restore children. In many instances, when the slightest action of the heart has been perceived, it would be advisable to keep up a friction or rubbing over the body, for at least an hour. Cases are stated, and many of them of infants still born, being restored by warmth and gentle rubbing, even when no signs of life had appeared for an hour or more after their birth. This should therefore encourage you to persevere, by every possible method, for the restoration to life a still born infant.

There are instances in which the child is born of a dark purple cast, in which the breathing is scarcely perceptible, and where death ensues in a few minutes. When these appearances take place, the infant has generally some defect in the formation of the heart and lungs. Doctor Hossack advises that a bath be made of *oak bark*, four ounces of which is to be boiled for a few minutes in about two gallons of water. When this bath is prepared, add to it a pint of spirits of any kind, permitting it to become pleasantly warm, bathe the child up to the neck in this water. If it is convenient you may add to this bath occasionally, a table spoonful of spirits of hartshorn so as to render it stimulating. When the child shows symptoms of recovery, take it out of the bath and wrap it in warm flannels; and should the infant be taken in the same way again, you must immediately make use of the bath again, after again warming it.

TREATMENT OF

NEW BORN INFANTS.

According to the old custom, the moment the child was separated from the mother, it was plunged in warm water, or washed with spirits of some kind, and well rubbed with a towel, to remove the mealy matter which adhered to it, and to prevent its taking cold, and perhaps to harden its skin. These foolish and dangerous practices, have caused the death of thousands of infant children, or produced other consequences highly detrimental to their constitutions. The consequences always are, that by washing and rubbing the child, you irritate and inflame the skin, which is at this time so tender, that nature in her wisdom has covered it with this *mealy matter* to defend it from injury in entering the world, and to preserve it from irritability and inflammation afterward.

An infant born in the winter season, has more of this *mealy covering* than if born in the summer; it is also more thickly covered with it at the arm-pits, the bends of the joints, and so on, which are more liable to rubbing or fractional injury during labor, than other parts of the body; and in addition to these considerations, this covering is intended to protect the infant against the action of the atmospheric air. This covering is perfectly natural, and should always be permitted to remain until nature herself removes it. This will be done in a day or two, without assistance or artificial means, by which the skin will be left white, soft, and beautiful, and the child exempted from innumerable diseases—diseases which by the old custom of washing and rubbing would almost invariably insue. By the old custom, the skin is greatly irritated and inflamed, then becomes of a dark red color, and afterwards breaks out with those eruptions or pimples which usually appear on children called the *red gum*.

Every person of common sense must know, that the application of spirits of any kind, especially when rubbed on the head and body of a grown person, will produce smarting and give pain. Now I ask what must be the consequence to an infant, whose skin is so delecately tender, that nature herself has shielded it from the atmosphere, until it will bear the change without injury. In many cases of grown persons, the application of brandy to the head, and washing the body with it, have been known to produce inflammation of the brain, or lungs or bowels: the evaporation from the surface being so great, as to produce a degree of cold sufficient to stop the perspiration or sweat. In infants this evaporation produces inflammations of the bowels, or of the lungs, and sometimes of the membrane which lines the *nostrils*, by which the child is afflicted with a disease called the snuffles.

The proper plan, and the one now practiced in the different lying-in hospitals throughout Europe and the U. States, is simply the following. Cleanse the face with tenderness and caution, with a little milk and water made pleasantly warm: then cover the body with thin muslin, over which is to be put the flannel. In a day or two the mealy covering will entirely peal off, and nature in due time will exhibit a healthy, delecate and beautiful skin, free from every disease, and entirely exempt from all those painful and eruptive diseases to which infants are usually subject, from the old method of treatment.

MECONIUM.

When a child is first born, its bowels are filled with a dark colored greenish matter called by physicians *meconium.* In a short time after its birth, or as soon as it commences sucking the *first milk* from the mother, which milk seems by nature to be intended to remove this dark colored or greenish matter from the bowels, for it is almost immediately discharged by stool. This is the reason, and I think an amply sufficient one, why children should be put to the breast as early as possible after their birth. Sometimes the milk in the mother's breast is rather slow in coming: or from some particular cause, the child will not suck the breast, and consequently it will not discharge by *stool* this matter from the bowels which I have described. It will then be necessary to give it something to open the bowels, such as a little molasses and water, which should be given frequently until the bowels are properly opened. Or you may obtain from any doctor's shop, a small piece of *manna*, about the size of a walnut, and dissolve it in a gill of boiling water; and when it becomes cool, give the infant a tea spoonful frequently, or until it operates freely. Or you may, if these remedies fail, give a tea spoonful of the best castor oil, which will remove the *meconium* immediately. The two first being the most simple remedies, should always be used first. Sometimes but the cases are not frequent, this necessary discharge is prevented from passing, owing from the fact of the fundament from some defect or other cause, being stopped up. Such cases require the immediate aid of an able physician, to examine and remove such difficulties or obstructions.

ORIGINAL IMPERFECTIONS.

Immediately after the birth of an infant, examine its body and limbs, and particularly its private parts: because childdren are not all born perfect in this respect. The passages of infants are sometimes closed up with this slime or tough matter, which require the aid of surgical operations to open them, before they can pass either their *stools* or their *urine*. Great care and attention ought always to be paid by parents to these examinations. Sometimes the parts which decency forbids me to name, are entirely closed up by malconformation or deformity of those parts: these cases however, are very rare and unfrequent; and I need not tell you, that in them no human assistance can afford relief.

RUPTURES are very frequent among new born infants, particularly about the navel. When these ruptures are very early observed, they may speedily be removed by bathing the belly frequently with cold water, and attending to the child's bowels; in other words keeping them regularly open. If the rupture should be at the navel, apply a piece of adhesive plaster, so as to give support to the parts; but by no means apply a bandage, which will do injury to the delecate and tender parts by the pressure. The fact is, that the constant application of cold bathing, as the infant advances in age and strength will always remove these early ruptures.

TONGUE TIED. In this case the tongue is confined to the roof of the mouth, by a small cord which prevents its motion. Sometimes indeed, the tongue is so confined that the infant cannot suck. But I have sometimes known children cut for it where it did not exist: therefore great caution ought to be used in this operation, although it may seem a very simple one. If the physician or other person, who cuts this small cord does not understand it properly, or cuts it carelessly, so great a quantity of blood may be lost as to prove fatal to the child. As many women are very uneasy, respecting their children being tongue tied, I will inform them that they are often alarmed unnecessarily, and have their children operated on when they are not tongue tied. A very simple method of discovering its situation by putting the end of your finger in the child's mouth; if it is able to clasp it with the same force it would the nipple, or the end of the tongue moves, it does not require cutting.

HARE LIP. There are different kinds of hare lip—and not unfrequently, both lips are disfigured by the opening or space extending along the roof of the mouth. When this is the case, it has a very unsightly appearance; and the operation of closing the lip cannot be performed, however skilful the physician with any probability of success. But where there is but one opening, or even double, provided it does extend to the roof of the mouth, as I have described, the cure or operation can be performed without much difficulty. You will bear in mind, that an operation (which means endeavoring to close up the lip,) ought never to be performed on an infant until it is a year old, as the lip requires strength to bear the operation, by which it is to be removed. In some cases but they are very rare, the infant is unable to suck; if this is the ease the operation may be performed; but at this early stage I should consider the success very doubtful. The method used in the country of sewing it up is highly improper. The operation to be performed in closing up the lip, where the fissure or opening does not extend beyond the upper part of the gum, is as follows:—At any silver smith's shop have two silver pins made something longer than a common pin, and without any heads to them. With a sharp knife pare well the edges of the opening: then with one of these pins, pierce the lip at the upper side entirely through, in a slanting direction; then pierce through on the other side in the same way. You will recollect to take a good hold, so that it will not easily tear out; then with your thumb and finger, close together the edges that have been cut; now you are to wind tight round these pins some silk, which has been properly waxed, so as to draw it together that it may heal. In six or seven days, or perhaps earlier, it will heal or adhere together; then draw out the pins and dress it with any simple ointment or salve, and if properly performed, the scare in a few years will scarcely be perceptible.

The feet of infants are sometimes deformed, by what are called *club feet:* if this is permitted to go on without immediate attention, the deformity will be very great, and cannot be removed after the infant is a few months old; the bones of the feet become hard and firm, whereas at an early age, or immediately after birth, they are in a soft grisley state. When if proper means are used, the foot or feet by gradual compression may be reduced to their natural form in a few months, if the deformity is not graet; but in some cases a longer time will be required.

EXERCISE OF CHILDREN

AND

PURE AIR.

If you are desirous of preserving your children's health, and giving them good constitutions, give them exercise and let them be frequently in the open air, so as to accustom their bodies to the various changes of the atmosphere. By no means keep them in a close room, or cooped up as if you were afraid they would catch cold at every gentle breeze. I have never seen children thus confined whose health and constitutions were not, through life, extremely delecate, and subject to colds and various diseases, which, by a contrary course, they would have entirely escaped. As an evidence, take two children, let one be clothed in flannel, and protected from the slightest exposure or change of weather; feet constantly supplied with stockings and shoes, and not suffered to go out in the least damp or inclement weather. While the other is moderately clothed, perhaps hardly enough to cover it with decency; no shoes or stockings; exposed to all kinds of weather, even during our inclement winters, without a shoe to its little feet. The first will be pale, thin, weakly, and of a delecate constitution through life, subject to colds on every change of weather; perhaps not attaining the age of manhood, before a breast complaint commences its ravages. While the other, full of strength, vigor, and a cheek like a rose, with a healthy constitution, exempt from colds, and free of every disorder, reaches a good old age without an hour's sickness. Are we not furnished daily with evidences of this fact. Why then take pains to throw obstacles in the way, when, if children were permitted to exercise freely, and not so much unnecessary care bestowed on them after a certain age: or in other words, when able to run about themselves, parents would be blessed with a more healthy and vigorous offspring, and have very little necessity for Doctors or medicines. By the use of cold bathing, or in other words, washing the child in cold water, you will, in a great measure, prevent the galling, and excoriation which frequently occur about the groins and privates, in the neck, behind the ears &c. which are produced by the sweat or urine. The parts after being washed in cold water, should be suffered to dry, and a little fine starch dusted upon it, this will very much relieve the child.

THE SNUFFLES.

This stoppage of the nose is quite common to young children. It frequently prevents them from breathing freely, and they cannot suck or swallow without considerable difficulty. This is quite a simple complaint, which will be speedily removed by giving the infant a purge of castor oil; about a tea-spoonful is the dose; and bathing its feet or body in warm water, pleasantly warm; and for a few days keeping its head a little warm. A little lard or sweet oil may be rubbed upon the nose and around the nostril.

THE RED GUM.

The red gum breaks out in small pimples on the skin, generally of a red, but not unfrequently, of a yellow appearance. This complaint appears principally on the face and neck; but it sometimes breaks out on the hands and legs, and the pimples contain. not unfrequently, a white clear matter. It would be highly improper to use any means outwardly to remove it, for by so doing, you might suddenly drive in the complaint, and thereby destroy the life of the infant. The child while laboring under this disorder, should be prevented from being exposed to the cold air. The only danger in this disorder is driving it in; when this is the case, the infant is greatly distressed in the bowels, screams and cries constantly; and not unfrequently has fits. In the management of this disorder, you are to keep the infant's bowels open with a little magnesia and rhubarb: for the dose of either of these medicines, (see table;) or a tea spoonful of castor oil may be given. Should the disorder suddenly disappear, and the child become sick from it, put it immediately in warm water, and give it one or two drops of antimonial wine, in a little sage tea. This may be repeated every hour or two, until a moisture is produced on the skin, and the pimples or eruptions brought out again on the body.

YELLOW GUM.

This is a disorder similar to the jaundice, and takes place with some infants a few days after their birth: it is known by a yellow tinge of the skin, high colored urine, and a constant desire to sleep. This simple complaint can be removed by a gentle puke of one or two grains of ipecacuanha, mixed with a little warm water, and in a short time followed by some mild purge.

THRUSH.

The thrush or sore mouth, is a very common disease in early infancy. The child suffers a great deal of pain in sucking, and frequently this complaint is attended with some fever. This disorder appears in small white spots on the tongue, corners of the lips, and inside the cheeks, and by degrees spreading itself over the whole inside of the mouth and throat; and in some cases, extending down through the stomach and canal. If the white spots on the tongue resemble coagulated milk, or in other words, look as if the child had been eating curds and that some of them remained sticking to the tongue, you will know by this appearance that the *thrush* or sore mouth is commencing. The thrush is produced from acidities in the stomach and bowels, occasioned from some particular quality of the milk, which disagrees with the infant, or from improper food. Those children who are raised by hand, are more subject to this complaint, which shows plainly, that it is the food which disagrees with the stomach and bowels, and brings on the thrush or sore mouth. The remedies are then very plain and simple; attend to the stomach and bowels first, before you use any astringent washes; after which it will be proper to use a wash for the mouth, made of a little borax, honey and alum, dissolved or mixed in a small quantity of sage tea. Then with a rag tied to a stick, rub or wash the mouth with this preparation, two or three times a day;

regularly persevering in washing, while any appearance of the disease remains. To regulate the stomach and bowels, give equal quantities of magnesia and rhubarb; [for the dose of either of these medicines refer to the table.]

CONSTIPATION.

Constipation means costiveness or being bound in the body, so that the infant cannot pass its stools. This complaint is sometimes hereditary or natural to the child; when this is the case, and it does not exceed proper bounds, it may not require the use of any remedy; but should the infant's health begin to suffer from frequent attacks of colic, flatulence, wind &c. it should be strictly attended to, as it may produce convulsions or fits, inflammation of the bowels, or other diseases of a difficult and lingering nature, thereby establishing this costive habit of body for life.

If the predisposition descended from a mother of the same habit, or in other words, if the mother herself is subjcet to being bound in her body, the child may be relieved for a short time but it will again return. When this is the case, the mother if possible should change the quality of the milk by being attentive to her diet, and to take occasionally some mild purge, which will alter the quality of her milk; for this purpose, there is no medicine superior or more innocent than magnesia or epsom salts, of equal quantities mixed and ground very fine in a mortar. Of this, take a tea spoonful or two in a tumbler of cold water of a morning on an empty stomach. When the constipation originates from the child's food it must be changed; and simple medicines given occasionally, to act as a mild purge, such as magnesia, rhubarb, manna, sweet oil, or castor oil, either of these may be given: [for doses of either of these medicines see table.]—But if the costiveness is obstinate, a little aloes pounded fine and mixed with honey or molasses, will procure a passage or stool. Or you may give a laxative clyster, made of a little warm water, in which put a tea spoonful of lard, and with a clyster pipe or syring, throw or squirt it up the fundament. In administering clysters, you are to recollect that they should not be given hot, but milk warm, by giving them hot, you increase the disorder, and do serious injury to the child; this is a mistake which is often made, and the consequence both to children and grown persons, when clysters are given hot, is extremely dangerous. [For directions as to clystering see that head.]

COLIC.

Whenever the child cries, the general practice is to suckle or feed it, by which its little stomach is kept constantly loaded, and being unable to digest the food, colicy pains, griping and purging are the consequences. The suffering of the infant in such cases being very acute and painful, recourse is had to *Bateman's drops* or *Godfreys cordial*, and sometimes laudanum or paregoric, all of which contain opium, and relieve the little sufferer for a short time; when the colic or griping again returns.

"From my experience in the diseases of infants," says a distinguished writer, in the New York Medical Inquirer, "I am satisfyed that these complaints if not produced, are nevertheless cherished by the causes already mentioned. I have in my practice, been in the habit of administering ipecacuanha in the dose of one grain, so as to produce puking in imitation of that excited by nature; and I am happy in saying that in no instance did it fail to produce the desired effect; that in some obstinate cases it has acted like a charm, and that the parents declared that it must have contained opium.

"In cases of griping and violent pain in the bowels of infants, I have also found the application of the following anodyne plaster to the abdomen or belly highly beneficial:—Take of gum plaster three drachms; camphor half a drachm; opium twenty grains; oil of anniseed ten drops; to be made in a plaster and spread on soft leather.

"Professors, Meyer, and Reich of Berlin, employ as a principal remedy in cases of bowel complaints of children, one drachm of the diluted muriatic acid in three ounces of simple syrup, of which they direct a tea spoonful to be given about every two hours."

Colic generally takes place in early infancy, from the first six weeks to the tenth or twelfth month; and is easily known by the infant's suddenly screaming or crying, and at the same time drawing up its legs: if the complaint is severe, the child cannot urinate or make water. If the colic is slight, and arises from flatulence or wind, give one or two drops of peppermint, to which if necessary, you may add a drop or two of laudanum; at the same time, expose the infant's belly to a warm fire, rub it well with the following mixture.—Take three table spoonfuls of spirits in which camphor has been dissolved, add to this a tea spoonful of laudanum, and bathe the child's belly with it. You will also find the application of warm salt, or bathing in warm water, valuable remedies.

When the colic originates from acidity, as may be known by the bowels not being bound, and the stools of a green color and sour smell, in addition to the above means, you should give occasionally a dose of magnesia: [See table for doses:] this will correct the acidity, and assist the discharge of the offending matter from the bowels. You will find the infusion of rhubarb in small doses, given so as to keep the bowels gently open, whilst at the same time, it communicates tone to the stomach and bowels, and increases the *peristaltic action.* The infant must be kept warm, and a flannel roller be applied round the belly, which gives support to the muscles, and is a valuable assistant in diseased conditions of the intestinal canal.

SORE EYES.

Sore eyes are very apt to make their appearance a few days or weeks after the birth of the infant, which occasions them to be fretful and uneasy. and sometimes if neglected, may produce blemishes, or blindness. It is often brought on by exposure of the infant to large fires, or the imprudent practice of holding it to a lighted candle to keep it quiet. It is also caused by cold: and when the eyes are sore at a more advanced age, it may be produced by cutting teeth.—The remedies are, to avoid cold, and exposure to too much light, particularly the fire; bathe the eyes three or four times a day in cold water, or make the following preparation, with which you are to bathe the infant's eyes frequently through the day: about the size of a common pea of sugar of lead dissolved in a pint of cold water. If this should not relieve it, give it a purge of castor oil. The application of the lead water as mentioned, is generally successful, and a valuable remedy.

TEETHING.

Children suffer a great many complaints during the time of cutting *teeth.*—Some infants suffer much less than others: but all seem, during this necessary operation, to undergo pain and a disordered state of the system.

The symptoms which go before and accompany the cutting of teeth, are more or less violent, according to the manner in which the teeth comes through the gum, or in other words, the resistance which the gum makes; and to the irritability of the infant's constitution, &c.

When the child cuts its teeth in the most easy manner, the pressure on the gums, however slight gives pain, and produces an increased flow of the fluids furnished by the mouth; the child is fretful, and restless during the night, is constantly putting its little hands, or any thing that it can get hold of, into its mouth. The spittle which it is constantly discharging or slabbering from the mouth, when swallowed, produces sickness, gripes, and looseness; after a short time the corner of a tooth is perceived; but the pain and uneasiness still continues for several days, when a second tooth is cut.

During the time between the cutting of the lower and upper teeth, the child generally improves in health and strength; but in a short time is again subjected to the same uneasiness. In strong, healthy, or fat children, a fever generally, and that sometimes violent, comes on before, or about the time of cutting every tooth; the gums are swelled, and inflamed, the eyes much disordered, the belly bound, the skin hot; and the child cries constantly, and sucks with much pain: sometimes it is unable to suck, and its sleep is very much disturbed. Weakly and delecate children where teething is painful and difficult, lose their color, fret constantly, vomit or puke frequently, attended with looseness or purging, and become quite emaciated, or in other words, reduced to great weakness. I have discovered that those children I have last mentioned, pass through the painful and dangerous process of teething, much easier and with greater safety than those who are fat and robust: and have particularly remarked, that those children who slaver, (vulgarly called slobber,) must cut their teeth with the greatest ease.

The treatment during teething, should be a particular attention to the bowels, by keeping them sufficiently open: also paying a due attention to every circumstance likely to promote the general health of the child, such as pure air, exercise, strict cleanliness, food easily digested in the stomach, and taken in small quantites. As the difficulties are sometimes greatly lessened, and frequently entirely prevented, by a looseness coming on spontaneously, or more plainly speaking of its own accord, it must not be checked, particularly in children of a fat or full habit, but permitted to go on, unless it weakens the infant too much, or runs to excess, when it may be stopped by degrees. But if the child is bound in its body, you will recollect that it should take some laxative purge, so as to produce two or three stools daily, for this purpose, give two grains of calomel, to which add three or four grains of rhubarb or magnesia. If necessary, the operation of this medicine may be assisted by clysters: [for directions, &c. as to clystering, look under that head.] When fulness, and quickness of the pulse, increase of heat, flushed face, frequent startings, oppressed breathing, immediate fits of crying, &c. denote fever; the irritation on the gums must be removed. which is done by cutting or lancing the gum down to the teeth, for which purpose a *gum lancet* must be made use of.

CONVULSIONS OR FITS.

Convulsions or fits, are at all times alarming and dangerous, and require a very great variety of treatments: therefore, procure in such cases, a skilful physician. But as these fits are frequently very sudden, I shall direct the means which may be used before a physician can be obtained, and I will make some observations as to the general causes which produce them. It is not unfrequently the case, for convulsions or fits, to come on suddenly, in others the attack is gradual, and the symptoms so slight as to pass unobserved by the mother or nurse. In the former, the child, from being in the most perfect health, turns of a purple color; the features and eyes are changed, and the whole frame is violently convulsed or agitated. In a short time, these symptoms are followed by faintings, or medically speaking, by a suspension of the vital powers; after which, the child gradually recovers, but for some time remains stupid and drowsy. In the latter cases, the infant shows uneasiness, changes color suddenly and frequently, the lips quiver, the eyes are turned upwards, and it stretches out, the hands become clenched, when the convulsions or fits come on.

Fits are apt to be produced by any thing which affec's

the whole nervous system, or that which produces irritation on any particular nerve; and by the sudden striking in of any eruptive disorder, such as the measles, or any complaint which breaks out on the skin; from improper food, or irritating substances applied to the stomach or bowels, will produce this disorder. These convulsions frequently occur during the period of teething; but I have found from particular attention to the causes which produce convulsions or fits, that worms are very often the cause of this complaint. But if they take place frequently, and with great violence occasioned from pressure on the brain, or any cause in that organ, they generally terminate fatally, or cause the child as he advances in years to become foolish.

The treatment of convulsions or fits, must depend on the causes which produce them. If the sudden striking in of any complaint, as the thrash, measles, &c.; or the drying up of any eruption or discharge on the body, it ought to be brought out by putting the child into a warm bath, then giving a dose of *Godfrey's cordial*, or *Bateman's drops*, so as to produce to the surface. the complaint; if indigestion or improper food has occasioned it, give a gentle emetic or puke of ipecacuanha, or emetic tartar, [see table for dose.] If the bowels are stopped, or the fits are supposed to arise from irritating matter of any kind in the body, it must be removed by purgative medicines, as two grains of calomel, mixed with five grains of rhubarb or jalap, which if necessary assist with a clyster: [for the method of preparing and administering a clyster, read under that head:] but if produced by teething, then scarify the gums, or in other words, cut them down with a gum lancet immediately over the tooth, this operation ought to be performed daily, or until the tooth is through the gum, or the fits cease.

When worms are suspected to be the cause, from which the convulsions or fits are produced, the remedies recommended under that head must be employed.

CROUP.

This is a very dangerous complaint, and the rapidity with which it proceeds, requires prompt and immediate attention, or the disorder will prove fatal in a very short time. Of all the the diseases to which children are liable, *croup* is certainly the most dangerous. Every mother should understand the symptoms and treatment of this disease; as in many instances, before a physician can possibly be obtained. suffocation is the consequences. The croup comes on with a difficulty of breathing and wheezing, a short, dry cough, and a rattling in the throat when a sleep. In a short time, the difficulty of breathing increases, the face of the child is flushed, and the veins in the neck are very full of blood and throb or beat very fast. The voice and coughing has a very strange sharp sound, something like the crowing of a young cock; the child is very restless and uneasy, the body is hot and attended with great thirst, and the pulse very quick. Those in whom the face is much flushed, seem over-powered by a heavy sleep, from which they are aroused only by the violent fits of coughing. As the disease continues, the fits of coughing return more frequently, and are attended with an uncommon degree of agitation throughout the whole frame; the breathing becomes more and more noisy; and unless relief is speedily obtained, the infant will die by suffocation.

The remedy is an emetic or puke. The moment the complaint is discovered, put six grains of emetic tartar, into six table spoonfuls of warm water, give the child about half a table spoonful every ten or fifteen minutes. The intention is to keep up a constant sickness and vomiting or puking. But if it is a violent case, you are to bleed it from the arm, and put it up to its neck in warm water. But recollect you are to keep up the sickness at the stomach, and puking it freely. I have frequently, when the *croup* was severe, kept the child puking occasionally through the whole night, and using now and then, the warm bath, before relief could be given. In this complaint you will find the seneka snake root a valluable remedy; it must be given to the child frequently, made into a strong tea. After using the remedies I have already described, without success, and the disease is desperate, the best remedy is calomel, in doses of from forty to fifty grains, (do not be alarmed at this dose.) I know by experience in a hundred instances, of the lives of children being preserved by large doses of calomel, which must otherwise have proved fatal. Then let me urge upon you the necessity of laying aside your prejudices against this medicine, and not to slacken your hand in this trying moment if you wish to preserve the infant. So powerful and salutary is this medicine, that it frequently relieves the complaint in ten or fifteen minutes without recourse to any other means. It acts on the stomach bowels and skin. Smaller doses may be given where the complaint is not very alarming: when given in smaller doses, you may add a little *ipecacuanha*, say two or three grains with the calomel, from which much benefit will be derived.

The following simple remedy is highly recommended by Doct. John D. Goodman, an eminent physician of Charlottsville, Virginia. The simplicity of the remedy, and the facility of its application, entitled it to a trial.

"When children are threatened with an attack of croup, I direct [says the doctor,] a plaster covered with dry Scotch snuff, varying in size according to the age of the patient, to be applied directly across the top of the chest and retained there till all symptoms disappear. This remedy is found to be always effectual when applied to the first and second stages of the malady. The mode of treatment was from prejudice, neglected by me, and in one instance, in which very considerable difficulty, one of my children was rescude by the ordinary treatment. But on being urged to make a trial of the snuff plaster, I determined to make the experiment whenever opportunity presented. This was not long wanting; and when called to a child laboring under all the symptoms of the early stage of croup, such a plaster made by greasing a piece of linen and covering it well with snuff was directed to be applied to the chest. The event was most happy, the symptoms of irritation, and half crouping cough, ceased shortly after; the child fell into a profound sleep, with gentle perspiration, and by the next morning, was free from all distressing symptoms. The plaster was re-applied for a night or two following, and then discontinued. Since that time my family has been saved from a great deal of anxiety and alarm, to which previously they were subject, as we were obliged to keep Cox's hive syrup, tartar emetic and all other articles resorted to, constantly ready to meet the attacks of the croup, which were very sudden and frequent in cold wet seasons. Since then, we have found nothing necessary but the snuff plaster. If a child is heard to breathe hoarsely, or cough with any thing of the dreadful ringing sound of croup, it is only necessary to apply the snuff plaster, and we feel under no further anxiety. Instead of being obliged to watch with the child all the rest of the night when once the snuff is applied, we go to rest again, with a feeling of entire security, which we have never had the least cause to regret.

FEVER OF CHILDREN.

The various complaints to which children are subject, being as I have before mentioned of an irritative nature, will generally produce fevers, and although severe while they continue, are not frequently productive of danger if properly managed.

A disordered state of the stomach and bowels, teething, exposure to cold, striking in of any eruption, and in short, every thing which can excite an increased action in the heart and blood vessels, will produce more or less fever.—The treatment of these complaints has already been described. When these fevers take place, cleansing the stomach and bowels will be proper, for which purpose give an emetic or puke, followed by two or three grains of calomel, to which add four, five, or six grains of rhubarb; for the dose of either of these medicines, [see table;] after which *Bateman's drops*, *Grodfrey's cordial* or *paregoric*, at the same time bathing the child in warm water, will generally assist in lessening the irritability of the system and removing the fever.

SCALD HEAD.

This complaint begins in brownish spots on the head, and in a few days forms a scab, and discharges a thick gluey matter that sticks amongst the hair. The sores gradually increase until the whole head is covered with a scab, discharging this matter which is very offensive. You are to cut off the hair as close as possible, and wash the head well every night and morning with fresh lime water. This is easily prepared by slacking a piece of quick lime, of the size of a hen's egg, in a quart of water, and when settled, pour the liquor into a bottle and keep it corked for use.

CHOLERA INFANTUM.

OR

PUKING AND PURGING.

This vomiting and purging of children, called by physicians, *Cholera Infantum*, prevails during the heats of summer; it is a dangerous and destructive disorder throughout the United States. Of all the complaints with which childhood becomes afflicted in its earliest stage, this is at least among the infantile population of the Western country, the most destructive. When this disease commences, it is very rapid in spreading itself through the section of country or neighborhood in which it first makes its appearance. Its desolation or fatal termination, depends very much upon the season, section of country, and state of the atmosphere. This disorder generally shows itself before the middle of June, or about the commencement of our summer months, continuing its ravages through the warm season, gradually lessening in violence as the cool weather approaches. Its frequency and danger is always in proportion to the heat of the weather: children are subject to it from the third week after birth, to the second summer, at which period it is the most fatal to them.

Many distinguished physicians have been disposed to consider teething as the cause of this complaint. I am however convinced, that this is not the cause of *Cholera Infantum* or Puking and Purging. Yet in children laboring under the irritation of cutting teeth, I have no doubt this complaint is much more severe than it otherwise would be, and that it is more easily taken by them, and that the disorder is more apt to be fatal in its consequences, I admit. But that it is brought about by the causes which I have before mentioned, will be admitted by every physician who has taken the trouble to investigate, or in other words, to search out the original causes of this disease.

As I have before told you, the digestive organs in the early stage of childhood, are liable to constant irregularities and irritations: but what excites morbid irritations in the intestinal canal, is perhaps difficult for the most learned of the profession at the present day to determine. Yet, whatever influence the irregularities of diet, teething, or orther complaints may have in producing this disorder, I am assured from long experience, that the violent heats of summer, together with sudden changes, or exposure to a moist and unhealthy state of the atmosphere, are the usual exciting causes of *Cholera Infantum* or Puking and Purging.

Symptoms.—This disorder commences generally with a purging, but when severe, the child is seized with a puking and purging at the same time, when a few moments before it appeares in the full enjoyment of health. The discharge or stool is highly offensive, and colored with a dark or yellow hue; the stools now become frequent, attended with severe griping: probably the motions will be as often as fifteen or twenty times during the twenty-four hours. So soon as the operation commences freely from the bowels, the vomiting or puking begins to cease; over the region of the stomach the slightest pressure will give pain, being very tender and probably swelled; tongue white, thirst great, a constant craving for water between the times of purging which cannot be satisfied. The skin becomes dry, and from the child falling away, which it does with great rapidity, the skin is very much shrunk on the inside of the thighs: and while the feet are cold, the head and belly are hot; pulse small and quick, sometimes full; generally towards evening the child is better; but after a short time the purging commences again. Countenance pale, wan and languid; eyes sunk and dull; the child moans and sighs much; cannot sleep, is excessively irritable, sometimes attempting to bite its nurse, or rolling about its head, or constantly putting up its hands to its face; the stools become bloody. Even water itself will produce purging. The least jar or irregular motion gives it pain; noise and light cannot be endured. It will scream on barely being touched; The gums are black and swelled; the lips or their edges are filled with a dark scurf: inflammation takes place; the breathing becomes hurried and laborious; the pulse quick, weak, and irregular, and death closes the sufferings of one of the most painful and distressing disease.

Remedies.—When this complaint is about to make its appearance, which you will know by a purging, a white tongue, skin dry and hot, slight fever, attended with gripings, and occasionally accompanied with cramps of the abdominal and other muscles—nothing is of greater service than a gentle emetic in the morning, followed by a dose of calomel, mixed with a small quantity of ipecacuanha, at night. [For doses of medicines see table.] The emetic not only cleanses the stomach, but produces a soft moist state of the skin. The calomel and ipecacuanha as I have before described, will greatly lessen the severity of the disease, and not unfrequently entirely relieve it. But should there continue looseness of the bowels, with a dry skin and wakefulness, you are to obtain at any doctor's shop a phial of wine of ipecacuanha, which is nothing more than the ipecacuanha steeped or mixed in wine—of this medicine give the child a few drops through the day, in a little warm tea of any kind: this will produce a gentle moisture or in other words a moist sweat. At night give a dose of paregoric. [For dose of this or any other medicine refer to the table.] The warm bath, that is bathing the whole body of the child once or twice a day in warm water, will be found a valuable remedy and greatly assist the cure. Many children have entirely escaped this dangerous complaint by daily using the warm bath. By following the directions I have laid down, in a great many cases, the complaint will be so relieved as to render the further use of medicine unnecessary.

When the remedies which I have mentioned fail, which is sometimes the case, give occasionally a dose of calomel, to which add a little ipecacuanha. As soon as the medicine has purged the child, or in other words, it has had three or four stools, you are to give a little paregoric in which put a few drops of the wine of ipecacuanha. This moderotes the operation of the purge, and brings on a gentle moisture or sweat of the skin. You will find great benefit from covering the child's belly with carded cotton, over which you are to put a broad bandage, drawn moderately tight. The cotton thus borne will check the purging.—Should the child be *teething* when it takes this complaint, immediate attention ought to be paid to the gums, and cut if necessary, when the teeth cannot pass through them. It may be necessary for me to inform you, that if the emetic or puke which I have directed, should happen to act too severe, you can easily stop it by giving a dose of paregoric or laudanum, in a little tea made of cinnamon. So distressing in some cases are the effects of vomiting or puking—not from the emetic but from the disorder itself, that you will be under the necessity of seeking means to check it; for this purpose there is nothing better than weak lime water and new milk, in which put a few drops of laudanum or paregoric, or apply green peach tree leaves beat up, over the stomach and breast, this is a valuable application for putting a stop to bilious vomiting: sulphuric eather is also a good remedy. If these however should fail in removing the vomiting or puking, a blister applied over the pit of the stomach will scarcely ever fail. This last remedy should not be applied until a fair trial is given those which precede or go before it.

HOOPING-COUGH.

This complaint occurs only once during life, and is contagious or catching. It prevails in the Western country during the winter and spring months, and its being mild or severe, depends very much on the atmosphere. When the winter and spring is extremely cold and wet, the Hooping Cough is generally severe, but on the contrary, it appears under a much milder form.

SYMPTOMS.—Hooping cough commences like a common cold, and as it gradually advances, the breathing becomes more hurried and difficult, the voice hoarse attended with cough; great thirst; after a few days, a strange hoopping sound is made whenever the child draws a long breath, followed immediately by the cough. The agitation of the whole system is such at this moment, that the child lays hold of whatever is nearest, in order to support himself during the fit of coughing: after which he pukes or spits up a tough, frothy, slimy mucus, and is for a short time relieved.

The treatment is quite simple:—When you discover the child has taken it, give instantly an emetic or puke of antimonial wine: [See the table for dose.] And should this puke not lessen the severity of the complaint, you are to give a second puke, and if necessary, a third; if bound in the body, a dose of castor oil. To lessen the cough, give frequently the juice of garlic sweetened with honey, or a tea-spoonful of Sweet Oil, to which you may add a few drops of Paregoric or Laudanum.

The *Hooping Cough* is generally most severe during night: to allay or ease the cough, the use of Paregoric or Laudanum will be highly necessary. [For doses see Table.] I have found great benefit in my practice by using in this complaint the Tincture of *Assafœtida*—which is nothing more than a small lump of *Assafœtida* steeped for a few days in a little whiskey, or any kind of spirits—of this Tincture you are to give a few drops whenever the cough is severe, and you will find it to allay the irritation of the system, and mitigate or calm the cough.

Doctor Robertson, in the January number of the *London Medical Repository*, states that, of all the remedies he has ever employed in Hooping Cough, friction—which means rubbing—on the region of the stomach with the Tartarized Ointment, has been the most undeviatingly useful: for as soon as the pimples begin to appear on the breast, the disorder begins to abate. This ointment, is nothing more than Emetic Tartar mixed with a little hog's lard. [For a description how to prepare it, look under the head Tartarized Ointment.]

MEASLES.

The measles generally make their appearance in the spring season. It is a contagious or catching disorder, and like the hooping cough attacks but once during life.

Symptoms.—For a few days before they break out on the body, the child complains of sickness; seems dull and heavy; very great thirst; short, dry cough, with frequent sneezing, as if laboring under a severe cold; the eyes look red, and much inflamed. On the fourth day, the eruptions, or red pimples—which resemble flea bites—make their appearance on the face and neck, which soon extend to the breast, and then cover the whole body. In three or four days they begin to go off; at the same time, the fever.

which always accompanies the *measles*, begins gradually to decline. In some cases, the fever and cough will continue without lessening in their violence for several days or a week after the measles have entirely disappeared.

REMEDIES.—As soon as the sickness or drowsiness is observed, and you have cause to apprehend, from the symptoms I have already described, that your child is about to take the *measles*, open the bowels by castor oil, so as to procure two or three stools: the next evening—for it is at this time the *fever* is the highest—give a gentle vomit, or puke, of antimonial wine. You will find, by giving gentle pukes, that the child will be greatly relieved, by lessening the fever and oppression—this being the cause of the drowsiness and stupor. If the vomit should both puke and purge, so much the better, for the child will be the sooner relieved. When the fever and cough continue for a few days after the measles have entirely disappeared, a dose of castor oil will be proper, and which should be occasionally given during its continuance. About this time there is a dark, offensive matter remains in the bowels, that produces this fever, and which ought, and must be removed by means of these gentle purges. You will always know if the fever continues, by the dullness, thirst, and want of appetite. Sometimes the measles and hooping-cough, attack the child at the same time: when this is the case, a physician should be immediately called, as there is considerable danger.

The diet in this complaint ought to be low: such as mush and boiled milk, chicken soup, &c. The drinks are to be slippery elm tea, flaxseed tea, balm tea, &c. Nothing to be taken *cold* or *hot* but moderately *warm*. Exposure to cold or damp must be avoided, or the disorder may strike in, which would be very dangerous. Let the child be kept in a room neither hot nor cold, but of a pleasant temperature. And you are to recollect that spirituous liquors of any kind, administered in any way, is highly improper. Bleeding is sometimes necessary, when the inflammatory symptoms run high, or cough is very severe;

but it ought always to be performed if possible, under the advice of a physician.—Blisters applied between the shoulders or on the sides, will abate the cough, and may be safely used at any time during the complaint.

WORMS.

The worms which infest the human body, are the long-round worm, the maw, or thread worm, the tape or long-joint worm, and the fluke worm. The long round worm is called by physicians, *ascaris lumbricoides*, deriving its name from its slipperiness. It has three nipples at its head, and a triangular mouth in its middle. Its length is from four to twelve inches, and its thickness, when at its largest size, about that of a common sized goose-quill. The body is furrowed on each side, and the tail somewhat blunt. This worm is quite common in children, and not unfrequently it crawls out at the mouth. It is generally of a milky, brownish, or ash color.

The maw or thread worm,—called by physicians, *ascaris vermicularis*—has a blunt head; the tail of the male is blunt, but that of the female quite sharp and winding. It is generally from two to four inches long, quite small—about the size of a small thread—of a white color, and very elastic or springy.

This worm is generally found in the strait gut, or fundament—most commonly in children, but not unfrequently it is met with in grown persons also. They are frequently found in the intestines, or guts in the form of a ball, and so completely covered with a slimy mucus, as to prevent the medicines which are usually given for worms, from acting—or in other words—causing their discharge by stool. In women, they sometimes escape into the *vagina* or womb, and thence into the urethra, or canal through which the urine passes—and they are also found in the intestines of children.

The long thread worm—called, medically speaking, *tri-*

cocephalus dispar—is from an inch and a half to two inches long—of a clear white; the head is sharp; the body of the male is constantly in motion in a curved or winding form. The female is straight, with a blunt head and sharp tail; they contain a brown matter, and generally inhabit the large intestines.

The long tape worm—called by medical men, *taenia solium*—is from one to six hundred feet in length. It is gifted with the power to contract, or enlarge its diameter; that is. to draw up or increase its size at pleasure. It rolls itself into a round form, and falls from one side of the stomach to the other on turning, when in the recumbent or lying position. When cramped by the position of the patient, or by hard pressure over the belly, disturbed by food which does not agree with it, by medicine, or some disease proper to it, or tormented by the approach of death, it leaves its hold, leaps about and falls, as it were into convulsions or fits.

The broad tape worm—called medically, *bothriocephalus latus*—the head is longer than it is broad; scarcely any neck. Its body is flat; generally from ten to twenty feet long, and at its broadest part from a quarter to a half an inch across, and of a white color.

The fluke worm.—This worm is about an inch long, and of a dirty, yellowish, greenish, or brownish color; you will know it by examining the worm which infests the livers of animals, as the sheep, the hog, the goat, &c. being the same worm.

It is extremely difficult to say, what are the original causes which produce worms. It is therefore, impossible that any physician, however learned he may be, to determine with any kind of certainty, their origin. That improper diet, or food assists in producing *worms*, is correct; but this is only true so far as this improper food disorders the stomach and bowels, and weakens their action; for worms seldom occur if the action of the bowels is healthy, strong, and vigorous. "Few infants have worms until they are weaned, which is to be accounted for on the principle that the bowels are in better order during suckling than afterwards, when the diet is more varied and indigestible."

[For the learned and distinguished Robley Douglison, Professor of the practice of medicine in the University of Virginia. I am indebted for the highly valuable information on the subject.]

Climate, infancy, weakened state of the bowels, and improper food, favor the production of worms. That climate has a particular influence, and is favorable to the origin of certain worms is evident. A fourth part of the inhabitants of Grand Cairo have the *Tape Worm:* and, in Holland, according to Rosen it is quite common. In the United States is quite rare.

Symptoms.—The head is generally affected; the face is pale, and sometimes the color of bees-wax; the lower eye lid becomes of a leaden color; itching is felt in the nose, occasionally picking it; the saliva or spittle runs down over the pillow during sleep; the breath has a remarkable bad fœtor or bad smell; frightful dreams; the child cries in its sleep, and awakes with great terror; itching about the navel; creeping or tearing pain in the belly, or a pricking and gnawing about the stomach; constant hunger, and yet the system becomes weak; frequent itching of the fundament; frequent dry cough, with tickling in the throat, accompanied with low fever; these symptoms singly or together, denote the presence of worms.

Treatment.—A great many medicines are daily employed for worms. From long experience, and an extensive practice, I have had a fair opportunity of treating their virtues, at the head of which stands calomel, worm-seed oil, Carolina pink root, sometimes called Indian pink root, or pink root, and spirits of turpentine; all of which when properly given, are valuable medicines for expelling worms.

You are first to commence, by giving the child a suitable dose of calomel; [For which see table of medicine.] you are occasionally to repeat this medicine as long as the stools have a very offensive smell, and look unnatural. On the days between the administering the calomel, give the child a little aloes, pounded very fine, and mixed with honey. [For dose see table.] "I have never known a case of failure," says a distinguished physician, when the patient or child, was freely purged with calomel, and then given either the worm seed oil, agreeably to the directions on the phials in which it is sold, or the Indian pink root in tea." [For a descripton of this root look under the head Carolina Pink root.] The oil should be given on an empty stomach in the morning on a lump of sugar, and when the pink root is used make a tea of it, by pouring a quart of boiling water on a handful of the roots, of which you are to give a cupful night and morning to the child; and to cause him to take it more readily, you may add milk and sugar: by this means children will take it as soon as any other tea. Sometimes the pink root will occasion the eyes to be sore, when this is the case, you are to stop using it until the eyes are perfectly well; this is produced as is supposed, from some other root which grows with the pink root, and is frequently gathered with it. After using the pink-root for a week or ten days, give a dose of calomel or castor oil. In those species of worm which I have mentioned as uncommon in our country, their expulsion or discharge, is produced by spirits of turpentine in large doses, requiring the advice and attendance of a physician.

M. Cloquet, a distinguished physician of France, affirms, that he has seen the long worm, or the one to which children are most subject, evacuated or discharged by stool, after the belly had been rubbed with a mixture of ox's gall and common soap, oil of tansy or of chamomile, mixed with spirits in which camphor has been dissolved, or garlic; and by the application of a plaster composed of common yellow wax, litharage, assafœtida, and galbanum, applied to the belly.

Pure air, simple digestible food, exercise, and the use of all those means by which the system is strengthened, should be attended to; otherwise, as soon as they are expelled, they will again return. For this purpose, accasionally administer to the child or person subject to worms, a simple dose of Charcoal in new milk. According to the latest and most enlightened experience of the Medical Schools in Europe, Charcoal is highly recommended.

REMARKS.

I have now given a full and general description, of the important diseases to which the human body is liable, and of the various remedies to be used in their cure. The limits of my work, will now exceed those promised my subscribers, by nearly one hundred pages, the surplusage of which I present to those subscribers, with sentiments of gratitude for the liberal and generous support I have received. Even with this extra number of pages, my work will not permit me to describe every trifling plant or root, nor would it even be necessary for me to do so. I shall therefore, proceed to describe as far as practicable, all the *valuable roots, plants,* and so on possible to be included in the work. I have observed in several books purporting to have been written for the use of families, descriptions of many plants and roots, merely calculated to fill up and increase the size of such works, without being of any benefit as medicines, or even affording any useful information to the reader. I shall therefore, mention only such as are truly useful as medicines, and whose virtues are highly important in the cure of diseases. Should my book be beneficial to mankind, and meet the approbation of my countrymen, I will, with the permission of the ALMIGHTY, endeavor to be still useful to my fellow creatures, by adding a second volume which will contain such information, as for want of room, I have been unwillingly compelled to leave out of this volume. I will also endeavor to notice, all the new discoveries which will have been made throughout the world, in the cure of various diseases to which the human race are liable, and such roots and plants as may be found worthy of attention.

SENEKA SNAKE ROOT.

This root possesses more virtues than any one used in medicine; and of all the roots used in medicine it is by far the most valuable. It is now more than eighty years since its virtues were made known to physicians, by Doctor *John Tenant*, who learned its use from the *Senagaroos* tribe of Indians. By rewarding them liberally, he obtained their secret remedy against the bite of the *Rattle Snake*, which he called snake root on that account. According to their practice, it was applied both outwardly and inwardly; either chewed and applied to the wound, or in the form of a poultice. Doctor Tenant thought the Seneka a certain remedy against the bite of the Rattle Snake, but it has since been doubted. A reward was given to the Doctor for this discovery, by the Legislature of Pennsylvania. The Seneka was recommended by him, to be used in *pleurisy;* and in this disease it is a truly valuable remedy, *after* the free use of the *lancet* and the *warm bath*. Sir Francis Millman, Doctor Percival, and many other distinguished physicians, have borne testimony in favor of its powers as a *diuretic* in *dropsies*—diuretic means whatever acts on the urinary organs, so as to produce an evacuation of the water from the bladder freely. In *Croup* this is a valuable medicine: and the discovery of its being such, is due to Doctor Archer, of Hartford county, Maryland, who first discovered its great efficacy in Croup, that frequently unmanageable disease. My practice is, in the first instance to employ the *lancet*, in the next the *warm bath*, and in the next the Sencka Snake-root, as directed under the head of croup. Given as a *strong decoction*, which is made by pouring on one or *two ounces* of the best root coarsely pounded with a hammer, about a quart of boiling water, which is to be stewed down to half a pint or less, in a close vessel over a slow fire:—a tea spoonful every hour, or indeed every twenty minutes to a child as the case may be dangerous or otherwise, will answer the effect in croup. It is of infinite service if it pukes the patient when given in this way; because it brings

KK

on a discharge of mucus or tough slime from the mouth and throat, which almost always relieves the person afflicted. It is proper if the case is a dangerous one, to give a dose of calomel with the snake root, adding to the calomel a small portion of ipecacuanha; in fact, in this disease when very dangerous, I give large doses of calomel when I resort to this remedy: in simple and gentle cases of croup, an emetic of ipecacuanha, and the warm bath, will frequently give relief. A strong tea made of this root, and given as in croup, is an excellent remedy for the hives, or for *rheumatism* of an inflammatory nature; and in violent colds, it is an admirable medicine to promote perspiration or sweating. Used in these cases, the best form is that of a handful of the root to a quart of boiling water, giving a wine glass full of the decoction every two hours, if a grown person, and increasing or lessening the quantity as seems necessary.

The virtues of this root in obstructions or stoppages of the Menses or monthly discharges, are absolutely incalculable; and every woman should return thanks to the Author of all *Good*, for giving such virtues to this root as are possessed perhaps by no other, in relieving this diseased state of the female system, which of all others is probably the most dangerous. When the menstrual discharge is looked for and does not appear, four ounces of the decoction above described ought to be taken in the course of the day, indeed, as much ought to be taken as the stomach will bear without sickness.—Without sickness to puking is induced, which is sometimes the case when the stomach is weak and irritable, add in the tea or decoction some cinnamon, or calamus, or angelica, or a little ginger; either of these in addition, will cause the stomach to retain the decoction: There is no danger in the seneka snake root, for I have frequently given it in *very large doses* in croup. The only difficulty is, that it sometimes passes off by stool, without being productive of its usual benefits in female cases—the remedies for which will be spoken of under the proper heads. But in *Dropsy*, this purgative effect of the seneka snake root is of great and important service, as well as in its active and powerful influence on the urinary organs. In all dropsical swellings it ought to be used very freely, and will always be found a medicine of high and inestimable value. I will close the notice of this great root, by observing that it has the confidence, of the most distinguished physicians of the United Stats, as well as those of Europe. The discoveries of its virtues in Female Obstructions, is due to Doctor Hartshorn of Philadelphia, one of the best of men, and a man whose heart is devoted to the cause of suffering humanity.

SASSAFRAS.

A particular description of sassafras is unnecessary, being known and found in every part of the western country. The root, bark, or flowers made into a tea, is used considerably by the people in the country. It cleanses any impurities of the blood, and if distilled, affords a valuable oil which is a good remedy in rheumatism. It ought to be rubbed on the afflicted parts in small quantities: and if taken inwardly a few drops are to be given on a lump of sugar, being highly stimulating. The oil rubbed on *wens* is considered a good remedy, and frequently removes them entirely. The sassafras bark mixed with the sarsaparilla makes a good diet drink for cleansing impurities the blood, &c.

SARSAPARILLA.

This root was first brought into notice by the Spaniards, in the year 1563, and was for sometime afterwards, considered a certain cure for venereal diseases; [see that head, where you will see venereal described.] It however, afterwards proved unsuccessful, either from want of proper attention, or from want of knowledge how to treat the complaint.

This little root has excited a great deal of inquiry and discussion of medical men, throughout Europe and the United States, as to whether it really is or is not, a cure for this wretched disease, the *venereal*. It has fallen several times into almost entire neglect, and as often been again revived into use. It has however, lately been brought forward, with a much higher reputation than it ever held before, and if used in the manner I have described in venereal, may be relied on as a certain cure. Years of practical experience have convinced me of the fact, even in the worst of the complaint. I will go still further, by asserting that the virtues of this root, are not yet fully known and duly appreciated: and I sincerely regret that the limits of my work will not permit me to go more fully into the great benefits I have witnessed from its use in chronic affections of the liver—[for a description of which disease, see diseases of the liver.]

In scrofulous sores, in all diseases of the skin, and for cleansing the blood, it will be found valuable. In rheumatism, gout, and to stop the effects of mercury, or to remove any bad consequences which have been produced by its use, the sarsaparilla is also good. In weakness of the stomach called dyspepsia, [see under that head,] is an excellent remedy by giving tone and strength to the stomach and bowels. The method of preparing it, is by simply boiling after washing it clean, in the proportion of an ounce of the root, split and finely cut up to two quarts of water, which must be boiled down to a quart, and suffered to get cold before it is taken. Take of it from a pint to a quart daily, or as much as the stomach will bear. The bark of the root contains the virtues. You must obtain it sound: and recollect always, that it looses its powers by being kept any length of time. The tea should always be made fresh every day. Sarsaparilla grows plentifully in the western country, and may be found along creeks, and on the banks of rivers. It is a small running vine when torn from the ground, and extends some distance from the head, which is of a dark brown color on the outside, and a pale white within. When cut into short pieces it splits easily, and has a very bitter taste. The main vine is about the size of a common goose quill. It is a native of the Spanish West Indies, from whence it was formerly imported, until discovered to be also a native of the United States.

The imported root is not quite as large as ours, and is of a darker color and much wrinkled on the outside. It may be considered as one of the most valuable roots in the western country, and although possessing great power, is entirely innocent. It ought most certainly to be used, in all cases in which mercury has had any effect on the system, or in which there is the least doubt that any infection lurks in the system connected with veneral.

JAMESTOWN WEED.

Sometimes called *jimston, thorn-apple, stink-weed:* and, by the learned, usually called *datura stramonium.* Whether this plant is a native of the United States or not, cannot at this late period be known; nor is it material that the fact should be ascertained, because it is now found in every part of the American Union; from the state of Maine to the Mexican Gulph, and from the Atlantic Sea-board to the Rocky, or Oregon Mountains. It was first noticed by the original settlers of Virginia, at *Jamestown,* from which circumstance it took the name which I have adopted. Beverly, who in very early times, wrote a history of the first settlement of Virginia, thus speaks of its effects on a party of British soldiers, who had eaten of the leaves of the Jamestown weed as boiled greens. "One would blow up a feather into the air, whilst another would dart straws at it with great fury: another would sit stark naked in a corner of the room, grinning like a monkey, and making mouths at the company: whilst another would caress and paw his companions, and sneer in their faces. In this frantic condition they were confined, under the apprehension that they might destroy themselves, though it was observed that all their actions were those of innocence and good nature. They were by no means cleanly, and would have wallowed in their own excrements, had they not been prevented. After the lapse of ten or eleven days, their senses again returned, without their being able to remember any thing that had occurred in the interim" I will give, for the satisfaction of my readers, some account of the first discovery of the medical properties of the Jamestown weed, and also adduce several cases in proof of those medical properties, abridged from the account of Doctor Storck, whose authority may be relied on.

"In the month of June, July, and August, I observed in the neighborhood of Schoenbrun, says the Doctor, great quantities of the Datura stramonium, or thorn apple. I well knew that this plant was altogether disused in medicine, because several authors had pronounced it highly dangerous. On the 23d of June, 1760, I went out very early in search of the weed, and gathered a large quantity of it, and resolved to give it a fair trial, notwithstanding all I had heard and read respecting its poisonous effects, and of its producing insanity or derangement of the mind. I next cut off the roots and threw them aside; then beat the leaves, branches and stalks, in a large marble mortar, and pressed out about one gallon of the juice. This I evaporated to the consistence of an extract, over a slow fire in a glazed vessel, often stirring it with a wooden spoon to prevent its burning: and the extract, when it became cold, I found to be a black brittle mass. I laid a grain and a half of this extract on my tongue; dissolved it against the roof of my mouth, and swallowed it down. It neither produced disorder of my body, nor the least derangement in my intellectual faculties.—After making several experiments on myself, and perceiving no manner of disorder, I concluded that the extract could be safely given to patients in samll doses. We happened at that time to have a case in the Hospital, in which it might be presumed this *Extract* of the *Thorn-apple*—which the reader will please to remember we call James-town weed—would be of service. Before using it, however, I consulted both ancient and modern writers, and all to no purpose.—They had all laid it down in explicite terms, that it would disorder the mind, destroy the ideas and memory, and produce convulsions. These were all dreadful effects:—but, notwithstanding, a *query* suggested itself to my mind in the following form. "If the

Thorn-apple by disordering the mind, causes madness in sound persons, may we not try whether, by changing and disturbing the ideas and common sensory, it might not bring the insane and persons bereft of their reason, to sanity, or soundness of mind, and by a *contrary* motion, remove convulsions in the convulsed." This motion, I confess, was far fetched, yet it was not without some good success. The experiments I made were as follows:

"CASE 1st. A girl twelve years of age, had been disordered in her mind two months; she answered confusedly when asked any questions, and what words she did utter, were very imperfectly articulated. She was sullen and refractory, and could be prevailed on by no means, to do any thing. All the medicines she had taken had produced no effect. I gave her half a grain of the extract morning and night; and made her drink after each dose, a cup of tea, or some veal broth. On the third week she began to be less sullen; returned more rational answers, and spoke distinctly. In two month's time—continuing the use of the same medicines, and giving three doses each day—she began to reason extremely well, and said her morning and evening prayers with a clear and distinct voice; gained a good memory and gradually recovered her understanding.

"CASE 2d. A woman over forty years of age, was afflicted with vertigo or dizziness in the head, and could find no relief from any medicines: she became gradually disordered in her mind, and finally a degree of *madness* accompanied her vertigo. She was brought to our hospital. The medicines first prescribed gave her no manner of relief. She began to be raving and furious: rose out of bed in the night, and by her bawling, disturbed and frightened the other patients—some of whom she would forcibly pull out of bed. "In this situation, I gave her," says Dr. Storck, "*half a grain* of the *extract* of *thorn apple* twice a day. The first day she became more composed, but in the night she turned as furious as ever. The third day, I gave her one grain of the extract morning and evening, and all the symptoms became milder. She made some noise indeed in the night, but soon fell asleep again. On the fourth day she began to give more reasonable answers, but soon fell again into raving fits. Her days and nights then became calm and quiet. On the eighth day, I gave her one grain of the extract three times, and continued these doses until the fourth week, when all her fury was laid. Her madness went off; her soundness of mind, speech, and judgment returned: and she slept as soundly as any of the other patients—yet the vertigo frequently and suddenly returned upon her as before, and at times with such violence as to make her fall down as if in a fit—but, *she always retained her presence of mind.* It was enough for the purpose of my experiment, that the extract of thorn-apple cured her madness; and perceiving that the vertigo was not removed, I forebore its further use. She lived five months in the hospital:—All the functions of her mind were good and sound, but the vertigo returneed gradually stronger, and the fits of it became more frequent, until at length a true fit of *apoplexy* carried her off. I dissected her, and found many of the blood-vessels of the head distended or swelled, and one of them turned bony for an inch and a half; besides which—says the Doctor—I found the two anterior ventricles of the brain distended greatly, and filled with many *hydatides* of different shapes and sizes.

Hydatides are little animals, formed like bladders, and distended with a watery fluid. All the *viscera* in the rest of the body were in a very sound state. From these discoveries made after her death, it appears that the vertigo of this patient was an incurable disease: and it also appears, that the *extract* of the *Thorn-apple—Jamestown weed*—not only laid her rage, but cured her madness, without producing any bad symptoms."

I have accompanied the *discovery* of the medicinal virtues of the Jamestown weed by Doctor Storck, with the two preceding cases, to prove clearly to my readers, that in the beneficence of his mercy, the great FATHER OF THE UNIVERSE, has clothed our soil with means, powerful means, of curing our diseases, with which we are measureably unacquainted, and with the medical properties of which it is our duty to become familiar. There is, in my opinion, nearly as much folly and stupidity in importing costly drugs at enormous expences from foreign lands, while we have their equals at home, as there would be in importing *bricks* and *timber* from Europe to construct our habitations. Industry and science alone, can develop the immense resources of this unrivaled country, and these we are personally, morally, and *politically* bound to employ.

Every part of the Jamestown weed exclusive of the root—of which we know nothing from experiment—when taken in considerable quantities operates as a strong *narcotic* or stupifying poison. This is however no valid objection to its medicinal use and properties; because some of our most powerful medicines, such for instance as *opium* and *aquafortis*, invariably destroy life when injudiciously taken. I am not alone in considering this plant as possessing high and invaluable medicinal powers; it has been spoken of in terms of high commendation by many of the most distinguished physicians of the present age, among whom are Barton, Fisher, Biglow, and King of Connecticut.

Among the Indian nation the leaves of this weed are made use of, especially in cases of wounds, bruises or contusions, ulcerations, and the bites of reptiles. The *extract* of this weed procured in the manner above stated by Doct. Storck, is valuable in various cases of the chronic kind: by which I mean those of long standing: also, in all those kinds of epilepsy, commonly called fits—those especially, which give warning of their coming on, or those which occur at regular times. It is also a better medicine than any thing yet known, for lessening the violent pain in *sciatica* or hip gout. The leaves of the dried plant, smoked as we do tobacco, are of great use in attacks of spasmodic asthma, which means phthisic accompanied with cramp. In making use of this medicine internally, the dried and pounded leaves may be given in doses of a single grain. If the first dose produces no sickness nor vomiting, you may give a grain of the leaves three times a day, and even increase the dose each time, until the effects are felt, or relief produced. The *extract* however is always to be preferred, given as before described by Dr. Storck the real discoverer of the medicine. The bruised or wilted leaves are valuable in painful tumors, and indeed in most swellings accompanied with pain. They are in these cases, to be applied externally, and in such quantities as to preserve their moisture against the fever of such tumors. The ointment made from the bruised leaves, is also valuable, and is made by boiling them in lard or tallow, straining it well and setting it off to cool.

In the abridged extract from Dr. Storck, I have shown the value of this medicine in *mania, madness,* or *phrenzy,* and I now say that, the value of his discovery in 1760, notwithstanding what has been said against it, has been amply substantiated by experiment of many distinguished men of the present age, among whom are Barton and Fisher—infact, Barton's experimental testimony alone, would be quite sufficient: and, here I wish it to be distinctly noticed by those affected with *epilepsy,* or fits, that this testimony is clearly in its favor, as a most powerful remedy, even in deplorable cases—he has proved the fact from actual experiment. I wish the reader also to bear in mind the following facts with regard to the value of simple medicines:—First; the most learned sometimes decry their use, because there is not scientific mystery enough about them to excite the astonishment of the common people; and second, because they are often abused by quacks and pretenders, and men who have not perseverance and resolution enough to give them a fair trial.

DOG WOOD.

The *dogwood* is so common throughout the United States, as to require no description whatever; it is infact to be found in every forest of the country.—The *dogwood bark* is generally considered equal to the Peruvian bark: but I conceive it greatly superior, not only on account of our always being able to procure it fresh from the tree, but because the Peruvian bark is old before it reaches this country, and nearly if not always *adulterated.* It is among the best *tonic* or astringent medicines to be found in this or any other country. The bark of the root of the dogwood tree is the strongest; next in strength to which is the bark of the *body* and *smaller branches.* In all *intermittent fevers*—by which I mean all fevers which go off and return again—it is an excellent remedy; and the only reson why it cannot be given in other fevers, is that when given in actual fever, it increases the pulse, and by so doing does mischief: hence you will see the necessity of never giving it except when the fever is entirely off. In cases where it produces pain, or griping of the bowels, a few drops of laudanum will remove the difficulty if given with the bark. In most cases, the dose in powder—which is the best way of giving this bark, is from thirty to thirty-five grains: and in some particular cases, mentioned under the proper heads—an addition of the snake root is to be made in the proportions of thirty grains of the dogwood bark to six grains of the snake root, pounded to powder. The wood itself of the dogwood tree is considerably used by Dentists—by which I mean tooth cleaners and setters, in putting in artificial teeth. The young branches stripped of their bark, and rubbed with their ends against the teeth, render them extremely white and beautiful. These are tooth brushes of nature's presenting, and are infinitely better than those made of *hog's bristles* and filled with *snuff*, and such other delightful aromatics! The negroes of the Southern States, and those of the West Indie Islands, who are remarkable for the whiteness of their teeth, are in the constant practice of rubbing them with the small branches of the Dogwood, or of some other tree which will answer the purpose. The ripe berries of the Dogwood, in spirits of any kind, make an excellent bitter for common purposes, and one well adapted to persons of weak stomachs, taken in the morning. All the Indian Nations use the flowers at the proper season, in warm tea, or in spirits, as a remedy in windy colic. The dogwood is an excellent remedy—boiled strong as tea or decoction—for *Horses* having that destructive disease, the *yellow water:* a distemper which carries off thousands of that useful and noble animal every year. Horses having the yellow water, should be bled freely every day, and given nothing to drink but strong dogwood tea. The powdered bark of this tree makes an excellent ink, and the process is very simple:—Take half an ounce of the powdered bark, two drachms of copperas, two scruples of gum Arabic, or cherry-tree gum, and put them into one pint of water; mix them together, and in a few days it will be fit for use. The medical virtues of this bark were discovered as early as the year 1787. It is an astringent, and also a stimulant, and the internal use of it renders the pulse always quicker, and often fuller than it naturally is.

PINK ROOT OF CAROLINA.

This is a medicine of highly and justly celebrated reputation for worms, and was learned from the CHEROKEE INDIANS at an early period of the settlement of this country. This plant grows plentifully in Tennessee, and is indiginous to all the Southern States, particularly South Carolina, where it is found in such abundance as to have given a name to the plant, I have frequently seen it brought to Knoxville for sale, and have been informed from good authority that, large quantities of it are to be found in almost all parts of the uncultivated country. Its growth is very rare in the state of Virginia; in fact, it does not grow wild in any of the states North of the city of Baltimore: it is, however cultivated in the gardens at the North.

This plant grows in rich soils on the borders of woods. Its time of flowering is from May to July, and grows from six to twenty inches high. Its root consists of a multitude of fibres, or threads forming together, a large cluster or bunch. This root is of a yellow or straw color, when you first take it from the ground, but becomes black when dried and old. It is so common in all countries where it grows at all, as to need a very slight delineation or description if any. From the root there arises several four-sided stems or stalks of a purplish color, on which are narrow leaves of some length opposite to each other; the flower is of a carmine or crimson color, a little inclined to yellow on the inside.

Carolina pink-root was first brought into notice among physi ians, by Doctors, GARDEN, LINING and CHALMERS, all of whom speak very highly of it as a medicine for worms. The root and plant yield all their virtues to water: in other and plainer language, you get all their strength out of them by steeping them in boiling water, or *making a tea of them.* When the root becomes old it looses much of its strength, and should always be had fresh from the ground if possible. When made into a tea, it has a sweetish taste, and will therefore be easily taken by children.

Of the dried and pounded root, the dose is about fifteen or twenty grains for children between six and eight years of age, and half that quantity for children under six years old. To a grown person, and to a person nearly grown one drachm, or two drachms may be safely given, the common mode of given it to children is as a tea, made in the proportion of one ounce of the root and plant to a pint of boiling water, of which from one to three table spoonfuls may be given to a child, and about half a pint to a grown person. If no effects follow, the doses may be increased accordingly. I usually give it as a tea to children for breakfast, in milk and sugar as they take it more readily in this way. *It must not be continued if it affects the eyes of the child,* which it sometimes does. After its use for eight or nine mornings, give a good dose of castor oil; and if no worms follow, give a dose of calomel. [See the table for doses.]

The *Carolina pink root as to its medical effects,* is not entirely confined to worms; it is sometimes given in fevers which arise from what physicians call *ascidity in th prime-via;* which means mucus or slime in the stomach and upper bowels: and the late professor Barton, recommends this medicine in the "protracted remitting fever of infants, which is supposed to lay the foundation of *hydrocephalus*," or in other words dropsy of the brain.

ALUM ROOT.

This is a native of all the North American forests, from Georgia to Maine, and from the Atlantic Ocean to the Oregon or Rocky Mountains. It is a very strong vegetable astringent; by which I mean that when applied to the human body, it makes the solids harder and firmer, by contracting their fibres. As a powerful astringent, it is usually employed in all cases of weakness and irritability, and report speaks favorably of its virtues. It is generally used in external applications more than as an internal remedy: in piles for instance, or *hemorrhages* from any part of the system; by which I mean spontaneous bleedings.

GINSENG.

This root is called by the people in the country generally, for shortness *Sang*. It is found in great plenty among the hills and mountains of Tennessee. and brought into Knoxville daily for sale. Some few years back it was used as an article of commerce, and sent to the Eastward in wagons as a commodity of foreign export, and offered considerable employment and profit to the gatherers of it who resided near and among the mountains. It has latterly however, fallen in price and value as an article of exportation, and therefore but little of it is brought in for sale.

This root was exported to China, and afforded to the shipper a handsome profit—generally selling it in the Chinese dominions for its weight in silver. The Chinese attributed great virtues to this root: so many indeed that at the period of 1748, the price at Pekin is said to have been eight or nine times its weight in pure silver. They considered it as a sovereign remedy in all diseases incidental to their climate and country, and had no confidence in any medicine that was not combined with it: and such was its astonishing reputation, that it was rarely, if ever administered to the poor, on account of the highness of its price. They chew it and take it in strong decoction so as to get all the virtues from this precious drug. These people are remarkable for their superstitious prejudices, civil, moral, and religious: as a proof of which, they set a higher value on those roots which have a resemblance to the human form, and ascribe greater powers to them than those of a different shape.

The ginseng has been fully tested by the best physicians in the United States, and they ascribe to it nothing more than its being a pleasant bitter, and a gentle stimulant for strengthening the stomach. It gives all its strength and virtues by being steeped in whiskey, or any other kind of spirits.

TOBACCO PLANT.

Called by the learned, *Nicotiana Tobacum.* This very common plant, was found in cultivation by the Indian nations, when the continents of North and South America were first discovered:—these however are not the only regions of the globe in which it is found to flourish; the East Indies have long been known to produce it. To describe the tobacco plant would be entirely useless; it would answer as little a purpose, as to describe on paper the countenance of an *old friend*, with whom we had long before shaken hands, and become perfectly familiar. I shall therfore consider it in no other light than as a medical drug.

I shall first notice tobacco as a remedy for worms. I do not recollect ever to have tried it myself, but Doctor Barton expressly says—and his authority can in all cases be relied on, that "tobacco leaves pounded and mixed with vinegar, and applied as a poultice to the breast and belly, will frequently *expell worms* in cases where very powerful remedies have been resorted to in vain. In cases also, where poisons of any kind have been taken into the stomach, and emetics given internally, and prove deficient in their operation, the tobacco poultice as just described, if applied to the stomach, will act powerfully and force it to discharge the contents. In cases where the bowels are obstinately constipated, in other words, where great *costiveness* exists, the leaves of the tobacco plant cured in the usual manner, stewed in vinegar and applied to the belly, will be attended with signal success, when the most powerful purges internally taken have failed.—The last mentioned application of tobacco leaves stewed in vinegar, is a good remedy in what physicians called *ascites*, or dropsy of the belly, of which there are two kinds. One kind is where the dropsical water is lodged in the great cavity enclosing the intestines, or guts, &c.,—this is called *ascites abdominalis* by medical men. The other is where the water is lodged in the membrane, suck or tube about the womb, and is called *ascite sacatus* by physicians. I will for the satisfaction of the reader, abridge a case of the latter kind, from a letter of Dr. Cutbush, physician of the American Marine Hospital at Syracuse. The subject of the disease presumed by Dr. Cutbush, to be dropsy, was a young woman brought to him by her parents. Some of her former physicians—*thirty-three* of whom had been consulted in her case, were of opinion that here disease was a collection of water in the womb; others, that it was dropsy of the *ovaria;* these are the parts taken out of the female swine when spaying: others that it was an enlarged liver; and others, still, that it was an *extra-uterine fetus* which is a cause of *conception* in which the child is not in the womb where it should, be, but in the cavity of the belly outside of the womb. On examination, Dr. Cutbush discovered a large tumor, or swelling in the abdomen or belly, which extended diagonally across it from the left to the right. The swelling or tumor, which was unusually great, had a number of inequalities on its surface, which could be easily felt, and which, when pressed upon, produced extreme pain; no fluctuation or movement of water, however, could be discovered on such pressure. The case was new to him; and in addition greatly perplexing, because the first physicians of Naples had given contrary opinions respecting it, and had also disagreed in their practice. She had been under the free use of mercury twice—once at Naples, and once at Syracuse: at the latter place, mercury had been given in large quantities by a surgeon belonging to Lord Nelson's fleet, without any beneficial effect. "From this history and examination," says the doctor, "I entertained no hopes of relieving her; but the solemn entreaties of her parents determined me to make a trial of a remedy which I had found useful in obstinate tumors, and which finally proved the disease to be a *dropsical* affection of the womb itself, of the right *fallopian tube*." These tubes extend from the sides of the womb towards the *ovaria*—which I have before explained—and are supposed to grasp them in sexual communication. "I directed the leaves of the tobacco plant, recently collected, to be stewed in vinegar, and applied to the abdominal tumor." The first application produced sickness at the stomach, puking, vertigo, or swimming in the head, great depression of muscular strength, copious sweating, and a loose state of the bowels. Her pulse became low; and the violence of the symptoms induced the Doctor not to continue the application long. On the succeeding day it was repeated twice—morning and evening—and produced the same symptoms but less violent, and attended with an immoderate *flow* of *water* from the vagina or womb. This remedy was continued twenty days, and the patient was completely cured. No medicines were given, except a little opium and some wine occasionally.

In cases of dropsy, generally the tobacco plant has been found very serviceable. When given in proper quantities, it acts as a powerful diuretic—or in other words, it produces a great flow of urine—entirely disproportioned to the quantity of liquid taken into the stomach. This is a conclusive proof that it acts upon, and dislodges the dropsical fluid from the system. In cramps, or spasms it is also productive of much benefit: being well known to produce great relaxations of the muscular powers, and unusual prostration of strength—on which account, it also may be given with advantage in cases of *tetanus*, or locked jaw, and in fact, in all cases where there appears to be a derangement of the muscular energies, local or relating to a particular part, or general, and involving the whole system. When tobacco is to be taken internally, by the stomach, it ought either to be in the *extract*, as described by Doctor Storck, or in *infusion*. The infusion is made by steeping an ounce of tobacco leaves in a pint of boiling water, and giving it by the tea-spoonful with much caution. One, two, or three table-spoonfuls, in half a pint of warm milk, or thin gruel, will generally produce relief, if given in clysters, in cases of colic or very obstinate costiveness, where all other medicines have proved ineffectual. If these quantities produce no relief, and there is no sickness of the stomach, the clysters must be repeated every half hour, gradually increasing the infusion until one or the other of these effects be produced. In this way, the dangerous effects of tobacco may always be avoided. I will record a case in which obstinate constipation of the bowels was relieved by an infusion of tobacco, when all other remedies had utterly failed. In the city of Charleston, South Carolina, some years since, and before reading medicine, I was attacked at night with severe colic, which terminated in obstinate constipation of the bowels. The pain was so excruciating that I was compelled to send for a physician: it was Doctor Witterage, a gentleman equally celebrated for his philanthropy, and his profound knowledge of medical science. During a period of ten days, apprehending an inflammation, and consequent mortification of the bowels, this gentleman resorted to almost every known and powerful remedy, *without effect.* As a last resort—of which he candidly informed me, recourse was had to clysters made of tobacco.

The first, which was a weak infusion, had no effect; and the Doctor directed my nurse to give me a stronger one at midnight. Her fatigue caused her to fall a sleep, and it was neglected till morning. By this time—the tobacco having remained in the water all night—the infusion had become unusually strong, in which state a clyster of it was given. The immediate derangement of my feelings and sensations, and the horrible nausea and sickness of the stomach I suffered, are absolutely indescribable. I perspired at every pore, and so entire was the prostration of my muscular powers, that I had to be held on the close-stool. It was with difficulty that I could draw my breath. In a few minutes, by an almost unconscious effort, an extremely fetid discharge took place from the bowels, of the color and consistence of molasses, when I was entirely relieved. Subsequent experience has taught me to believe that, had this great and good man applied tobacco leaves, stewed in vinegar, to the abdomen, whilst I was under the operation of medicines taken by the stomach, I would much sooner have been relieved from my miseries. In concluding this subject, it can scarcely be necessary to advise my readers, that the tobacco plant is an active and powerful medicine, and dangerous when used to injudicious excess.

THE UVA URSI.

Sometimes called the *Bear-berry*, the *Bear's Whortleberry*, and the *Wild Cranberry*.

The Uva Ursi—sometimes designated by the names I have noted above—is a native of the mountains and cold regions of Europe, and it is said of the northern parts of the United States. It is presumed, from numerous and well authenticated experiments, to be the best remedy ever yet discovered, in all diseases of the urinary organs, whether of the kidneys, ureters, or bladder, and is therefore entitled to no ordinary consideration as a medicine. The dose usually given, of the powdered leaves of the *Uva Ursi*, in any kind of syrup, is from twenty to thirty grains, three or four times a day, which may be doubled in quantity, in cases of extreme urgency and danger. The description of this plant, given by the celebrated Galen, which is considered the most accurate one on record, is in *substance* as follows: It is a low shrub, which grows and spreads itself near the surface of the ground, and has *pensile*, or hanging branches; bark of a reddish or pink color, and is thickly set with oblong, oval, and entire fleshy leaves. The flower is oval shaped, and broader near the base than the mouth which has an edge scolloped into five divisions, with small, blunt, and curled points. The fruit is a roundish, red-colored berry, similar in appearance to the small wild cherry, and contains *five* hard bony seed, with plain sides, and *no more*. It is an *ever-green*, and produces fruit every two years. Every part of this shrub, particularly the bark and leaves, has a bitter and astringent taste. I am thus particular in the description of it, because the Bilberry or Red Myrtle, is often mistaken by good *Botanists*, for the Uva Ursi—they being so nearly alike as scarcely to be distinguished from each other. The only distinguishing characteristics which can be depended on are these: The flower of the Uva Ursi has ten *stamina*, more commonly known by the name of *antlers* or *uprights*, and the berries contain five seed only, while the other—the Bilberry or the Red Myrtle—has only eight *stamina* in the flower, and sometimes twenty seed in the berry. I have some doubts, notwithstanding the opinion of the celebrated Doctors, *Biglow* and *Chapman*—for both of whom I entertain a high respect—that the real and genuine Uva Ursi of Galen, is not a native of any known and inhabited part of the North American continent: and that its having been measureably brought into disrepute, like many other medicines, has been owing to the fact of other plants being mistaken for it, and used medically in its stead. Galen says that it is a rare plant, and is only to be found in the coldest countries, and in the neighborhood of mountains covered with eternal snows; and that he never met with it but upon two of the highest mountains in Europe, one of which was an Austrian Alp called *Gans*, and the other a Styrian Alp called the *Snowy Mountain*, six leagues from Marianstein. We have no such mountains in North America, unless the Oregon or Rocky Mountains west of the Mississippi of whose botanical productions we know little, perhaps nothing. But whether the Uva Ursi is an American plant or not, it can always be had genuine in the shops, and my principal motive for mentioning any doubts respecting its being a native of this country, is to guard those afflicted with diseases of the urinary organs, against the use of spurious or useless plants in its stead. The following case abridged from a work of high authority, will show the genuine Uva Uursi in its true light.

CASE 1st. "A man about sixty years of age, had been about *twenty years* afflicted at times with a difficulty of making water, which was usually voided by single drops, accompanied with exquisite torture, a fœtid smell, and much mixed with blood. Sometimes there was a total suppression of urine, which could only be relieved by the catheter. He first took proper laxatives for the relief of the bowels, and then commenced taking *half a drachm* of the Uva Ursi every morning. This prescription was continued for seven complete months; by which time his urine became more free and full of mucus, but not so fœtid as before; and the pain which had tortured him for so many years *was quite gone:* he slept well; and had a good appetite; grew strong; walked well; and made water without any pain.

CASE 2d. "This was also a man about sixty years of age, who had for a long time been afflicted with exquisite pains, and a suppression of urine to so great a degree, that for *seven weeks* he had never passed his water but by the help of a catheter. Half a drachm of the powdered leaves of the Uva Ursi was given him every morning and gentle doses of paregoric at night; and after six days he had no further use of the catheter. Having persevered in the use of the medicine for fourteen weeks, he was restored to perfect health.

CASE 3d. "A man came to us, whose name was Christian: he was afflicted with *hydrocele* or dropsy of the *scrotum* or bag, for which he had taken medicines usually given in such cases. When this course was finished a defect in the urinary system began to threaten, insomuch that in a short time his urine became of a white color; was passed with great difficulty and pain; and as soon as discharged had a very bad offensive smell. The catheter being introduced repeatedly, evidently proved that there was a calculus or stone in the bladder. The Uva Ursi was therefore given in the quantities before noticed; by which in a short time so great relief was obtained; that not only a due retention of urine took place, but it was also passed without difficulty or pain, in smell and color perfectly natural: "And I assert it," says the writer, "that by continuing the use of this medicine two months, every calculus sign and symptom was entirely removed; although by sounding him again, the calculus or stone was still found in the bladder." This is the first, and the only person among all that I have seen, who frequently made water of a healthy appearance while a stone remained in the bladder. How it came to pass, and by what means, that the patient should obtain such benefit from this plant, as to be entirely exempt from pain, and all other inconveniences, when a stone still existed in the bladder, I must confess myself entirely unable to explain.

SLIPPERY ELM.

This tree deserves great attention, as being among the best remedies in our country. I have mentioned frequently, that in many diseases it should be used as a poultice, and in many others as a clyster. I shall now describe the valuable properties of this tree more at large. The inner bark must be used, and that of the young tree is preferable. As a poultice, nothing is superior, particularly in old sores or ulcers, burns, and wounds—particularly gun-shot wounds. During the Revolutionary War, our surgeons used it with the happiest effects. They applied poultices of it to fresh wounds, and always produced immediate suppuration, in other words, discharge of matter, and a quick disposition to heal. When any appearance of mortification was evident, the bark was pounded and boiled in water, and made into a poultice. When applied, it produced immediate a surprising change for the better. In dysentery or consumption the inner bark boiled in water and drank freely, will be found a valuable medicine. It is cooling and soothing to the bowels. It may be made into a fine jelly, which if taken freely, is a certain and astonishing remedy in all bowel and breast complaints, and may be freely administered to children. This mucilaginous bark is so nutritive, that it supplies the Indians with food in times of scarcity. It is one of the most cooling and pleasant remedies and I may add, that it is not only one of the most valnable articles we have, but deserves the confidence of every person who practices or administers medicine.

JERUSALEM OAK.

From this plant which grows plentifully throughout the State of Tennessee, and which is too well known by almost every person to require a description. The oil called *worm seed oil* is made. This oil has for some time attracted a considerable share of popular favor, as an antidote against worms in children. It is sold in almost every store, under the name of "Wormseed Oil." And persons who purchase this oil or medicine, should be careful that they are not imposed upon: because it is very often adulterated with *Spirits of Turpentine* by which they are always disappointed in their expectations of benefit.

In its pure and unadulterated state, there is no medicine preferable to the oil made from Jerusalem Oak for expelling worms from children; but it must never be given when the child has fever: because it will in that case, increase the fever, the oil being highly stimulating and inflammatory. When the oil is administered from eight to ten drops must be given to a child two years old, on a lump of sugar--it ought to be given three times a day for three days in succession; after which you must give a good dose of calomel, say five or six grains, or a dose of castor oil, the calomel however, is the most certain to produce a full discharge of worms. If no worms are discharged, and they are still suspected to exist in the system, repeat the dose again—and again, until you bring them from the child. A wine glassful of a *decoction* of the Jerusalem Oak made by boiling it in milk, in the proportion of a handful of the leaves to a quart of milk, is a dose for a child, but the pure oil is by far the best.

PENNYROYAL.

There is no description necessary of this plant, as it grows in almost every garden. In slight stoppages by cold, of a female's monthly discharges; generally called *Menses*, Pennyroyal tea will generally remove the obstructions. The tea must be made strong and sweetened with honey, molasses or sugar, and drank as warm as possible, at the same time bathing the feet in warm water. It is probable however, that in obstructions of the menses which have existed for any considerable time, more efficient and powerful remedies than pennyroyal tea must be used. I will also, mention that the American pennyroyal is a different plant from that known in England by the same name.

DITTANY.

This handsome little plant belongs exclusively to America: and is known to almost every farmer and his family in the country. 'It grows plentifully in Tennessee. The dittany is always found in dry soils, and in shady and hilly places; it is used in slight fevers as a tea: every old lady in the country has more or less used dittany tea in colds. It is excellent to relieve nervous head-aches, and is a good remedy in hysterical affections of women. In South Carolina and Georgia, the dittany is given frequently by infusing the leaves of it in hot water and administering it as a tea, drank as warm as possible to produce sweating.—The medicinal virtues of dittay are much the same as penny-royal, mint and sage: it is a perfectly innocent plant.

MAY APPLE.

Sometimes called wild lemon, duck's foot, *Ipecacuanha*, and by the learned, *Podophyllium Peltatum.*

This plant which possesses very important medicinal virtues is presumed to be an exclusive production of the North American Continent: it is every where found in abundance on congenial soils, from the State of Main to the Mexican Gulph, and from the Atlantic sea-coast to the Oregon Mountains. In the language of the learned, it is a perennial herbaceus plant; in other words the roots do not perish by the frosts and snows of winter. The May Apple is well known to almost every person in the United States: —it has a plain upright stem, of a yellowish green color, about twelve or fourteen inches in height; two large horizontal leaves at the top, between which, and in the fork when in bloom, there is a white flower which is succeeded by a yellow acid fruit. Respecting the different properties of this plant, the reader is desired to recollect that *the fruit is good for food,*—the leaves poisonous—*and that its medicinal virtues* are *wholly confined to the root.* The season proper for gathering the root is late in the fall, when the leaves begin to drop: if gathered in the spring it is comparatively good for nothing. The Indians dry it in the shade, and use it in powders.

The American May Apple-root is an excellent, gentle, and effective purge, and is presumed by many celebrated practical physicians to be greatly superior to the jalap obtained in the shops. Practical experiment has proved that this root operates more gently as a purge than jalap: that it operates a much longer time; and that it is by no means so drastic and griping as jalap. It is also preferable to Jalap in other respects; it is less nauseous and more easily taken; less irritating to the stomach and bowels, and may be more easily used by delecate females, and persons having weak and sensitive stomachs. It may be given with much advantage in what physicians call *colica pictonem*, or *dry belly ache*, sometimes a dangerous complaint; in intermitting fevers; and particularly *dropsy*, on account of its producing continued and large evacuations. Taken in a small dose, say of ten or twelve grains in powder; it is a gentle and easy laxative. Twenty-five or thirty grains usually operate with activity and power; and where griping is apprehended, the mixture of eight or ten grains of calomel will be of advantage.

CANCER ROOT BEECH DROPS.

Called by the learned *Orobanche Virginiana*.—This plant is the natural growth of every part of the United States: is usually found under the beech tree, and is of a sickly yellow or pale pink color, and entirely without leaves. The root which appears blunt and round at the bottom, and is covered with twisted and matted fibres on its lower end, is of a yellow color; the stems and branches are finely furrowed; and on the ridges formed by these furrows, there will be found dark purple, white and yellow stripes. Between the root and the first divisions of the stalk, there are blunt pointed and bud-like scales, which stand out from the surface: and similar ones, but more resembling buds, are scattered along their branches nearly to their tops. The top grows from eight to fifteen inches high. The reason for my being thus particular in the description of this plant will be presently seen.

From the best information I can collect respecting the history of the *cancer root*, it appears to have been originally a cure for cancers, used by the Indians, and communicated by them to a Surgeon of one of the Pennsylvania regiments many years ago, stationed at what was then called Fort Pitt. The physician to whom the secret was communicated by the Indians, afterwards came to Philadelphia, and advertised for the *cure of cancers*. He had been the student of Doctor Rush, who speaks thus of the application: "It gave me great satisfaction to witness the efficacy of the Doctor's application, in several cancerous ulcers, the cures he performed were complete. But, when the cancers were connected with the *lymphatic* system, or accompanied with a scrophulous habit of body, his medicines always failed, and in some instances did evident injury." The word "*scrofula*," is derived from *scrofa*, a hog, because this animal is subject to a similar disorder, which means King's Evil. The physician who had the secret from the Indians, died in 1784—and it was supposed the secret had died with him: but Doctor Rush procured from one of his administrators some of the powders, and found them compounded of the dried and pounded Cancer root and Arsenic: the proportion of Arsenic—of the pure white kind, was not more than *one fortieth* part of the whole compound. Most of the cures effected by these powders, were situated about the nose, forehead and cheeks, and upon the surface and extremities of the body. Cancers, taints of the fluids of the body, or those which affect the whole lymphatic system, must be cured by diet and internal medical remedies. Dr. Rush says that the powders compounded of cancer root and arsenic, in the proportions I have mentioned, and applied in the proper cases of cancer, produced inflammation which separated the sound flesh from the cancerous ulcer and its roots, and that he therefore preferred the application of those powders, to the use of the knife in all such cases. I will conclude these remarks by observing that the cancer root is a valuable remedy in old and obstinate ulcers, in which it has often been known to succeed, when all other applications had failed:—It must be gathered in the month of September.

POPLAR.

Sometimes sailed the *white wood* and sometimes the *American poplar:* the learned name of this tree is *Liriodendron Tulipiferia.*

This tree, as every reader of this work must know, is a native of the United States, and is so generally found in all parts of the country, that a description of it would be entirely unnecessary. It is sometimes called the *tulip tree*, from a supposed resemblance between its blossoms and those of the tulip. The first physicians of the United States and many distinguished men in Europe, have borne ample and uniform testimony respecting the valuable medicinal properties of the poplar. Its virtues reside in the bark of the root, branches and trunk, that of the root is presumed to be most powerful. It is a valuable medicine in all intermitting fevers, and particularly in ague and fever, and has been found of great benefit in dyspepsia or indigestion, in gout, in dysentery, and in *chronic rheumatism.* I say in chronic rheumatism, which is always without fever: because if given in acute rheumatism, where there is always some inflammatory fever, the poplar bark being a stimulant, will increase the fever instead of diminishing and subduing its violence: and here I wish the reader distinctly to bear in mind that, for the above reasons, stimulants can never be given in fevers which continue without intermission, and that they can always be given with safety and benefit, when there are periodical sensations of fever. For the same reason, also peruvian bark is never given in paroxysms of fever. The reason why poplar bark is beneficial in chronic rheumatism, and several diseases of the same character, is presumed to be because it is a powerful sudorific, or active agent in producing sweat, if given in tolerably strong decoctions. Given in powders, especially, if mixed in equal quantities of pulverized dogwood bark, it is equal to the best peruvian bark, and is to be given in the same quantities. "In pulmonary consumption, attended with hectic fever, night sweats, and diarrhœa, when combined with laudanum," says Dr. Young, "it has frequently abated these alarming symptoms. I effectually cured a man fifty years of age, who was afflicted with catarrh and dyspeptic symptoms for five years, which had baffled the skill of the best physicians, and the most celebrated remedies, by preserving in the use of the *poplar bark for two weeks;* and I can assert, from actual experience, that a more certain, speedy, and effectual remedy in *hysteria*, or hysterics, cannot be found in medicine, than the poplar bark combined with a little laudanum. I have used no other remedy after cleansing the primæ viæ—[by which the Doctor means the stomach and upper intestines, or first passages,] in *cholera infantum*, for more than two years: [cholera infantum, means a disease of children, attended with griping and purging, and sometimes with puking.] I have never known it fail—continues the Doctor—in a single case of worms which has come under my observation: I have prescribed it to a child when convulsions had taken place. After giving a few doses, several hundreds of dead *ascarides* were discharged with the stools." Ascarides in plain english, are all kinds of worms which are found in the human intestines, from the stomach to the rectum and fundament. The dose for a grown person, of the powdered poplar bark, is from a scruple to two drachms: it may also be given in decoction or in infusion: but when given in substance, it is most beneficial. The dose should be decreased in quantity in proportion to the age of the patient. The time for collecting and drying the bark, is the month of January or February.

SPICE WOOD.

Otherwise called *Allspice bush*, *Spice berry*, *Fever bush*—and by the learned *Laurus Benzoin*.

It is altogether unnecessary to describe the Spice wood; it is known to nearly every person of any intelligence in the United States. It is used as a medicine in the middle and Southern States, as well as the Western country, and operates in giving tone to the stomach, and strength to the general system: and when given in *intermittent fevers*. either in the pounded bark, or in tolerably strong decoction, it is generally attended with success. Doctor Barton alledges in some of his works—I have forgotten which—that, a decoction of the twigs in water, has often been given to children *for worms*, and that it is considered a good remedy in such cases. As a proof that the Spice wood possesses considerable medicinal qualities, the Indians make use of it in several of their complaints; but in which of them particularly, I am unable to say. The dose of Spice wood in decoction, is about a pint in twenty-four hours: and when used in the powdered bark, one drachm must be taken three or four times a day, in a glass of wine, or in any other liquid with which it will mix When taken freely as a tea, it produces copious perspiration, or sweating.

BONE SET.

Sometimes called *Thorough wort*, *Cross wort*, *Indian sage*, and perhaps, more properly, by the Indians, *Ague weed*:—The learned name of it is, *Eupatorium Perfoliatum*.

The Bone-set is a valuable plant, and cannot be too highly prized as a medicine. I regret to say, that at this time, most of its medical virtues remain unknown. It has been used in the hospitals of New York with great success, given either as a tea or in powder. The limited size of my Book, prevents me from writing at large on the great virtues it possesses: but I will merely make this remark, that it is endowed with more real and genuine virtues than any plant now known. The stalk is heavy, rises from two to four feet, perforating or bearing the leaves at each joint. The flowers are white, and appear in July and August. The leaves at each joint are horizontal, teethed and rough, from three to four inches long, about an inch broad at their base, gradually lessening to an acute point, of a dark green color and covered with short hairs. It is a native of the United States, and is every where to be found in Tennessee. It is generally found in abundance, on the edges of ponds which are surrounded with thickets of brush wood; in low and damp wood-lands; on the banks of small water courses creeks and rivulets, which are deeply shaded by the close foilage of the trees; and is sometimes in open meadows, and waste-lands. I do not know what the name *bone-set* was derived from; nor do I think it very material that the reader should be informed; because real wisdom and useful intelligence, have much more relation to the *nature of things*, than to the *mere names* of things. The medical properties of this plant, are various and powerful: nor do I believe there is a one which is a native of the soil of our country, more entitled to the attention and experiments of medical men. The whole plant is extremely bitter to the taste, and in some degree astringent; by which I mean that when it is applied to the tongue, or any other part of the body, it contracts the fibres and surface without any voluntary exertion of the muscular power. It is a strong tonic or strengthener to the stomach: and always when used internally, produces an increased discharge from the skin, which when condensed on the surface is called sweat; in these respects, from well attested experiments, its medical virtues are unequivocal as well as powerful. It can always be given successfully and without danger, in violent *catarrh* or *colds*, even when attended with some fever; because its stimulant effects are too slight to increase the fever, while the other qualities of imparting strength and causing perspiration, are in active operation. I wish the reader particularly to notice, that I mention the beneficial effects of the bone-set plant, in cases of violent *catarrh or cold*, because it is a dangerous forerunner of *phthisis*, or *pulmonary consumption*, in very many instances, and ought always to be removed immediately if possible. This plant is also an excellent remedy in ague and fever: which is the reason of its being called by the Indians, by a name which in their language signifies *ague weed*. It is also a valuable remedy in all intermittent and remittent fevers—always acting as powerfully and beneficially as peruvian bark. In fact, I think it in many cases, preferable to the bark, because it can be given when there is *considerable fever*: in which condition of a patient, the bark cannot be administered without great danger. For this reason also, I mean because it never increases fever it can always be given, and has been repeatedly administered successfully, not only in remitting bilious fever, but in typhus or yellow fevers. Dr. S. G. Hopkins of New Jersy, a physician of much celebrity, in an extensive practice of several years: during which intermittent and typhus fevers were very prevalent, gave the bone-set freely in warm decoction with great success. By giving the bone-set tea very copiously, he always produced sweating to allay the fever; and in dangerous cases, pushed the remedy so far as to produce *emeses*, or vomiting; and also purging. He related to several of his friends, that many of the farmers in his vicinity, without calling in a physician, had by the liberal use of a strong preparation of the bone-set tea, given warm, entirely succeeded in curing themselves and their families, of both intermittent and typhus fever. The truth is, that in low typhus which is very dangerous, and always attended with an unusual dry hot skin, the bone-set is an inestimable remedy. It is always used with the best effect, in a warm decoction of the flowers and leaves, which ought to be dried in the shade, and kept for use: the warm decoction is generally preferable to the plant in subtance; and from one to two table spoonfuls.

given every half hour, will in most cases produce sweating without causing so much nausea of the stomach as to produce vomiting. If the fever is broke, and you wish to give strength to your patient, give the bone-set in the powdered leaves and flowers, from twenty grains to a drachm, from three to six times in the lapse of twenty-four hours. Used in decoction as above stated, it is also a valuable remedy in *yellow fever*, as has been proved by repeated and well attested experiments. The bone-set is also very efficacious in removing acute rheumatism: [For a discription of which look under that head.] but it ought to be employed in this disease after blood-letting, to reduce the inflammatory action.

With the above commentary on the important uses of this plant in medicine, I recommend it to the serious attention of my readers. It affords another proof that Providence has given us the means of curing many of our diseases, without resorting to the adulterated drugs of foreign lands.

COMMON BLACK BERRY BUSH.

Called by Botanists, *Rubus Villosus.* This root is every where known, and therefore requires no description. It is eminently useful in all such diseases as are to be treated with astringent medicines: the root particularly is powerfully astringent, and when used medicinally is generally made into a tea. When the ripe fruit itself is employed, it ought to be given in the juice, or made into a syrup, or jelly. The tea or decoction is made by boiling a handful of the bruised roots in a pint and ahalf of water, until it is reduced to a pint: thus prepared it is given with success in diarrhæs and dysenteries, a small tea cupful every two hours, and has often been known to effect cures when many other remedies had failed. In the disease called by physicians, *Cholera Infantum*, known by painful gripings, and purgings in children, a weak decoction of the black-berry root may be given with good effects. But as these purgings may in many cases, be considered as the *efforts of nature* to remove the caues of disease, it ought to be given with much caution, and not until proper evacuations have been made to remove offensive matter from the stomach and bowels. In fact, it ought to be given in no case of dysentery or cholera infantum, until all offending matter, if any is presumed to exist, be removed by gentle pukes and purges. Black berry syrup made from the ripe fruit ought to be kept prepared in all families and given freely in all cases of derangement of the bowels.

BUTTON SNAKE ROOT.

This is a native of all the Southern States, from the seaboard, to the Mississippi: the root has a sharp arromatic, and very bitter taste, and whenever chewed it produces a considerable flow of saliva or spittle. A tea or decoction of it taken internally, produces a discharge from the skin, and expectoration from the throat and lungs. By many physicians of reputation, it is held in higher estimation than senoka snake root, which it very much resembles in its effects.

THE HOP.

This is a native of both Europe and America, and is found wild in the wooded tracts of the Western country, as far as the white population has extended:—there are large quantities of it on the uncultivated bottom tracts of all our rivers. Beside the bitter and strengthening properties possessed by the hop, used in beer and malt liquor as a common drink, it contains considerable narcotic powers, by which I mean those qualities which produce *sleep*. The qualities which produce sleep, are supposed to reside in the risinous part of the hop blossom, and can easily be extracted by alcohol or spirits. Bitters made from the hop blossom, are very useful in nervous debility or weakness, and where persons are recovering from sickness and cannot sleep.

CHAMOMILE.

The tame species is a native of Europe, but may be cultivated in most parts of the United States, and partienlarly in the mild climate of Tennessee. It is perenniel: that is to say its roots do not die by the frosts of winter, but shoot forth and blossom through succeeding years. The flowers are generally used for medical purposes, and sold in the shops: the single ones are the best, because they are the strongest. Infusion in water extracts the medicinal properties of the chamomile flower, which drank cold, is highly useful as a tonic: in other words it will give tone and strength to a weak and irritable stomach, repair a debilitated or lost appetite, and operate favorably on such young females as labor under what are called *green sickness:* which means a retention or stoppage of the menses. It also operates as an anti-spasmodic: that is to say, it relaxes the involuntary contractions of the muscles of all parts of the body, and particularly of the stomach, in what is commonly called cramp: it is also of service in all the nervous weaknesses in females. When taken warm and in considerable quantities, it aids materially in the operation of emetics or pukes, &c. &c.—The chamomile flowers when steeped in old whiskey, or any good spirits, and taken two or three times a day, in moderate quantities, is an excellent medicine to give tone and strength to a weak stomach, and restores the appetite. For women given in *hysterical complaints*, is a valuable remedy.

CHINQUEPIN.

Every person who resides in the western country knows what this is: It is sometimes called the dwarf chesnut, and grows in all parts of the middle and southern states, and in nearly every part of the Western country. Its bark is used with success in intermittent fevers, or such as periodically go entirely off; for like peruvian bark, if given while there is fever, it will increase it, and aggravate the symptoms. And like peruvian bark, and perhaps it is equally as good, it imparts tone and strength to the stomach, and consequently to the whole system.

FOX GLOVE.

Called by physicians *Digitalis Perpuræ*, is biennial, which means that its root lives two years in succession: to my knowledge is not a native of the United States, but may be cultivated with success, in all the states south of Pennsylvania, as has been proved by repeated experiments, and particularly in Kentucky and Tennessee. The leaves have a bitter, and nauseous, and acrid taste: Their medicinal properties may be extracted either by pure water, or alcohol or spirits.

The general virtues and properties of the Fox glove are *narcotic*, by which I mean they induce sleep,—and also *sedative:* which means that they diminish the animal energies of the system without destroying life; for instance, when the Fox glove is given in due quantities, it diminishes in a remarkable manner, the force and frequency of the pulse. From its producing the latter effect on the circulation of the blood, the exercise of common sense will teach any person that it must be beneficial in all kinds of hemorrhages, or spontaneous bleedings, whether the lungs, the womb or any other part of the body. From the same reasoning, and numerous experiments, it is also manifest that in diminishing the frequency of the pulse, and the irritability of the system, it may be beneficially employed in all *inflammatory diseases*, as a substitute for depleting remedies, such as bleeding, purging, &c. which always materially weaken the system—The inflammatory complaints upon which it acts beneficially, are of the brain and the lungs, and indeed of the viscera generally. It is also of much use in the early stage of *phthisis* or pulmonary consumption, in some cases of which it merely operates as a palliative remedy, while in others it wholly removes the disease, particularly when given seasonably and cautiously until its effects are felt in the head and stomach, or both. Chronic coughs, by whicih I mean coughs which are seated and of long standing, where no actual and positive injury has been done to the lungs, have often been strikingly and decidedly relieved by the fox glove. In *Dropsy* it is also considered an excellent remedy, particularly in that kind called *anasarcous;* which means where the dropsical water is diffused between the skin and flesh or rather in the cellular system, and not in the great cavities of the breast and belly, and so on. When you intend to give the fox glove, you ought always to evacnate the stomach and bowels in the first instance, by tolerably strong purgatives.

The first dose of the dried and pounded leaves of the fox glove ought to be but one grain: if you give of the tincture. you may give from ten to fifteen drops; and if you give of the infusion, you may give the half of a fluid ounce. You may increase these doses gradually, by adding one sixth part at a time, given three times a day, until nausea or sickness of the stomach, and vertigo or dizziness of the head ensues. It is not safe to proceed further with the fox glove, after the head and stomach have become affected as I have described. And here it may be proper to remark, and I wish it *distinctly to be borne in mind* by the reader, that when the medicine is taken incautiously, and in improper quantities, it becomes a poison, and is followed frequently by alarming and dangerous consequences.

IPECACUANHA.

This root is a native of Spanish America: and in the Spanish language it means *vomiting or puking* root. The word ipecacuanha, is implied to several other roots which produce vomiting or puking to any extent. The preper or *Botanical* name of this root is *raicilla:* I have however, adopted the name, *Ipecacuanha*, by which it is most commonly known to physicians. This root was first brought into Europe about the middle of the last century, but did not come into general use until about the year 1686, when it was introduced into the practice of medicine by Helvetius, under the patronage of Louis XIV. The ipecacuanha is one the mildest and safest emetics or pukes with which we are acquainted, and has this great advantage; that if it should fail to puke, it passes off by purging or sweating; and further if by accident an over dose is taken, it is attended with no danger, as the whole of it is vomited with the contents of the stomach as soon as it operates.—The vomiting or puking is promoted by drinking freely of warm water.

The genuine ipecacuanha in its dry state, is a small wrinkled root, about the size of a hen's quill, variously twisted, and marked with projecting parts, apparently like rings ash colored. Its taste is sickening and slightly bitter, with little smell, and covering the tongue with a kind of mucilage. On breaking the root, the outer bark is very brittle; and it is in this brittle part, that the activity and power of the root as a puke resides—the centre being nearly destitute of any medicinal virtues. This root is generally sold in the shops as a powder, that being the form in which it is used as a vomit or puke: The powder is the color of common ashes.

I have now described to you the important ipecacuanha, or the medicine which is now used throughout the world under that name; and I may justly remark that it stands at the head of the vegetable emetics, for the promptness, efficacy, and safety of its operations.

In powder, which is the manner in which it is generally given, full vomiting or puking will be produced in a grown person, by a dose of a scruple or half a drachm: or you may put a drachm into six table spoonfuls of warm water, and give a table spoonful occasionally, until it operates: or you may steep it in wine, and give it in small doses, until the effect you desire is produced.

The medicinal uses of this powder, when properly applied, are very great and valuable. In addition to its acting as a vomit or puke when given in small doses, so as to produce nausea, which means sickness of the stomach; it generally produces moisture of the skin, or sweat, or evacuation of the bowels: and still in smaller doses, it generally stimulates the stomach, increases the appetite, and assists digestion. In small doses, it acts not only as a diaphoretic, which means sweating, but as an expectorant, which means a free discharge of tough mucus and spittle from the mouth and throat. It is also a valuable medicine when given in small doses, to stop spontaneous bleedings from the lungs and womb.—These bleedings are called hemorrhages.—In intermittent fevers, it has generally succeeded in stopping them, especially when given about an hour before the coming on of the fever: and also when given so as to produce vomiting at the time of fever, or end of the cold stage. Great benefits are often derived from this medicine in continued fevers; and particularly in the commencement of typhus fever, an emetic or puke of ipecacuanha followed with a sufficiency of this medicine in very small doses, to keep up a gentle moisture or sweat, will if attended to in the early stage of this complaint, probably at once cut short the disease, or greatly lessen the severity and symptoms of the fever.

Wine of ipecacuanha is sometimes substituted for the powder: it is however better suited to children. As an emetic or puke, the dose for a grow person is one fluid ounce, which is about half a large wine or stem glass full. [For a description of this wine of ipecacuanha, look under that head.]

COMMON TANSY.

Tansy is perennial or perpetual, and grows wild by the sides of roads, and the borders of fields, but is most frequently cultivated in gardens, both for culinary and medicinal purposes. It flowers in July, and frequently in June. The leaves are generally used as a medicine, and when steeped in whiskey, or any kind of spirits, makes a moderately warm and highly valuable bitter for weak stomachs, very beneficial to children in preventing worms. It should be given to them in the morning, on empty stomachs. Some physicians have spoken highly of its virtues in hysteric disorders, particularly those proceeding from a deficiency, or suppression of the menses or courses. An infusion or tea made of tansy and drank freely, has been strongly recommended as a preventive of the return of gout.

SAGE.

This valuable garden herb was once supposed by the ancients, to prolong the lives of those who would frequently use it. They dedicated it to the following maxim:—"How can a man die in whose garden there grows Sage' in allusion to its many virtues. It is too well known, and too much used to require a description. It makes an excellent tea to produce a sweat or moisture of the skin, and by adding a little lemon juice or vinegar, so as to make it pleasantly sour, is a good remedy in fevers.

RUE AND BALM.

Rue is also a garden herb; the leaves which made into a tea, will produce perspiration or sweating, quicken the circulation, and remove obstructions of the blood. It is invariably to weak and hysterical constitutions.

Balm is also a garden herb, and affords a pleasant tea to be drank in fevers. When drank freely, it will produce perspiration or sweat, and, of course is good in slight fevers.

AMERICAN COLUMBO.

This stately and elegant plant is a native ef the United States, and is found in abundance in both Kentucky and Tennessee. It has various names: such as columbia, Indian Lettuce, Columbo root, Marietta Columbo, and wild Columbo. The stalk grows from eight to ten feet in height: it is strong, Juicy, and fleshy; nearly square and furrowed at the sides, and sends off its leaves, which are of a deep green color, at intervals of six or eight inches, to something more than half its length, and smaller leaves and flowering branches to the top. The root is biennial, that is, it lives two years: it is large, full of knots, plump and full, and of a yellow color. The leaves are occasionally apposite to each other, and usually grow from four to eight together: they are something sharp, and sometimes oblong: in other words oval or egg shaped, and sharp at the points. The flowers grow in clusters, and are of a greenish yellow, or cream color.

The Columbo root, which is the only part to be used —is a mild pleasant and highly valuable bitter, acting as a powerful tonic or strengthening medicine. It is valuable in dyspepsia or indigestion; and in diarrhæa or looseness ef the bowels, arising from a redundancy of bile. It will generally check vomiting or puking, and will always be found beneficial in colic, or cramps of the stomach, want of appetite, and cholera morbus, which means puking and purging: it may be taken in substance, by which I mean powdered,—a tea spoonful every three or four hours: or as a decoction or tea, a wine glassfull three or four times a day: or you may steep the root, say two ounces in a quart of old whiskey, which must stand for a few days, that the spirits may extract the virtues from the root. This valuable bitter may be used three or four times a day, in doses of a table spoonful or more: and adding a few drops of peppermint to this preparation, it is a good remedy to moderate the puking which sometimes occurs with *pregnant women*.. All persons who are subject to lowness, or depression of spirits, instead of resorting to more dangerous stimulants, should use this columbo bitter freely.

BLOOD OR PUCCOON ROOT.

Sometimes called *Indian paint*, and *Redroot*, but learnedly denominated *Sanguinaria Canadenis*.

This plant is a native of North America, from the Canadian Provinces to the Gulph of Mexico, and perhaps of no other region of the globe. It is not only a plant peculiar to the continent of North America, the virtues of which are so well known to the Indian Nations, but its root is perennial: in other words it is not destroyed by the frosts and snows of winter. It generally grows about a foot high in rich wood lands, and varies in thickness from a quarter to three quarters of an inch in diameter—which means across. It is generally about the size and length of a finger; fleshy and round, and the end of the root has the appearance of having been cut off by a dull instrument, or as if it had been broken off in removing it from the ground. The out side color of the root is brownish, but on being cut, the juice flows of a blood-red color.

The puccoon, flowers early in April, bearing but single flowers on each stem. The blossoms are white; the stems perfectly naked; the upper side of the leaf a pale sickly green, and the veins which pass through it, of an orange color. The flower-bud is of a faint or delecate rose color: the seeds which are round and pointed, are very numerous.

The leaves and seeds of the *Puccoon plant*, which is the name I have adopted, like the seeds of the *Stramonium*, or Jamestown weed, are poisonous and must never be used.

The root seems to contain all its medicinal qualities; and is closely allied in its effects on the human system, to the *Seneka snake root,* and in some of its effects to the *Digitalis Purpuria,* or fox glove. A decoction or tea, as it is usually called, made of the puccoon root is highly recommeneded in the treatment of old and indolent ulcers, which simply means old sores that do not seem inclined to heal, and the dried and pounded root applied a few times, in some cases of ill-conditioned ulcers, with callous edges, and an itcherous or itching discharge, seldom fails to produce a healthy state of the sores.—it is an excellent remedy in croup, and must be given in doses sufficient to produce vomiting, or puking; some physicians rely on it wholly in croup. It is also an excellent remedy in dropsy of the chest, called by physicians *hydrothorax,* given in doses of sixty drops of theJuice three times a day, and increased until nausea or sickness of the stomach follows each dose. This root in powder from twenty to thirty grains, is an active emetic or puke. Dr. Barton one of the professors in the Phyladelphia Medical College, thinks it nearly equal to the Seneka, or Rattle snake root, in cases of ulcerous sore throat, croup, and hives, and diseases of this nature. It is a valuable medicine to produce a determination to the surface, by which I mean sweating; and also in colds; pleurisies rheumatism, and other inflammatory disorders. When used for these last diseases, it should be used as a tincture, which is the root steeped for several days in spirits of any kind, and given in doses of ten drops every two or three hours, until a moisture or sweat is produced on the skin. This tincture is also valuable in jaundice, in torpor of the liver, attended with a colic and yellowness of the skin, a disease common to southern climates. The Puccoon rootmade into a tincture, and gradually and cautiously used, will be found a valuable medicine in stoppages of the menses or courses in women. I have used it with great success in my practice, when every other medicine usually resorted to had failed. My usual method of preparing it, is to steep about a handful of the roots sliced, in half a pint of old whiskey, letting it stand five or eight days when the tincture is fit for use, beginning with, ten drops, and gradually increasing the dose, as circumstances may require. But you may give it in a decoction or tea, a handful of it to a quart of boiling water, a table spoonful of it every two or three hours, as the situation of the patient may require.

This root powdered very fine, and snuffed up the nose, is said to be a certain cure for *polypus;* a fleshy teat, or grisley substance, which grows in the nostril gradually increasing in size until breathing becomes difficult, and which sometimes unless removed, ends in suffocation. I have lately made experiments with this root, in a disorder called *tetter worm;* and in several instances succeeded in curing it when other valuable remedies had failed. Steep the sliced root in strong vinegar ten days, and wash the part affected two or three times a day. I shall conclude my remarks on this valuable root by observing that it possesses a great many valuable qualities which are probably yet unknown. The best time to collect it for medical purposes, is when the seeds are ripe, which is about the beginning of May.

SENNA.

I shall first describe to you, the foreign or imported Senna, generally used in the practice of medicine; after which I shall describe the American plant Senna, which on almost numberless trials, has proved to be but very little if any, inferior to the imported, or that sold in the shops, and mostly used by physicians. I have used them both, and can discover no difference. This affords another proof of a bountiful Providence, in bestowing on this people a plant of so much value, and one which before its discovery here, we were compelled to import from Egypt. Here I again repeat what I have frequently said in this work, that all that is required of us are industry and attention, and we will discover in a few years, thousands of medicinal plants in the Western country, superior in every respect to the foreign, by which we will have this further advantage: we will always have them fresh, and in full possession of their virtues.

The leaves of the senna are alone used in the medicine. The imported plant grows in Turkey, Syria, and Persia. It is commonly called Alexandria Senna, because it was once imported exclusively from the city of Alexandria in Egypt. This medicine was originally received from the Arabians: and large quantities of it are now brought from Nubia, which is known in Egypt by the name of the Valley, or Country of Barrabas, it is a narrow valley through which the Nile flows, where the view is confined on two sides alternately, by a lofty chain of mountains, Senna is the chief production or commodity of this country. It is not cultivated, but grows naturally on the sides of the hills and ravins. Each person has the right of gathering what grows in his district. The crops are annually made; the productiveness of which depends upon the duration of the rains, which fall periodically every year. The first and most fruitful crop, is that gathered at the termination of the rains, the second crop is small. No expense attends the preparation of the plant, which merely consists of cutting and spreading them on the rocks to dry. The senna is then put up in bales of one hundred pounds, and the slave merchants convey them by camels to Sienna, and Darao, where they are sold for elven or twelve francs a bale, which is about two dollars and twenty-eight cents. They are then carried to the Farmer general at Cairo,—an officer appointed by the government to examine and purchase them. The sum fixed by him is from thirty to thirty-three francs—which is about eight dollars and twenty-seven cents. They are then sold by him to the European factors or merchants, for one hundred and six francs each bale, which is equal to twenty dollars and fourteen cents, and by them exported to the different quarters of the world. American citizen, why will you pay such accumulated and enormous expenses to foreign goverments and merchants, for an article which is furnished plentifully by the soil of your own country?

The demand for this article from Europe every crop is, generally from about fourteen to fifteen hundred quintals, of one hundred pounds each. The great demand for this medicine, both in Europe and the United States, has induced the Egyptian merchants to mix with it senna of an inferior quality, which sometimes occasions it to fail in producing the immediate effect intended. Although this *fraud*, when practiced, does no serious injury, it frequently disappoints us in the active operation of the medicine. The inferior Senna, although producing eventually the same effects, is much slower and weaker in its operation.

AMERICAN SENNA.

Having given you the history of the European, I shall now proceed to describe to you *our own* Senna, which grows abundantly in the United States, and particularly in the Western country. In fact, it is found plentifully about Knoxville, and on the shores of the Holston river. I have told you that I had used both, and could perceive no difference in their operation—and I now repeat the fact, that it may be the more forcibly impressed upon your mind. Notwithstanding this, those who prefer the foreign Senna to our own, may easily gratify their prefference, as the imported kind is now cultivated in North Carolina, and is found to flourish abundantly. It is evident that we do not obtain the pure plant from abroad: and I have shown the manner of adulteration: why, then. should we not cultivate the foreign plant sufficiently for our own consumption, if we must and will have it? The wild senna of America, is a most beautiful plant. I will describe it in as plain terms as possible—knowing at the same time, that it is very difficult, if not utterly impossible, to delineate in mere language, what can only be known to the eye. It has frequently several stems from the same root: these stems are generally either entirely smooth, or furnished with a few straggling hairs. The larger sized leaves, I believe, are mostly confined to the larger branches, and are disposed in pairs opposite to each other, on the sides of those branches which run out nearly a horizontal direction from the stem. The flowers are of a bright orange color, and are usually found on small sprays or sprigs, which shoot out in the angles formed by the stems and larger branches.—Near the top, the flowers are attached to the main stems. The stems rise from four to two feet in height. The leaves are rather long, green above, and pale underneath: *they should be gathered about the last of August for use.*

Dr. BARTON, an eminent physician, and professor of Botany, in the University of Philadelphia, informs us that he had some experience with the American Senna, during a term of practice in the Marine hospital of that city. "I have says, the doctor, for some months past, substituted the American for the Alexandrian Senna, and very frequently employ it.' I have also in a single instance, used it in my own family. I have had reason to confirm the high character, which the American plant has maintained.

But, reader, whether you may prefer the imported or the American Senna, which I consider equal in their medicinal powers, the following remarks are applied to both, or to either of them.

The senna is a valuable purge, and when good, is active in its operation, and at the same time quite innocent. Senna is seldom given by itself, but is always mixed with Manna, a description of which will immediately follow this plant. When you enquire for senna as a medicine at a doctor's shop, always ask for a dose of Senna and Manna, because these two medicines are always given together. Sometimes a little salts is mixed with the senna and manna, especially if you wish to make the operation sure and active. In fevers, first giving a good dose of calomel, follow it up with senna, manna and salts: senna has but one fault; it is apt to gripe during the operation: this can always be prevented, however, by adding a little ginger. But I believe from an extensive experience, that after calomel to remove bile if the following mixture be made up and given, it is superior and more innocent than any medicine now known as a purge. Take of senna and manna, each *half an ounce:* of ginger *one drachm;* of salts *one ounce,*—pour on these medicines a pint of boiling water; cover over the vessel in which you make this tea, so as to prevent the steam from escaping. This tea is to stand until it becomes cool. You are to give of it to grown persons one gill every hour or two until it operates freely. According to the age of the person, you are to give this tea in smaller doses, and as it is quite innocent; it may be given to children occasionally in small doses until the desired effect is produced, which is a free operation as a purge. If you wish it to act as a very mild and gentle purge, you may leave out the salts. I repeat in order that you may remember it, that whenever the bowels are obstructed, or whenever you require an active and searching purge, senna, manna, and salts, in the proportions I have just mentioned, adding thereto a little ginger, are superior to any means of operating on the bowels now in use.

MANNA.

The word manna means a *gift,* it comes from a Syrian word *mano,* being the food supplied by the Almighty to the children of Israel in the wilderness: or it comes from the word *mahna,* what is it? an exclamation by the Israelites on its appearance; so say the best authorities.

The manna, or medicine so called, and that which is mostly used by physicians, come from Naples on the Mediterranean Sea. The best manna is in long flakes, moderately dry, brittle and crumbling, of a pale yellowish color, and considerably transparent; in other words you can partially see through it. It is moist, very sticky, and dark colored, it is considered of inferior quality, although not less purgative. The manna is principly collected in Calabria, Apulia, and Sicily, in the warmest season of the year, from the middle of June to the end of July. Various trees afford it: particularly a kind of ash, called Manna ash. It flows from the trunk of the tree when tapped, similar to the juice or sap of our sugar tree when used in the same manner. The liquor first flows from the tree like a white froth, extremely light and of agreeable taste. The heat of the sun in a few days, hardens it to the consistence we find it. Manna has something the taste of sugar, and is sickish and searching on the tongue. Its great resemblance to sugar both in appearance and taste, induces children readily to eat it, in its effects it acts on them as a mild purge. Manna is, however a very feeble purgative medicine, requiring large doses for a grown person, say an ounce or two: for this reason as I have before told you, and so directed, it must always be mixed with senna and salts. It ought never to be given alone, except to *small children*, as a mild and opening medicine. [See table of doses.]

WHITE WALNUT.

During our Revolutionary War, when medicines became scarce, the physicians of the army employed the inner bark of the *white walnut* as a purge. In the dose of from ten to twenty grains, it operated well by evacuating the bowels thoroughly, and was much resorted to by them as a purgative in all *billious cases of fever*. By the addition of eight or ten grains of calomel, the efficacy of the white walnut may be greatly and beneficially increased. As I have stated to you, the medicinal virtues of this bark, are confined to the *inner bark:* and the proper time for getting it in the full possession of its virtues, is about the month of June, because the bark is at this time considerably more powerful than at other periods.

I have used the white walnut in may practice, and always found it among the best purgative medicines possessed in the Western country, and have very often been surprised that the article is not kept in the family of every farmer in the country. The manner of extracting the virtues of this bark is very simple:—It is merely to be boiled in water several hours, then strained and boiled again, until it becomes about as thick as honey. Two, three, or four pills, which it can be made into with a little flour, make a dose of this extract. One or two of these pills taken at bed time, is a valuable remedy in the removal of costive habits of body, which occasions head-aches, colic, &c. &c. By increasing the dose, these pills are good in dysenteries and billions fevers, and will be doubly beneficial, if combined or mixed with a little calomel.

RHUBARB.

Rhubarb, properly so called, is the root of a plant designated by the learned, *Reum Palmatum.* It is a native of various countries of Europe and Asia, and might be cultivated with perfect ease, perhaps, in every part of the United States.

Attempts has been successfully made to introduce the culture of this valuable drug in England; and it appears from authentic accounts, not only that immense quantities of it may be produced there, but that the English root is fully equal to the best Rhubarb obtained from Turkey, or China. The greatest difficuly seems to be in drying it properly. Its cultivation is by no means difficult: it is merely to sow the seed in a light soil in the spring; to transplant the smaller roots the next spring in a light soil, well trenched, and set them about three or four feet a part. The third year the plants will produce the flowers: but the roots are not to be raised for use until the fall of the sixth year. This is the whole process of rearing the Rhubarb: a process which I am convinced every American farmer is fully equal to.

The cultivation of this valuable medicine in the United

States, ought to be considered an object of high individual and national importance. That our climate throughout the different States, particularly the Western States, is fully equal to its production, there can be no doubt, as has been fully ascertained by an actual experiment.

That it will grow in Tennessee I well know: because it is now flourishing in abundance in the garden of Mr. Woods fifteen miles from Knoxville. The root was originally purchased by Mrs. Woods, from some drug store in Knoxville, and planted for the purpose of experiment, which has perfectly succeeded.—I mention the fact, in order to prove conclusively, with how much ease we might become independent of foreign countries for thousands of medical drugs which are annually draining our country of immense sums of money. Such experiments as that made by Mrs. Woods, ought to be made by every person who has opportunity and leisure. They are duties the American people owe both to themselves and their country.

There are three varieties of Rhubarb found in the drug shops: The Russian, the Turkish, and the East Indian Rhubarb; the two first, the Russian and the Turkish, resemble each other in quality and appearance, while the East Indian is a somewhat different character. The best Russian and Turkey Rhubarb is in roundish pieces, with a large hole in the middle of them. The East Indian or Chines Rhubarb, comes to this country in long flatish pieces, seldom if ever, having holes in them. The Turkish Rhubarb is the best, and is generally used in this country.

The marks of Rhubarb being of a good quality are, the liveliness of its color when cut: its being firm and solid, but not flinty or hard; its being easily pulverable, which means reducible to powder; and its appearing when powdered, of a fine high yellow color; and when chewed, by its imparting to the spittle and tongue, a deep saffron color.

Rhubarb is one of the mildest, best, and pleasantest purgatives, now in use in this or any other country; because with its purgative power, it is also astringent and strengthening, and in this it certainly differs from almost every other purgative of the same class known in medicine. It is superior to nearly all other purges for another reason; it may be taken with opium, and act on the bowels as well as if taken without it. This is a vast advantage; because where purging would be connected with great pain, its being combined with opium relieves the pain, while the Rhubarb is left free to do its duty. The operation of Rhubarb is slower and milder than any other purges, but it is very certain in its effects, when given in proper doses. It may always be given with innocence and safety, in all cases of extreme weakness, where a purge to open the bowels becomes necessary, and where violent and severe purging would be highly improper.—You will find this medicine very valuable and safe, as it always acts with much gentleness in relieving the bowels. It is a common and proper purge for children, even at a very early period of life, and in every situation where their bowels become disordered, partienlarly in dysentery or lax, because it leaves the bowels in a favorable state, after removing the offensive matter from them. It is also an excellent purge for grown persons laboring under this complaint. In small doses, say from two to six grains, it is excellent for the stomach when laboring under indigestion, generally called dyspepsia; and must be given in such small doses, so as not to purge, but to act as a tonic or strengthening medicine.

There are various ways of giving Rhubarb; such as in *tincture*, which means steeping it in any kind of spirits, but the best and most certain method of giving this medicine, and obtaining the virtues of it fully, is to give it in fine powder. A dose for a grown person is, from about a scruple or twenty grains, to half a drachm mixed with honey, molasses, or any kind of syrup. The root chewed as tobacco, and swallowing the saliva, or spittle is an innocent and efficient way of taking it, for keeping the bowels gently open, particularly with those persons who are subject to habitual costiveness, indigestion, and those long trains of nervous diseases which afflict men and women, who are subject to derangements of their systems from costiveness. In such cases, if they will chew the root of the Rhubarb, it will act as a moderate purge, and gently open their bowels, at the same time, it will act as a tonic or strengthening medicine to the stomach, by which they will always obtain relief.

INDIAN PHYSIC.

This plant is a native of the United States, and as its name imports, was a great favorite among the Indian nations. It is almost every where found in the Western country, inhabiting shady woods, and the rich sides of hills and mountains, from the Lakes of Cannada to the Floridas. The number of stems proceeding from the root of this plant varies considerably: sometimes there is but a single one, and occasionally there are many. The stems are branched above, say about two or three feet from the ground; they are round and commonly of a reddish color. The leaves are of a deep green, long and pointed, and the flower nearly white. The root of this plant which is all that is used in medicine, is perennial; that is to say it is not destroyed by the frosts of winter. It is composed of several long brown slender shoots, which run out from the bottom of the stem to some distance under the ground. This root possesses many of the virtues of the ipecacuanha, and is much used by the country people as an emetic or puke. Given in the dose of thirty or thirty-five grains in the powder, for a grown person, it is an easy, safe, and certain emetic; and if you give it in what are called broken doses, of six or seven grains about every two hours, it will act as a sudorific: in other words, it will produce sweating. If you give it in infusion or weak tea, a handful to a pint of boiling water, of which you may take a small tea cupful every fifteen or twenty minutes, it will produce vomiting. The active power of this root, seems to reside exclusively in the bark, which in addition to its emetic qualities, probably possesses considerable tonic powers.

AMERICAN IPECACUANHA.

This singular and very useful plant is exclusively a native of the United States, and may be found in great plenty, in the middle, southern, and western States. It nearly always grows in loose, moist, and sandy soils, and is very often found flourishing in beds of almost pure sand. The leaves of this plant vary so much in shape and color, and in fact the whole plant itself varies so much in its different states, that it is often mistaken by those unacquainted with its habits, for several distinct species of plants. The stems are numerous; they are nearly white below the surface of the earth or sand, and of a reddish color, or a pale green or yellowish hue above it. The leaves are opposite to each other, and generally of an oval form; I say generally, because they are sometimes of a long oval, sometimes pointed, and not unfrequently linear. In the month of May, while the plant is in flower, the leaves are very small, but as it advances in age, they become greatly increased in size. The seeds of the flower are only *three in number*, enclosed in a triangular or *three-square capsule*, or case. I mention these things particularly because they afford the best possible means of knowing the plant. The root is perennial, in other words, it is not killed by the frosts of winter. It is from three to seven feet in height, and from half an inch to an inch and ahalf in diameter or across, and of a yellowish color; sending off towards its upper part many smaller roots, about the size of small quills.

I believe and am sustained in the opinion, by several high authorities, that the American Ipecacuanha, the plant just described to you, is superior in its medicinal properties to any other species known. The root of this plant alone is to be used; if the stems and leaves possess any medicinal virtues, they are yet to be discovered by experiment. It is a powerful emetic, both safe and certain in its operation, and is applicable to nearly all cases in which emetics are required. In small doses, of from five to ten or fifteen grains, it is an excellent emetic or puke; but if given in doses of twenty grains, it operates downwards as an active purge. Larger doses produce in addition to the above effects,—heat, vertigo, which means swimming in the head, and great prostration or loss of strength.

Dr. Barton gives us the following experiment on the American Ipecacuanha, which I transcribe for the contemplation of the reader. "A portion of the dried root was finely pulverized, (*powdered.*) and administered with caution to several patients. I at first, commenced with small doses of three, four and five grains. In these quantities the powder produced nausea—sickness of the stomach, determination to the skin—sweating, as small doses of Ipecacuanha do. On increasing the number of grains to ten, vomiting was produced, with occasionally an operation on the bowels. Fifteen grains I found sufficient to produce full vomiting in most cases; and in a single instance, having given the powder to an extent of twenty-five grains, I had reason to be alarmed at the violent cathartic—purgative effect which ensued, and continued for *fourteen hours*, attended with distressing sickness at the stomach. I have tried the American root in various combinations, and can confidently assert that, in all the instances it has proved equal, if not superior to the imported Ipecacuanha. It has some advantages which the foreign article does not possess: Its occasional purgative effect is nothing more than what follows the foreign medicine. This view of the subject derives peculiar importance, from the well known fact, that the imported Ipecacuanha is rarely if ever good, and perhaps seldom genuine."

In this plant, or rather root, for that alone is to be used, we see another instance of the bounty of Providence, in furnishing us with an article possessed of great medicinal virtue, the production of our *own soil.* And here again I repeat that, we have only to develop the resources of our own country, to become completely independent of foreign lands for all our useful medical drugs: even Opium, as I shall show you in the proper place, can be made here in sufficient quantities for our own consumption. We are in fact, paying enormous sums annually, for what nature and our own exertions would furnish us. Foreign ipecacuanha adulterated and inferior to our own, is costing us *three dollars* the pound, while we can have our own for nothing.

BUTTERFLY WEED.

OR

PLEURISY ROOT.

The Butterfly weed or Pleurisy root, called by the learned *Asclepias Tuberosa*, is a native of every State in the American Union, and abounds particularly in the southern and western States. It flourishes best, and grows to the greatest perfection, in light sandy soils, and is frequently found under fences, and near old stumps in grain fields. From twenty to thirty stalks, the size of a pipe stem frequently rise from the same root, and stand in almost every direction. These stalks are round and woolly, and of a reddish brown color on the sun-side. The leaves are placed very irregularly, and are spear, or tongue shaped, and covered with a fine down on the lower side. The stalks rise from one to two feet in height, and spread to a considerable extent; and at the extremities of the branches are found clusters of small shoots on which are found the flowers when in bloom—which is about the month of July or August. The clusters of shoots from the end of the branches, as also the flowers, resemble those of the common silk weed, for which this plant is sometimes mistaken. There is, howover this difference between them, and it ought to be particularly noticed; the flowers of the silk weed are of a *pale purple hue*, while those of the butterfly weed are of a *beautiful bright orange color*, and are succeeded by long slender pods, which contain the seeds. The seeds have a delecate kind of down or silk attached to them.

The root of the Butterfly weed is spindle, or carrot shaped, of a light brown color on the out side, and white and coarse within. It has long been celebrated in the Southern Atlantic States, and particularly in Virginia and the Carolinas, not only as a powerful remedy in pleurisy, but in pneumonic discases generally: by which I mean diseases of the lungs. This root possesses one remarkable power: given in proper quantities it affects the skin, and produces copious perspiration or sweating, without heating the body. Given in the simple form of a decoction or tea, it often produces sweating, when all other remedies have failed in their effects. The powdered root sometimes acts as a mild purgative on the bowels; but it is more particularly, and inestimably valuable, in producing expectoration, or the throwing off of mucus from the throat and lungs; in causing perspiration or sweating when other remedies failed; and finally in reducing obstinate feverish affections. Its efficiency and power in fevers, have been attested by many of the best physicians in the United States. In feverish affections proceeding from inflammation of the lungs, in colds recently taken, and in diseases of the chest generally, this root is an excellent remedy. It is to be given in a strong infusion or tea: say a small tea cupful every two or three hours. Many families have long resorted to this root as a *domestic medicine*, to relieve pains in the stomach, indigestion, colic; and so on, and for these reasons call it *wind root.* Doctors Chapman and Biglow, whose testimonials alone in its favor would be sufficient to establish its reputation, for the virtues I have ascribed to it, speak in very high terms of the medicinal powers of this root.

"As a diaphoretic,"—or medicine which sweats, says Dr. Chapman—I think this root is distinguished by great certainty and permanency of operation; and has this inestimable property, that it produces its effects—sweating—without much increasing the force of the circulation, raising the heat of the surface, or creating inquietude or restlessness. On these accounts, it is well suited to excite perspiration in the *forming stages* of most of the inflammatory diseases of winter—and is not less useful in the same cases, at more advanced periods, after the reduction of the feverish action by bleeding. The common notion of its having a peculiar efficacy in *pleurisy*, I am inclined to believe is not without foundation; for certain it is, that it very much relieves the oppression of the chest in recent catarrh—cold in the head and throat—and promotes perspiration in protracted inflammations of the lungs."

JALAP.

This plant was originally found a native of Mexico, near the celebrated city of *Xalapa*, from whence it derived its present name Jalap. It has since been discovered growing plentifully near Vera Cruz, and in our own countries of Florida. And, on the authority of Dr. W. P. C. Barton, I take upon myself to assert, that it is also certainly a native of the State of Georgia. The root of this plant alone is used for medical purposes: and when of a good quality, comes to us in slices, which are solid and heavy, and of a dark gray color, having little smell, and scarcely any taste. When swallowed, however, it affects the throat with a warm and pungent sensation.

This root is a powerful laxative medicine or purge; its activity resides principly, if not wholly, in the risinous part, which, even when taken in small doses alone, will sometimes gripe severely. The great activity of jalap as a purge, causes it to be much used in the onset, or commencement of bilious fever. Combined with calomel in the proportion of ten grains each, was the purge generally given in Yellow Fever by the great Dr. Rush, of Philadelphia, and which caused his students to give him the ludicrous nick-name of "*Old Ten in Ten.*" Used as what physicians call a Hydragoque, by which they mean any medicine which will expel water from the cavities of the body, the Jalap root is entitled to all the praise that has ever been bestowed on it, by the medical profession: yet I am induced to believe, from actual experience, and the practice of other physicians, that it produces a better effect in all dropsical cases, when combined with *cremor tartar.* Ten grains of Jalap with one drachm of cremor tartar, constitute probably, one of the best medical prescriptions ever known, where long continued purging is required in the cure of a complaint. The dose of Jalap when uncombined with any other medicine, is from twenty to thirty and even up to forty grains. Our common May Apple root, has sometimes been called the Jalap of the United States. But I am of the opinion above; that the Jalap of Mexico is a native of the state of Georgia, and probably of all the southern States. Perhaps this would be an inquiry worthy of the attention of the lately established *Medical Board* of Tennessee, especially if they intend to remunerate the country for the privileges granted to them by the Legislature.

PRICKLY ASH

OR

TOOTHACHE TREE.

The Prickly Ash is a native of the United States, and also of the West India Islands, where it sometimes grows to the height of sixteen feet. There are two kinds of Prickly Ash in the United States, which I believe possesses the same medicinal powers: one is called the Ash-leaved Zanthroxylum, which grows in the Northern States, and particularly in the States of Pennsylvania and Maryland, and the other is known by the name of the Prickly Yellow Wood, growing abundantly to the South and South-west of the States I have mentioned. The fresh juice obtained from the root of the Prickly Ash, is an excellent remedy in that painful complaint called *dry belly-ache.* This discovery, like most others of importance, was the result of accident: it was made by watching a female slave in one of the west India Islands, who collected the root in the woods, and gave two spoonfuls of the juice every two hours, to a negro suffering severely under this colic. The medicine caused a profound and composed sleep, for twelve hours, when all sense of pain, and other distressing symptoms had vanished. The cure was rendered final by giving an infusion of the juice as a diet drink.

The most important discovery, however, relating to the Prickly Ash, or Yellow Wood tree, is the following: The juice of the root preserved in spirits of any kind, given in doses of about a wine-glassful, has repeatedly *removed the most obstinate epileptic fits.* I do not know precisely the manner in which this preparation ought to be managed, but would give it in the dose of a wine-glassful morning and evening. The leaves and rind of the Prickly Ash, or Yellow Wood, in their taste and smell, resemble those of the lemon, and possess a similar volatile oil. The bark has a separate acrid, or hot and biting principle, which it will communicate either to water or spirits of any kind: this acrid or biting principle, however, is not perceived when the bark or liquid is first taken into the mouth; it gradually makes itself known, by a burning sensation on the tongue and fauces, sometimes called the valotine arch, or cavity at the root of the tongue. Chewing a small quantity of the bark, produces a great flow of saliva, or spittle, and is very often used in this way to cure the tooth-ache.

The bark of the Prickly Ash has also acquired a considerable name as a remedy in chronic rheumatism, by which I mean rheumatism of long standing. Taken in full doses, it produces a sense of heat in the stomach, and a strong tendency to perspiration, or sweating, and consequently much relief in rheumatism. The dose is twenty grains of the pounded bark, to be taken three times a day; or you may boil an ounce of the pounded bark in water. and take this tea, or decoction in the course of the twenty-four hours. In the West India Islands this strong decoction of the bark is used with great suncess, as a wash for old and foul ulcers, which it always greatly cleanses, and disposes them to heal up. The West India people also mix the pounded bark with what are called the dressings of such old sores. The value of this remedy for old ulcers, is attested by numerous instances of its success, to be found in the London Medical and Physical Journal.

INDIAN TURNIP.

The Indian Turnip is a native of every part of the U. States: it grows in low rich meadows and woodlands, to the height of from two to three feet, and is too well known to require a very particular description. The leaves are but three in number, of a roundish or oval form: The stalks is of a purple color, and the berries of a bright and beautiful scarlet. In its recent state, that is when first dug up, the root is exceedingly hot, sharp, and biting to the tongue: and on being swallowed, a sharp acrimony is sensibly felt about the fauces, or cavity at the root of the tongue.

Of all our American roots, the Indian turnip has the highest reputation in country practice, as a remedy in pulmonary or consumptive complaints: it is also given with considerable success in asthma, and in coughs of long standing.—My own experience has convinced me, that it is among the most valuable of our expectorants, or medicines which cause a dislodgement of mucus from the throat and lungs, and that it is a good remedy in croup and hooping cough. The green or recent root, boiled in hog's lard to the consistence of an ointment, has been found very useful in tenea capatis, or scald head, in which I would always recommend its use. When given in consumptive complaints, the fresh root should be boiled in sweet milk. When the dried root is to be given, it must be finely grated in sweet milk—one root in half a pint of milk, and well boiled before it is taken. Some acrimony or sharpness should be perceptible to the throat and tongue:

the root has probably lost its powers. The ointment I have mentioned above, is valuable also in some diseases of the skin: such as ring-worm, tetter-worm, and so on.

WILD CHERRY TREE.

This tree is so very common as to require no description. The bark of this tree, or the bark of the root, which is still better, combined with the bark of the dog wood, when employed in the cure of ague and fever, bilious fever, and other diseases where tonic or strengthening medicines are proper, is by no means inferior to the best peruvian bark. Combined with Virginia snake root, in the proportion of one part of snake root to four parts of this bark, it is an excellent remedy in intermittent fevers of an obstinate character, and long standing. You may either give it in powder, in the same dose that you would peruvian bark, [See table of doses.] or you may give it as a tea or decoction. It has also been found very useful in dyspepsia or indigestion, and in consumption of the lungs. Infused plentifully in strong round cider, it will in most cases remove jaundice, especially if preceded by a dose or two of calomel: and a strong decoction of the bark is an excellent wash for old and ill conditioned ulcers. It is a singular fact, that the leaves of the wild cherry tree will poison cattle: nor is it less singular than true, that the distilled water of the leaves is a powerful poison to most animals. This effect seems to be dependent on the presence of the same poisonous principle which exists in peach kernels, and other substances of a similar kind, lately shown to the *Prussic acid*, the strongest poison known to us.

AMERICAN CENTAURY.

This is a very elegant little plant, a native of the United States: and is no less valuable for its medicinal virtues, than admired for its simple beauty. The root consisting of a few thick yellow fibres, generally sends up but one single stem, which grows from a foot to eighteen inches high: this stem is smooth and foursided, and where the branches shoot off, it has generally two leaves, which grow opposite to each other: indeed the leaves of every part of the plant grow opposite to each other, and are oval and sharp at the points. The flowers are very numerous growing at the points of the branches, from two to five in number, and are generally of a beautiful pale rose color. This plant is in full flower in the month of July.

Every part of this little plant is a pure strong bitter, and parts with its medicinal qualities to both water and spirits, it has no astringent powers. On stomcahs that are weak, it exerts a strengthening influence, and is considerably used in the southern States in intermittent fevers. In fact, by the best practitioners in the Union, it is generally administered in fevers. Dr. Barton says "it was often employed with much benefit in the city of Philadelphia, in 1793, in certain stages of the yellow fever. On the whole, Centaury may be confidently recommended for its pure bitter, tonic, and strengthening virtues. It ought to be taken as a decoction or tea, and always taken cold: it may be taken in powder, in doses of from ten to twenty grains, but I think not with the same advantage.—In relaxations of the stomach, and general debility of the system, mixed with calamus, angelica root, it forms an excellent and strengthening bitter.—This root is called by country people *Centry*.

HORSE MINT.

Horse Mint grows very abundantly in all parts of the United States, and is so extremely common as to require no description. A tea made either of the green or dried leaves, will stop vomiting or puking, especially in bilious fevers. It will also act in simple cases, as a valuable remedy for promoting or bringing on the menses or courses of women, when they are obstructed. In this instance it may be placed on a footing with Rosemary, Pennyroyal, and many other simple herbs. All this, however is well known to every old lady in the country.

PEPPERMINT.

Peppermint is originally a native of Europe, but it is now cultivated in almost every garden of the United States. The roots of the peppermint should be transplanted every three years, otherwise the plant is apt to degenerate into the flavor of the spearmint. This plant is certainly so common, that a description would be entirely unnecessary. From this plant the oil is distilled, which, when mixed with alcohol or proof spirits, make the essence of peppermint old in the shops.

Peppermint is a warm stimulant to the stomach, and through that medium to the rest of the body, holding a first rank in the list of medicines called *carminations:* which mean those medicines which dispel or scatter the wind from the stomach and bowels. It is also beneficial in allaying spasmodic affections of the stomach and bowels: removing the sickness of the stomach; dispelling flatulence or wind, and in removing all colicy pains. It is very often beneficial when cramp takes place during the operation of an emetic, or puke. The green leaves, stewed in spirits, or hot water, and applied to the pit of the stomach as warm as they can be borne, will often stop puking when some of the best remedies fail.

GINGER.

Ginger is a perennial plant originally found in the East Indies, but at present cultivated in all the West Indian Islands. I think it highly probable, that the ginger would grow well in all the southern and western States, particularly in Louisiana, Alabama, Georgia, and South Carolina. In the West India Islands, it is cultivated very much in the manner that we cultivate potatoes in this country, and is fit for diging once in every year. There are two sorts of ginger, the black and the white. The black ginger consists of thick and knotty roots, of a yellowish grey color on the outside, and an orange or brown color in the inside. The white ginger is not so thick and knotty as the black, and is internally of a whitish grey or bright yellow color. The white is firm and resinous, more pungent or sharp in its taste than the black, and consequently a higher price. Pieces which are worm eaten, soft, light, and easily broken, you are always to reject.

Ginger has a fragrant smell, and a hot, biting, aromatic taste, and is very useful in cold flatulent or windy colics, and in all eases of looseness and weakness of the bowels or intestines; it does not heat the system so much as the different kinds of pepper, but is much more durable in its effects. Some time since, the powder of ginger, taken in very large doses in sweet milk, was considered a very valuable remedy in gout. I have never tried it myself, and therefore cannot say as to its correctness, but the experiment would be an innocent one, and is very easily tried. I think it unnecessary to say any thing more on the subject of this root; every old lady in the country, is acquainted with its general character, and medicinal virtues.

OPIUM.

Without this valuable and essential medicine, it would be next to impossible for a physician to practice his profession, with any considerable degree of success: it may not improperly be called, the monarch of medical powers, the soothing angel of moral and physical pain.

PP*

"Charmed with this potent drug, the exalted mind,
All sense of woe delivers to the wind:
It clears the cloudy front of wrinkled care,
And soothes the wounded bosom of despair!"

There are two kinds of this drug known in commerce, distinguished by the names of the *Turkish* and *East Indian* opium. The Turkish opium is the best: it is considerably solid and compact, possesses some degree of tenacity or stickiness, and when broken, leaves a shining fracture. It is of a dark brown color: and when first taken into the mouth, produces a nauseous bitter taste, which soon becomes acrid, with some degree of warmth. The best kind of Turkish opium is in flat pieces, and generally covered with leaves used in packing it, and has nearly double the strength of that brought from the East Indies.

The East Indian opium is not so solid as the Turkish being sometimes not much thicker than tar, its color much darker, and its taste more nauseous and less bitter. By these distinctions, which are obvious to even tolerable judges, you will easily know the Turkish opium from that of the East Indies.

Opium is combined, or in other words mixed, with more medicines for the cure of diseases, than any other drug known to, or used by medical men.—In every patent medicine sold in the shops, especially for the relief of pain in diseases, opium forms the principal portion. *Bateman's drops* and *Godfrey's cordial* both of which have sustained their characters for near a century, have opium for their bases or principle parts, and they are certainly valuable medicines. Were I to trace back the use of opium as a medicine among mankind, it would probably be found among the Greeks; but the limits of my book will not permit me to go minutely into its history; suffice it to say, that this valuable, singular, and astonishing drug, seems capable of changing our very nature to a more exalted state of being, at the same time that it holds in due and proper subjection, without imparting it, the rationality of the human mind.

Opium is made from the white poppy, which is or can be cultivated in all our gardens: it is probably a native of the warmer parts of Asia. Some attempts have been made to cultivate it extensively in England, but the climate of that country seems to present an insuperable obstacle to its being cultivated as a productive object of commerce. The United States, however, and particularly the more Southern and Western portions of the Union, on the score of climate and soil, present no difficulties in the cultivation of opium, in amply sufficient abundance for the consumption of all our citizens. This is another proof, among several others which I have adduced, evincive of the independence of our country in the production of important medical drugs, if we will only employ industry and enterprize; the fact is, that enormous sums of money are yearly expended for opium, which go into the pockets of foreign ers, that we could very easily produce from our own soil. The leaves, stalks, and capsules of the poppy, which capsules mean the cases containing the seeds, abound with a *milky juice*, which must be gathered when the seeds are nearly ripe.

The manner of collecting this juice is as follows:—After the sun has gone down, or about the twilight of evening, make several incisions or cuts, lengthways, on the surface, of the capsules or poppy pods. As I have just told you, this is to be done when they are not quite ripe; and is the best performed with a knife made for the purpose, having four or five blades. The milky juice which flows out from these cuts during the night, must be collected the following day, after a sufficient time has been allowed for the milky fluid to become inspissated or thickened by the heat of the sun. It is now to be collected by a thin iron scraper, made for the purpose, and put into an earthen vessel. This is the whole secret of opium making, a secret which every man in this country ought to know and profit by, and the ignorance of which has already cost our citizens millions of money; the price of foreign opium in our eastern cities, much of which is of an inferior quality, is about four dollars the pound. The operation of cutting or scarifying the poppy pods, in the manner I have mentioned, may be repeated every evening, or as long as the pods will furnish the milky juice. When a considerable quantity of this juice is collected, you have nothing to do but to work it with a wooden knife or spoon, until it becomes of a proper consistency or thickness, and to enclose it in the leaves of the plant itself, or in tobacco leaves.

"A paper has lately been read, in the *Harrisburgh Medical Society*," says the Medical Recorder, "on the cultivation of the poppy, and the manufacture of opium. The author, which is Dr. Webster Lewis, of Lewisburgh, York county Pennsylvania, has transmitted a specimen of his manufacture of opium, equal to the best foreign opium of the shops. After many unsuccessful experiments, he has fallen on a mode of cultivation and preparation, both easy and profitable. The plan will be put in operation in the ensuing season, by several other members of the society, to whom he has presented some of his best seed " And, with regard to the cultivation of opium in the United States, the following extract of a letter from a gentleman in England, to a citizen in the United States will throw much light on the subject. "Let me entreat you to make an experiment on the cultivation of opium. I caused great increase of this article at Patna; it used to sell at 225 rupees the cake, of 160 pounds: and has been sold for 300 lately. The company sells to the amount, annually I presume, of fifteen millions of rupees, two and six pence sterling, amounting to one million eight hundred and seventy-five thousand pounds sterling: *I know it can easily be produced in America*, and is the best article of commerce that can be sent to china." If these representations be correct, of which there can be no doubt, the cultivation of the white poppy, and the manufacture of opium, are not only easily practicable in the United States, but would afford an immense revenue to the citizens as an article of commercial exportation: and the fact is, if the real state of the case were truly known, that we yet remain in comparative ignorance of the multiplied and inexhaustable resources of our own country.

There is a considerable difference between the effects produced by wine or spirituous liquors, and those produced on the system by opium. The excitement of pleasureable sensations produced by wine or spirits, is acute and powerful while these sensations last, but they are of extremely short duration. The one is a flame which soon subsides, and leaves nothing but the ashes of self reprehension and bitter reflection behind it; while the other affords a steady, agreeable and permanent glow of pleasure, physical and intellectual, which last from ten to twelve hours. But, the principal distinction between these stimulants of the human system, lies in this: that wine or spirits disorder and confuse the intellectual faculties, while opium in all its forms, if taken in proper quantities, introduces order, harmony and pleasureable serenity among them. Wine or spirits unsettle and cloud the judgment, and deprive us of our intellectual self possession: while opium on the contrary, produce a just equipoise between our intellectual strength and sensibilities, arouses all our dormant faculties, and disposes them to harmonious and pleasureable activity: and with regard to the temper, moral energies and physical sensations in general, opium produces that sort of simple and vital animation, cordial warmth of feeling and sensibility, which we would almost suppose to have accompanied man, in his primeval and unfallen state. Wine or spirits if taken to any excess, always lead men to the brink of absurdity and extravigance, and beyond a certain point, invariably produces a distraction of the mental faculties; while opium, on the contrary, soothes our irritations of feeling, concentrates our intellectual energies, and robs pain and misfortune of their stings. This however, is but one side of the picture. Opium, as I have already told you, although a very valuable medicine in many diseases, and also always producing those agreeable sensations I have attempted to describe, when used to any considerable excess, especially if persisted in, has many disadvantages and miseries attending it. It is used by the Turks to great excess, because all wines and spirituous liquors are prohibited by the Mahomedan creed. Opium if habitually taken, in other words, when it is made use of as a stimulant or luxury, and not as medicine, affects the physical system in a terrible manner, and produces the same sufferings as those which arise from intoxicating liquors. When the pleasureable effects I have before described begin to cease, or the effects of the opium begin to die in the system, the feelings are as agonizing and dreadful as can possibly be conceived: the mind becomes weak, irresolute, heavy, dull, and languid, and the body averse to activity or motion of any kind, is not only disposed to sleep, but seems little affected by objects of pursuit which usually put it in motion. If the dose of opium has been very considerable, all these symptoms seem to increase, until tremors, convulsions, vertigo, stupor, insensibility, and total depravation of muscular strength succeed—when death usually closes the scene. All these symptoms appear singly or combined, in proportion to the comparative moderation or excess of the dose, and the peculiarities of the constitution of the person. Therefore, use not this drug, but as intended by the great Father of the Universe, the universal parent of mankind; because used as a medicine alone, it is an invaluable blessing, in the relief of pain and suffering, and in soothing and tranquilizing the system, with balmy and refreshing slumbers.

☞ Having under the head of each disease, mentioned particularly when it was necessary to make use of *opium*, or *laudanum*, which is nothing more than opium dissolved or steeped in any kind of spirits, for which look under the head *Laudanum*, I shall now close these remarks. Opium and laudanum, which are the same things in substance and effect, are always efficient in mitigating or subduing pain, in overcoming spasm or cramp; in fact they are the chief means employed by physicians in these cases. I have now as fully as the limits of my book will allow: described to you this great and effective medicine, which is valuable, and powerful, if properly used, innocent. In a small dose it acts as a stimulant; in a moderate dose it eases pain and procures sleep, and in an over dose, when the person is not in the habit of using it, the consequences will always be fatal. It is therefore evident, that this medicine should be used with great judgment and discretion. The average dose of *opium* is about one grain: and the dose of *laudanum* for a grown person, is about from twenty-five to thirty-five drops, in a little cold water. For a child about the period of birth, the dose of laudanum is half a drop; but the table of medicines to which you will please refer, will explain the doses of both opium and laudanum for all ages.

EXTRACT OF GARDEN LETTUCE.

This extract which produces the same effect as opium, ·'as discovered by John Redman Cox, Professor of the med-:al College of Philadelphia and published by him in the merican Philosophical Societie's transactions, in the year 806.

'he extract of our garden lettuce, which is the milky uice of this plant, is a valuable substitute for opium, and :an always be procured and kept for use, by every family in the United States, with the least possible troubled. It has the power of allaying pain, of producing sleep, of diminishing the too frequent action of the heart, and of repressing the inordinate heat of the system, without producing those unpleasant effects which are sometimes felt, by persons whose constitutions cannot bear the stimulous produced by the opium obtained from the Poppy. It always allays or quiets cough, and in this particular respect, it will always be found a most valuable substitute for opium. Garden lettuce is so common a vegetable, and so constantly used at our tables, that it may excite some surprise in my reader, that it should produce so valuable and powerful a drug as opium: but such is the fact. And here I may go a step further, and by no means exceed the bounds of truth by asserting that it is even superior to the imported opium. This is another plain proof, that the *Creator* has in his bountiful providence, bestowed on us a plant which is not only a succulent and nourishing food, but one which in the hours of pain and affliction, will soothe the pains of our suffering systems, and in sweet oblivion steal upon our senses, until the leaden wings of sleep render us unconscious of the cares of life.

If you will recollect, there are two kinds of *lettuce* cultivated in our gardens; one is the common *lettuce* and the other is the *ice lettuce*, both of which yield opium producing the same effects on the human system. The ice lettuce, however is the best, and yields the greatest quantity of milky juice. The following is the simple method of preparing this juice for medical uses. Take the leaves and stalks of the ice lettuce—and if you have not this kind you may use the other—when the plants are nearly ready to flower. Bruise them well in a mortar, and put them in a bag made of hemp: then press them strongly until they yield their juice. This juice is then to be evaporated in flat vessels, heated with boiling water; and the evaporation is to be kept up, until the milky juice of the lettuce is reduced to the consistence or thickness of honey. Twelve pounds of the stalks and leaves of the lettuce plant, of either kind, will yield about eight or nine ounces of opium. This is the whole secret of making opium from the lettuce, which every farmer in the country ought to know and practice.

PEACH TREE.

This valuable tree affords us not only a most delightful fruit, but its leaves, flowers, and gum, possess the most active and important medicinal virtues. I have also been informed, but never tried the experiment, that the bark of the Peach tree contains very active powers as a purge. The leaves and blossoms purge the bowels freely, and without the least griping, when taken as a strong tea, in doses of a tea spoonful every hour: and they also act as a mild purgative when taken as a syrup, prepared by boiling slowly their juice, with an equal quantity of honey, sugar or molasses, and given to children in doses of a table spoonful; and to grown persons in doses of a wine or stem glassful.

The leaves or flowers, or both made into a *strong tea*, and a gill taken every hour until it operates well on the stomach, bowels and skin, which it will do—puke, purge and sweat the patient, has very often relieved persons in the country when attacked by *bilious fever*. This medicine however, is to be taken for several days in such cases of fever, or until relief is obtained. I have been informed from respectable authority, that the bark of the Peach tree is valuable, both as a puke and a purge: and I well know from experience, that the gum of this tree will answer all the purposes of gum Arabic, which is an imported article, frequently mentioned in this book.

CASTOR OIL,

AND HOW TO MAKE IT.

This Oil, which is essential to the preservation of health in every family, is made from the seed of a plant called *Palma Christi*, which is a native of most countries lying within the tropics, and will grow and flourish in all temperate latitudes. In the process of manufacturing this oil, the outer coat or covering of the seed or been, must first be taken off: in the next place, you must bruise them in considerable quantities, and afterwards subject what may be called the *prumice*, to a pressure sufficient to throw out the oil. The oil thus expressed, is called *cola expressed oil*, and is by far the best. That extracted by boiling the bruised seeds in water; another process of preparing it, is more nauseous, of a much darker color, more easily becoming rancid or stinking, much more disagreeable to take, and more active in its operation on the system.

The *Palma Christi* will grow in any climate or soil in the United States: it rises to about ten or twelve feet in height, and is usually about the size of a common corn stalk, having very large and beautiful spreading leaves: Whether you extract the oil cold, or employ boiling water in the process, you must first collect the branches having the ripe seed on them, and expose them to the sun until perfectly dry. Then lay them on a scaffold or floor, and beat them with a light flail, to separate the hull or shell from the seed, after which to dislodge every particle of shell, you may pound them gently in a wooden mortar. Take care that you get all the covering off the seeds: because there is an *acrid skin*, which if intermixed with the oil, sometimes makes it operate as a puke, and always as a drastic or griping purge. It is not improbable that the oil obtained by boiling, is saturated or filled with the properties of this skin, which forms another of my objection to boiling the seed. If you prefer however, to extract the oil by boiling, you must put the seed divested of their covering, in a vessel of boiling water; in about twenty minutes a dirty scum will rise, which must be taken entirely off. The clear oil will then rise, which must be put into a vessel without water, and kept warm by a slow fire, taking care that it does not arrive at a boiling heat. As soon as it becomes clear and transparent from taking off the scum which arises, and which will make an inferior kind of oil, you must put the clear oil, when cold, into clean bottles and cork them well. The kind of palma christi which produces the finest oil, is the species of which the stalk is of a pink color. I neglected to mention in the proper place, that the quantity of water in the first vessel used, should be *three* measures to *one* of seed, which should be frequently stirred to prevent any portion from sticking to the sides and bottom of the vessel, would give the oil a burnt taste; you must also be careful that it does not boil over. The dose for a grown person is two table spoonfuls, for an infant, a tea spoonful, even at birth.

DIRECTIONS FOR PRESERVING

ROOTS, HERBS, FLOWERS AND BARKS.

Roots which are annual, or grow and die yearly, should be collected before they shoot out their stalks or flowers: roots which are biennial, or which live and grow two years, should be collected in the harvest of the first year, or in the spring of the second year; perennial roots, or those which survive the frosts of winter, should be gathered before the sap has begun to mount, or after it has returned to the root. When a root is worm eaten, or otherwise decayed, you are always to reject or refuse it: the medicinal virtues of such a root are destroyed.

You are now with a brush and some cold water, to cleanse the roots newly dug up, and to let them remain in the water as short a time as possible; after which you are to cut the small and useless fibres or strings from them, if there be any; and carefully to dry them in a moderate heat. Roots which consist wholly of fibres or strings, of which there are several kinds, the black or Virginia snake root for instance, are to be dried as soon as possible by a regular and moderate heat. But should the root be aromatic, which means spicy and fragrant, like ginger for instance, you are to dry it in a cool airy dry situation, turning it frequently in order that it may retain its virtues and fragrance. If roots that you obtain are thick and strong, you are to split them in thin pieces, and string them on a cord or twine so as to admit the air freely to them in drying; if they are covered, which is sometimes the case with a thick tough bark, peel them while fresh and dry them. Some roots are apt to loose their virtues by drying; when this is the case, you have nothing to do but to keep them buried in dry sand, which will preserve them in such a manner that they will always be fit for use.

Herbs and Flowers are always to be gathered in dry weather, and not until the dew is off. They are then to be dried in as short a time as possible, by the gentle heat of a stove or fire: for by this speedy method of drying, the herbs and flowers retain their virtues, which are usually destroyed by the common method of drying them in the open air, and in the shade. When herbs and flowers retain their virtues, they generally also retain much of their natural color.

BARKS and WOODS, for medicinal uses, are to be gathered in the spring or in autumn, and from the youngest and most vigorous trees, because their most active and powerful virtues are at those periods residing in them. If they are of the resinous kind, by which I mean *rosinous* merely, they are to be gathered in the spring; but if they are of a gumy nature, you must always gather them in the fall, or autumn. You are to recollect distinctly, that all decayed and injured parts of any of the articles I have mentioned, are to be entirely rejected. Persons are very frequently disappointed in the medicinal effects of roots, herbs, barks, &c. this is generally owing to the want of due care in obtaining and preparing such vegetable substances in due time, and in a proper manner.

SULPHUROUS FUMIGATIO'

OR

SULPHUR BATH.

I have frequently mentioned in the course of the preceding pages, that this bath was a most invaluable remedy in which this head is referred to: I shall now, therefore, endeavor to give as minute and as plain a description of it as possible, and in as common and plain language as I can find.

The fumes of sulphur were employed as a bath, and a remedy against many diseases as early as the time of the celebrated Hyppocrates. After falling into disuse for a very long period, this Bath has of late become a matter of general interest—especially since the experiments made by Dr. Gales in 1812—and since his publications on the efficacy of sulphurous Fumigations in the cure of many obstinate diseases. Dr. Gales made his first trials of this remedy, by placing a small basin of sulphur and nitre under the bed clothing of the patient, who was stripped naked, and exposed to the fumes of the contents of the basin: at the same time that these fumes were confined to the body by the bed clothes, and prevented from reaching the mouth and nostrils of the patient, by wrapping his neck and shoulders very closely with the clothing of the bed. This method was found, on fair experiments, to be imperfect and unsatisfactory; and he afterwards adopted in place of it, what he very properly called his Fumigatory Box, which I shall now describe:—

This Box is merely a wooden case, something resembling a *Pulpit,* in which the patient can sit upright in a chair, with his head above the top of the Box, and his shoulders immediately below it. Underneath this box, and connected with it, are the parts which are necessary for producing the fumigations to be applied to the naked body. The lowest story is the ash-pit: the middle one contains the fire, and the uppermost one, is the hearth for the Sulphur. The floor of the box itself, is immediately above the hearth for the sulphur, and is bored, or perforated full of holes, in order that the fumes of the sulphur, when heated by the fire below, may ascend through the bottom of the box, and completely surround, touch, and envelop the naked body of the patient. The top of the box is so constructed, that the hole or opening in the middle of it, closely embraces the neck, and effectually prevents the fumes of the sulphur in the box from reaching the mouth, nose, and eyes of the patient. This description, reader, is the whole secret of the sulphur bath, so much talked of, so little known and so rarely used in the United States. When the seat of the disease to be removed, is on the face or any part of the head, the vapor, or fumes of the sulphur from the box, may be applied to the part affected by means of a *flexible pipe*—by which I mean one that can be moved in different directions, like the leader of a Fire Engine, reaching from the box to any part of the face or head. This sulphur bath must be taken from fifteen minutes to an hour, according to the state of the patient, and the stubbornness of the disease to be removed. Immediately after taking it, the patient ought to retire to bed for an hour or two.

I have mentioned in this Book under the head Indigestion or Dyspepsia—that when the remedies there noticed, for Rheumatism have failed, recourse must always be had to *Sulphurous fumigation*, which I have now accurately and plainly described to you. The truth is, it is an active and powerful remedy in very many diseases besides rheumatism. It is an excellent remedy in *Psoriasis Palmaria*, which is a very obstinate species of Tetter, confined to the palm of the hand; also, *Psoriasis Scrotalis* in which the skin of the *scrotum*, or bag containing the testicles, is afflicted with heat, itching, tension, or tightness and appears of a red color. In cases where the skin of the scrotum, or bag is thus affected, the above symptoms are succeeded by a hard, thickened, brittle texture of the skin, and by painful *chaps*, *cracks*, and *excoriations*, or scalings of the skin, not easily to be healed by any other means than Sulphuric Fumigations. This remedy is also valuable in what physicians call *Psoriasis Inveterata:* which is known by universal scalings of the skin of the whole body, which becomes harsh, dry and much thickened. This disease commences with a few irregular, though distinct patches on the extremities. these patches next appear on different parts of the body: and lastly, they become what is called *confluent*, and spread over the whole surface of the body. The skin is then red, deeply furrowed, and so stiff, or rigid as to impede the movements of the joints: and so quick is the formation and exfoliation of the scales from the body, that the bed is frequently found covered with them.

I have now occupied more space under his head than I at first intended; but considering the vast importance of the Sulphur Bath, and its being likewise a *most valuable remedy* in cases where the human system has been charged with *mercury*, which requires removal, I think the space well and profitably occupied. [For a further description of this bath, see pages 145, and 550, 3d. vol. of the Medical Recorder:] the limits of my book preventing my giving a minute detail of this valuable remedy.

BLOOD LETTING.

Every person should not only know how to open a vein with a lancet, but should also be acquainted with the cautions that are necessary to be known for avoiding danger; because many cases may, and do occur, where medical assistance cannot be had in time, and where actual loss of life occurs for want of Bleeding.

To Bleed *in the arm;* you are to apply a ribband, or other broad ligature, an inch or two above the elbow joint, and to draw it so tight as to compress the veins of thearm immediately under the bandage, and to fill and swell them immediately below it. As soon as the vein rises in whichyou intend to Bleed, place the thumb of your left hand about an inch below the place you intend to pierce, or open with the lancet: and then with your right hand, holding the lancet firmly between your thumb and fore finger, making the incision obliquely, or slanting in the vein. without changing the direction of the lancet: because, by raising the handle, the point of the lancet would be so much lowered as to cut the under part of the vein, and perhaps dangerously wound an artery.

When you have drawn the quantity of blood intended, untie the ligature, or bandage, and close the orifice, or hole. To do this properly, you must place your thumb on the orifice, and press with a moderate force, so as to bring its sides, or edges together. The flowing of the blood will now be stopped and you must next apply a compress, made by twice doubling a piece of linen, about two inches square, and placing it between the thumb and the orifice; over this, you are to place another compress, or thick folding of linen, about four inches square, so as to fill up the hollow, or bend of the arm. When this is done, you are to confine the folds of the linen, by passing over them *crosswise*, both above and below the elbow joint, a ribband or broad tape, in the form of the figure eight, and to finish with making a knot over the linen. If the bleeding should continue, the bandages are to be taken off for a few moments, and while the thumb of the operator is pressed firmly on the orifice, or hole, so as to bring its sides, or edges together; the coldest water is to be poured on the arm, or the orifice, or the hole itself washed with sharp vinegar. If it is convenient, a piece of adhesive, or sticking plaster, placed over the orifice, will generally stop the flow of blood.

To bleed *in the foot*, a moderately tight bandage must be placed above the ancle joint: after which, you are to open the fullest and largest vein with a lancet, observing the same conduct I have laid down for you in bleeding in the arm. If the blood does not flow sufficiently, you will easily remove the difficulty by placing the foot in warm water. On removing the bandage above the ancle, the blood will cease to flow: and if it should not, the bandage I have described for the arm, a piece of court, or any other sticking plaster, will generally stop it.

TOPICAL BLEEDING.

To Bleed *topically:* that is to say, to bleed from some particular part of the surface of the body, you are to proceed in the following manner, if you employ *Leeches:* The part is to be scarified, or slightly cut in shallow gashes with the point of a sharp lancet, or by a *scarificator*, which is an instrument with a number of lancets, acted on by a spring. The leeches are to be previously prepared, by allowing them to creep over a dry cloth, or by drying them. In order to attract them, the scarified part should be moistened with a little cream or sugar; and if the blood about the surface should not induce them to fix themselves, you are to confine them to the place by applying a wine-glass over them—they will then soon take hold.

If you Bleed *topically*, by *cupping*, you are to proceed in the following manner: You are, in the first instance, to scarify the part in the way I have just told you, with the point of a sharp lancet, or with a *scarificator*, such as I have described it to you. When this is done, you must take a cup, and exhaust it of the atmospheric air it contains. This is done. by burning in and over it, some soft paper, dipt in spirits of wine, or any other kind of proof spirits. When the flame is nearly, or quite exhausted, and the air in the cup consequently destroyed, you are to place the mouth of the cup over the scarified part As the cup cools, it will stick fast, and as it were, suck the little scarifications, or gashes, and fill itself with the blood, in place of the air, which cannot get in. When the cup is full, it will easily be removed by raising one side of it. Burning the air, as I have told you, and applying the cup as I have described, may be repeated as often as you may think necessary; or dipping the cup in hot water and immediately applying it over the scarified part, will cause it to take hold or draw. This is the whole secret of cupping—about which so much has been said by medical men, and so little understood by the general community.

After bleeding in the arm, or wherever else a vein is opened, there is sometimes a swelling of the part, called by physicians *eccymosis*. Whenever this takes place, you must shift the position of the limb frequently, so as to produce a free discharge of blood from tumor, or rising. If this will not do, you are to double pieces of linen, dip them in brandy or other spirits, and compress them on the tumor by bandages. If neither of these measures will answer, the tumor, or swelling must be opened with a lancet, the coagulated, or congealed blood let out, and the sore treated as a common wound.

There is another effect which sometimes follow Blood-letting: which is an acute pain, felt on the first introduction of the lancet, and immediately communicated to the extremity of the hand or foot. Here you must apply cloths wrung out of sugar of lead-water to the whole limb, and renew them frequently. You must also resort to bleeding, cooling purges, and very simple food, for the purpose of preventing inflammation. If these measures do not answer, you are to give laudanum in considerable doses: and if laudanum also fails in producing good effects, you must divide, or cut the nerve, or tendon which was pricked by the lancet?

Sometimes an artery is wounded in bleeding. You will know this, by the tremulous, or pulsatory motion with which the blood flows, and by the blood being of a lighter and richer color than that which flows from the veins: and besides you will be unable to stop the blood by the usual pressure. The cure may be attempted, however, in the early stage, by compressions and bandages in the usual way, and by living on very low diet; but should these fail, a surgical operation must be performed, by taking up the ends of the artery, and securing them with ligatures, or ties until they re-unite, or grow together again or until the circulation of the blood can be again restored.

CLYSTERS OR GLYSTERS.

Language almost fails to express the great value of this innocent and powerful remedy, in very many diseases to which mankind are daily and even hourly subject; and I most sincerely regret to say, that it is a remedy not only too little known, but too seldom used in the western country, both by physicians and in families. This disregard for the great virtues of clystering, must either arise from the supposition that the operation is too troublesome, or from a false and foolish delicacy, which forbids the use of an instrument, by which thousands of lives have been preserved in extremely critical circumstances, and with which every mistress of a family should be perfectly acquainted, so as to be able to administer a clyster when required in sickness. And I do here most positively assert, and that too from my own experience, that hundreds to whom I have been called in cases of colic, must have died, had it not been for the immediate relief given by glysters; I will mention one strong instance to prove the correctness of my assertion, to which many others might be added, if the limits of my work would permit. While practicing in the State of Virginia, I was called on at midnight to attend a stranger, who had arrived but a few moments before in the mail stage. The gentleman was one of the Judges of the Supreme Court in the State of N. York. He stated to me that the colic had been coming on him for a considerable time before the stage stopped. By the time I arrived, his misery was so extreme, that he repeatedly exclaimed—"I must die unless immediate relief is given me!" After administering all the usual remedies which are enumerated under the head colic, without giving him much relief, I commenced administering glysters of water pleasantly warm; and on the first being thrown up the bowels, he received more relief than had been produced by all the other remedies I had tried. He felt an immediate exemption from pain, and after two or three more had been given, a copious discharge by stool followed, and he was entirely restored.

Glysters principly act by exciting the lower portion of the intestinal tube, and sometimes from the effect of sympathy. In the latter cases, the discharges are generally copious, or in other words of large quantity; and to produce these full discharges by stool, you are frequently to repeat the clyster of warm water, so tempered as to be pleasant to the feelings of the patient, and in such quantities as the bowels will bear. I have continued to use these injections of warm water for an hour or more in many instances, before I could subdue or overcome spasm or colic: and in cases of great constipation, which means that the bowels are so bound up that the patient cannot have a stool, the water is to be thrown up as far as possible, and the edges of the fundament pressed together as you draw out the pipe of the instrument, so that the clysters may be prevented from returning until it has produced the intended effect. When I have had cases of the kind I have mentioned, after throwing the warm water up the bowels as far as possible, I have always closed the fundament on drawing out the pipe, because without this necessary precaution, in very many instance, the water would return with as much rapidity as it was thrown up with. You will there see the necessity of following my example, and the directions I have just laid down; and you are in all cases of danger, to repeat the glysters of pleasantly warm water as often and in such quantities as the bowels will admit.

The best method of administering glysters in extreme cases, is first to give purgative medicines in the usual manner, and as directed under the different complaints mentioned in this work; when it becomes necessary to use glysters, to give them so as to assist the medicines taken into the stomach in their operation. For instance, when you give a purge in the usual way, you know that it will require some time to operate; now if you wish to hasten the operation of this medicine, give a glyster or two of warm water, especially in spasm, croup, or costiveness, and you will find yourself speedily relieved of the spasm or colic: because the water will soften the hardened excrements in the bowels, and assist in bringing off any undigested food which may have remained in them. Whenever a purgative medicine has been given, and you in proper time administer a glyster to assist its operation, the alimentary canal is soon completely evacuated or cleared of its contents. I have somewhere before told you, that there are hard lumps of excrements in the lower bowels, which require to be removed by the finger of the physician, or by an instrument calculated for the purpose: now your own good sense will always teach you, that these clysters will always soften the concretions or lumps of hard excrement alluded to, and give you relief by a stool.

In fevers and inflammations, any man of common judgment must know, that glysters made of slippery elm bark, which I have frequently directed and administered, must and will tend to cool the whole system, allay the heat and irritation of the bowels, and gently assist the medicine which had been given to operate. They will also produce a determination to the skin, which means a gentle moisture or sweat. I have told you that tepid or warm water always opens the bowels; but the very reverse of this practice is sometimes resorted to, in desperate circumstances, and with great advantages by some of the most distinguished physicians. In some cases of very obstinate constipation, the meaning of which has been sufficiently explained, relief has frequently been obtained, when all other remedies had failed, by a glyster of the coldest water, even of iced water. In such extreme cases, however, when all other means have failed, and the constipated state of the bowels likely to prove fatal, the last resort is, and you are only to adopt it in such cases, to dissolve from twenty to sixty grains of emetic tartar in water, and given as a glyster: Ipecacuanha may be used in place of emetic tartar, and is sometimes preferred for safety. In the numerous cases of constipation and colic, in which I have been called, and some of them very dangerous ones, I have never been compelled to use more than twenty grains of emetic tartar in the glyster I have mentioned; and even when this quantity is to be used, it ought to be administered under the direction of a physician, and never but in extreme cases, and as the last alternative. I shall here mention a remedy for *colic*, which has lately been discovered, and which is said to give immediate relief. Give by the mouth, fifteen grains of *calomel* and two grains of *tartar emetic*, which you are to mix with honey, molasses or any kind of syrup.

In common cases of *constipation*, when the bowels are not easily moved so as to produce a stool; or in *colic*, arising from indigestion, or from having taken some improper food in the stomach, or from having gone some time without a passage, if you wish to hasten the operation of a purge, or if the stomach is too weak to bear one, all that is required is a simple laxative glyster, made of two table spoonfuls of castor oil, or sweet oil mixed with the same quantity of molasses, and put into about a pint of pleasantly warm water, to which you may add a table spoonful of common salt, if you wish the clyster somewhat stimulating. This is a simple and innocent clyster, requiring nothing for its administration but the instrument for injecting it into the bowels, which will hereafter be described, with the method of making clysters, either simple or more active, as the complaint may require.

Glysters are frequently used in dysentery or flux, to soothe and quiet the bowels, relieve the pain, and restrain the too great frequency of the stools. In these cases, the clysters are to be mixed with some laudanum, and some mucilage, such as slippery elm tea. I have mentioned these things under their proper heads, and in such complaints as require their use: [See under the heads *Colic*, *Choleramorbus*, and *Dysentery*,] together with many other cases in which glysters are used.

There are many persons, both men and women who are constitutionally subject to costiveness: by which I mean being bound in their bowels as that they cannot have their regular stools. This costiveness arises from a variety of causes: such as diseased liver, indigestion, torpor of the bowels, and from improper food being taken into the stomach and bowels, and always produce spasms or colic pains: for remember this, that whenever your stomach and bowels are disordered, you will become costive, your head will be confused and otherwise distressed, your spirits will become low and dejected, and the whole train of hypochondriacal feelings and sensations will haunt you. All these last symptoms can easily be relieved, by a simple glyster, made of queal quantities of milk and water, and thrown up the bowels: for by this your bowels will be relieved of their load, which always produces irritation, and your mind and feelings soon experience an agreeable change. You who are always taking medicines to keep your bowels open, and whose stomachs are becoming exhausted and worn out by medical drugs, let me advise and entreat you as a friend and physician, who has witnessed throughout France the great and surprising benefits arising from this simple operation, to abandon the idea of constantly taking medicines. Your good sense must teach you, if you will give yourselves time for reflection, that they must and will eventually destroy the coats of the stomach, and vitally impair its powers; and that when you do really require medicines to subdue disease, your systems will have become so habituated to them as to require tremendous doses, or so completely worn down by their constant use, as to produce no effect. In France, there is scarcely a family unprovided with an instrument for glystering, which is always used when there is the slightest obstruction or costiveness of the bowels. These people mostly use a simple clyster of milk and water, and sometimes water alone: in summer they use cold water, and in winter, water pleasantly warm. It is to the warm bath, and to the common use of clysters, that are to be attributed in a great degree, the cheerful dispositions, the uniform health, and the practical philosophy with which these people bear the hardships and misfortunes of life: in fact, if you take from a French Physician the warm bath and glyster pipe, he cannot practice medicine with any kind of success. The importance of glysters, both in the hands of physicians and families, has become so well known, and is now so highly valued, as to call forth the commendations of the most eminent physicians of both Europe and America.

The old plan of administering clysters was by an assistant; it was both inconvenient and indelecate, and has been measureably superceded, except in cases of infancy and extreme weakness, by a new and valuable invention, called a self-pipe. The common method of using the old glyster pipe, is as follows:—You are to take a beef or hog's bladder, which has been blown up and suffered to dry; and after incerting and fastening a short hollow reed, or a quill in it, cut off at both ends of the barrel, you are to put the glyster itself in the bladder. The end of the reed or quill, or end of the glyster pipe of the shops, if you use one, is now to be covered with some oil or lard, and gently put up the fundament about an inch, by an assistant, and the sides of the bladder squeezed together gradually, so as to throw its contents as far as possible up the bowels: but a full description of the particular mode of glysteringe in this way, will be given in the sequel or conclusion.

The new invention consists of a pewter syring or pipe, called a *self-pipe:* the meaning of which is, a pipe that can be used without an assistant. It is so constructed as to be used by yourself, or by an assistant if you are so weak as to require one. The pewter syringe holds nearly a quart, and by a screw, a long pipe is connected to the syringe which holds the glyster itself. All that is required is to put the small tube in the fundament, and gradually to bear on the handle of the syringe, which, as you bear down steadily, throw the glyster up the bowels. The force with which the glyster is thrown up the bowels, depends on the pressure on the handle of the pipe. You are to recollect that force, unless it be very gently and steady, is never to be used; all you have to do, is to press gradually on the handle ot the syringe, by which yon will feel the distention of the bowels as the glyster is thrown up. When the glyster is to be thrown up by an assistant, the long pipe or tube is to be unscrewed, and a shorter one made for the purpose and screwed on, which is to be used as a common squirt, on which principle it acts. One of these pipes may be purchased at any drug shop, for about two dollars: and I trust from the great advantages to be derived from this valuable instrument, which in very many instances has even saved life, that no family in this country will be long without one. I shall now state the manner of administering a glyster, in such a way as that it may be understood by any person possessed of the least judgment.

In giving a glyster by an assistant, the patient is to be laid on the edge of the bed, with the bottom a little over the edge, and the knees drawn up near the belly. The clyster pipe is then to be taken, the finger placed before it to keep in the contents, and applied to the fundament. On pushing in the pipe, the finger is to be taken away. The pipe is to be pushed up very gently, the operator's hand near the thighs, a little backwards toward the backbone, and then the contents are to be forced out, by gently pushing the handle of the syringe with one hand, while with the other the syringe is firmly held; or if a bladder and pipe are used, there is nothing to do but to introduce the pipe into the fundament, as just described, and to gradually and gently squeeze the bladder, so as to empty the contents into the bowels. Glystering is one of the most powerful, innocent, mild and beneficial remedies known in the science and practice of medicine.

FRICTION.

Friction, in medicine, means the act of rubbing a diseased part with a soft brush, a course linen cloth, or with flannel, or by rubbing into the body or diseased part, oils, ungents, and other matters, in order to ease, relieve, and cure them. This exercise, or rubbing contributes remarkably to the health, particularly of sedentary persons: for it excites and kindles the natural warmth, diverts defluxions, promotes perspiration, opens the pores, and tends to dissipate stagnant humors. This operation is also particularly beneficial to the nervous, debilitated, and studious—being a useful substitute for other exercises. Hence I recommend to such individuals to spend half an hour every morning and evening, in rubbing their whole bodies, especially their limbs, with the brush or flannel. It ought, however, to be observed, that this practice will be of the greatest service when the *stomach* and *bowels* are empty. Lastly, I venture to assert that, the most important purposes to which friction may be rendered subservient in the animal economy, have hitherto been almost entirely neglected: I am convinced, from experience, that medicated frictions, or the introduction of the most active medicines into the human system, by rubbing them in properly on the surface of the body, is attended with the most happy effects, especially in all chronic diseases. Common sense appears to have long since pointed out this excellent method of administering medicines, even to the Indian savages, though it is little practiced in the United States, where the stomach is doomed to be the field of battle, for deciding commotions and irregularities in our complicated frame. But who is hardy enough to maintain that, the digestive organs was by nature destined to become the exclusive vehicle of drugs, and to serve as their common laboratory?

FLANNEL.

A kind of light porous woolen stuff, woven on a loom with two treadles in the manner of baize.

This, is unquestionably, one of the most useful articles of wearing apparel, and it is much to be regretted, that it is not more generally worn; as we are fully persuaded, that it would be the means of preventing many diseases.

The principal objection to the wearing of flannel appears to be, that it irritates the skin, and occasions disagreeable sensations: these, however, continue only for a few days, and the subsequent advantages thence resulting, amply compensate for such temporary uneasiness. Both young and aged would derive from it equal advantages. I do not, however, mean to insinuate that flannel next the skin should be universally and indiscriminately worn by infants and young persons; though it is an ill founded assertion of its adversaries, that it has a tendency to produce eruptions, as it evidently opens the pores, promotes perspiration, and thus removes the principal cause of cutaneous diseases, that originate from an obstructed and irregular state of the skin. There are, however, certain cases in which flannel cannot, with strict propriety, be used as an under dress. In order to enable the reader to ascertain whether its constant use be advisable or not, I shall point out the leading circumstances which may, in this respect influence his determination. It is a salutary dress to all those, in general, who have passed the meridian of life, or the 35th year of their age, though they should not have been accustomed to it from their infancy, to persons of a cold and phlegmatic habit, or leading a sedentary life, to such as are subject to fits of the gout, rheumatism, frequent colds and catarrhs: to individuals very susceptible of impressions connected with the vicissitudes of air, weather and climate; as well as to nervous patients, and those who have recently recovered from severe chronical diseases. On the contrary, the wearing of flannel next the skin may be injurious to constitutions so organized that they are liable to profuse perspiration on taking even moderate exercise: or to those who are already afflicted with scorbutic or other eruptions of the skin; or lastly, to all such whimsical and irritable persons as possess neither bodily nor mental vigor sufficient to overcome the first uneasy sensations which it occasions. But I am fully warranted to assert, from daily experience, that the habitual use of this beneficent texture, has essentially contributed to the recovery of numberless ricketty children, not less than to the saving of others who were born of feeble and enervated parents. In short, there is every reason to believe that, a more general adoption of this cloth might prevent many fatal inflamations of the throat, breast, lungs, &c. to which the poorer class of people are remarkably liable, and thus preserve the lives of multitudes who are constantly becoming a prey to our damp and changeable climate.

ISSUES.

Issues are small ulcers or sores, formed by artificial means, in various parts of the body, for the purpose of procuring discharges of matter, considered beneficial in many diseases. They were formerly considered merely as drains, to carry off noxious or foul humors from the blood, and were therefore opened as near the affected part as practicable. But, as it is now well known that they produce benefit, as well by sympathy as by acting as a drain, they are usually placed where they will be the least dangerous and inconvenient. The most proper parts to place them in, are between the ribs: on either side of the back bone; in the hollow above the inner side of the knee; in the outer and fore parts of the shoulder; in the nape of the neck; in fact, wherever there is cellular substance enough for the entire protection of the parts underneath. They must never be placed near any blood vessel of a large size: nor over a tendon or thinly covered bone; nor over what is called the belly of a muscle. There are three kinds of them; the seaton or cord, the pea or pepper issue, and the blister issue.

When you take off a blister, and wish to convert the sore into an issue, a discharge of matter can easily be kept up for any length of time, by dressing the part once a day with any ointment mixed with a little powdered Spanish flies. If the discharge is too small, put a little more of the Spanish flies into it; and if too large, put a little less into the ointment, or desist from using the ointment for a few days, until the discharge be sufficiently diminished. This is called the blister issue.

When you want what is called the pea or pepper issue, you must make an incision, or cut with a lancet, large enough to admit one or more peas or grains of pepper, or any thing else that will keep the sore running. When this opening is made with a lancet, or any other sharp instrument, the skin must be pressed or pinched up together, and the cut made of sufficient size to admit the substance to be put into it. The employment of caustic, however is the best mode of opening an issue: This caustic is the *lapis infurnalis* of the drug shops. The caustic must be made into a kind of paste, with a little soft soap or water. You are then to put on an adhesive or sticking plaster, with a hole in the middle of it; and in this hole on the skin you are to spread the caustic paste, and cover it with another sticking plaster, to keep the paste from spreading. In four days the place will become sore, and separate so as to admit whatever you may choose to place in it, for the purpose of keeping it running.

The seaton or cord issue, is always made when a large quantity of matter is required to be discharged: it is frequently put in the back of the neck, for diseases of the head and eyes, and between the ribs for complaints of the breast. The cord which is to be introduced, ought to be of cotton or silk threads, either not twisted together or very loosely twisted. A part of the cord must then be besmeared and smoothed with some kind of ointment, and passed through the eye of the seaton needle, and the needle fairly passed through the skin and part of the flesh, leaving a few inches of the cord hanging out on each side, to be moved backward and forward every day, for the purpose of keeping it running.

THE MALE CATHETER.

This instrument is used for drawing the water from the bladders of males, whenever there are obstructions to its natural flow from the body, arising from gravel and stone, or any other causes. The male catheter is sometimes made of elastic gum, and sometimes of silver: it is about nine inches in length, and hollow from the but nearly to the point, which is rounded and smooth, and about the average thickness of a large rye straw. It is slightly and evenly curved about an inch, and has an oval opening, or hole near the point, on one of the sides.—Being hollow and open at the but end, it has a handle which is fixed to a common sized wire, bent to fit the curve of the hollowed gum or piece of silver.—This is the Catheter so often used in the obstructions of the urinary organs.

Directions for using this Catheter.—When you are about using this instrument, the curved wire which is attached to the handle, is to be pushed fully into the gum elastic, or silver case, where it is to remain until you have introduced the point of the instrument into the bladder. You are now to take the penis of the patient near the head, between the thumb and fore-finger of your left hand; he ought to be lying on his back, on the edge of the bed, and you standing beside him. You are next to introduce the point of the Catheter well rubbed with sweet oil, into the urinary passage called the urethra, with the convex side of the instrument towards the knees of the patient; and while you are gently pushing the catheter down the passage of the bladder, you are to endeavor to draw up the penis on it. When you first introduce it, the handle of the catheter will of course be near the belly of the patient; but as the instrument descends the handle will be thrown further off, until the point enters the bladder; you will know when this is the case on drawing out the wire, by the flow of the urine.—If you cannot succeed while the patient is on his back on the floor, while his legs and thighs are held up by an assistant. If this position, will not answer, place him again on his back, and when you have got the catheter as far in as it will go, rub your fore-finger well with oil, and introduce it into the fundament: then endeavor to push the point of the catheter upwards with your finger, while you still press it forward with the other hand. Force is never to be used: vary your position as frequently as you please, and let the patient vary his; but always remember that you are to succeed by *humoring* the instrument, and not by force and violence.

THE FEMALE CATHETER.

This instrument is made, like the male Catheter, of elastic gum or silver: it is hollow, six or seven inches in length, and about the thickness of the male Catheter. Like the male instrument, it has a handle, and a wire to fit the tube. which is rounded and smooth at the point. From the open or handle end, the tube is nearly straight for three inches; here it curves gently, first downward and then upward, about half an inch. Like the male Catheter, where the end of the tube is introduced into the bladder, the wire is to be withdrawn, in order that the urine may flow off.

The operation of using the female Catheter is so perfectly simple, and attended with so little danger, that every female ought to understand and be able to practice it: first, because she can always operate on herself when necessary. and second, because if a Physician is to be sent for in every case of necessity for the operation, and he should reside at a distance, the delay might often be dangerous and fatal. You will please to recollect, that under the head, *outward parts of female generation*, I have been very particular, and perhaps it may be thought by many, too plain and explicit, in my description of those portions of the female system: which modesty usually conceals and forbids us to name, in treating on this subject of the use of the catheter, however, it will be easily seen, that without thoroughly understanding those parts, the relief of many diseases connected with the urinary organs would be impossible. And, besides, by explaining those parts fully, to which refence may always be had, females will always be enabled to relieve themselves, without an indecent and mortifying exposure of their persons to males who act as physicians.

Immediately under the *clitoris*, which I have before described, you will find, on close examination, a small orifice or opening: this is the lower end of the canal which leads to the bladder, and is only from two to three inches in length. Into this orifice you are to introduce the end of the Catheter, after rubbing it well with oil; you are then to push it gently inward and upward, without any force or violence, until the end has reached the bladder, when you must draw out the wire affixed to the handle, and the urine will flow off through the tube into any vessel prepared to receive it. This is the whole secret of using the Female Catheter, for a want of the knowledge of which, thousands of females have been compelled to submit to an exposure of their persons, and thousands more have lost their lives. where assistance could not be obtained. By a little attention to this subject, female friends, or even female servants, could easily give the required assistance.—By retaining the urine any length of time, the consequences are always dangerous, and very often fatal; because the stoppage frequently terminates in inflammation of the bladder. In a state of pregnancy particularly, the retention of the urine is highly dangerous: it not only displaces the womb, but often causes death. Therefore I advise you, in the slightest obstructions of this kind, always to send for a physician before it be too late.

DISPENSATORY

OR

CLASSIFICATION OF MEDICINES.

The medicines required for common and useful purposes, are very few in number, compared with the hundreds you see displayed in *Doctor's shops* for mere show, or because they possess some simple and innocent virtues. I assert it without fear of contradiction, that more than one half of the medicines now in use, could be very easily dispensed with, and not the least inconvenience be felt for the want of them. When you see an extensive drug store, filled with drugs, tinctures, essences, &c. &c. &c., it ought always to remind you of a dinner table, covered with many unnecessary dishes, where two of the substantial ones, properly cooked, would answer the same purpose. This hint will be sufficient to surprize you, that there are many different medicines which produce the same effects on the human system, and consequently that there are a great many which are absolutely useless; and the choice of which, even by physicians, depends not so much on the characteristics or nature of the disease, as on the particular caprice or partiality of the physician himself.

Under the head of each disease, I have mentioned the principle medicines now in use to effect the cure, and also those which are held in the highest estimation hy the most distinguished medical men. But as the classification of several that may be useful and possibly may have been omitted, may he useful to those who have but a limited range of selection, I shall proceed to classify and describe them, as minutely as my limits will admit.

You will recollect that when you are in the habit of taking medicine often, or any particular medicine frequently, your system will become so habituated to the effects, that larger and more increased doses will be required to produce the usual effects. This doctrine is proved to you, by those who have long been accustomed to the use of opium, spirits or even tobacco. Man is the creature of habit, and can easily bring his system to bear, by slow degress, medical drugs which would in the first instance produce death. By this rule you are to remember, that in giving medicine, you are to vary it in *larger* or *smaller doses*, according to the strength or weakness of the patient, as your good sense and discretion may dictate. What would at times only act as a good purge, would in other cases, and where the patient is weakly and delccate, be productive of fatal consequences. Therefore, always take the constitution, the state or condition of the person, and the particular character of the disease into consideration before you administer medicines.

EMETICS OR PUKES.

These are medicines which on being received into the stomach, produce vomiting or puking. They are called *emetics* by physicians, and are given in a great variety of cases, which you will see enumerated in the body of this work. Their operation will always be increased, and rendered much easier by drinking milk, or blood-warm water in considerable quantities after the first operation.

Ipecaculanha.—This is the mildest of pukes; the dose for a grown person, is from fifteen to twenty grains dissolved in warm water, say five or six spoonfuls: give one spoonful every ten minutes until it operates.

Tartar Emetic.—This is my favorite puke; you will always find it of superior efficacy in bilious fevers. It is the most generally used by physicians in producing full and copious vomiting or puking. A dose for a grown person is from five to six grains, which you are to dissolve in five or six table spoonfuls of warm water, and one table spoonful of which you are to take every ten minutes until it operates.

ANTIMONIAL WIN.—This is nothing more than Tartar Emetic dissolved in wine. The dose is two or three tea spoonfuls given every ten or fifteen minutes until it operates. Antimonial Wine is made as follows:—just dissolve forty grains of emetic tartar into a large wine glass of warm water, which is about two ounces of water. After the emetic tartar is dissolved, add to this water about half a pint of Teneriffe wine, after standing a few hours it will be fit for use.

In cases where an emetic or puke is necessary for children, antimonial wine is nearly always given to them, and that too at a very early age. I have never hesitated, when necessary to give to children when first born, to relieve difficult respiration or breathing, where there was an accumulation of phlegm. The dose in such cases ought not to be more than one or two drops; this medicine however, is so much oftener given to children of more advanced age. At any period under one year of age, and over four months, the dose when intended to produce vomiting, is from five to ten drops, according to the necessities of the case, which is to be repeated at short intervals of time. until the effect is produced. But in the dangerous disease called *croup*, and I wish you particularly to recollect this, a larger quantity of antimonial wine should be given, because there is in this disease a great insensibility to the operation of emetics. In an attack of croup, therefore, you need not be afraid to give a child six months old, from twenty-five to thirty drops every fifteen minutes.

WHITE VITRIOL.—Of all the emetics or pukes known in medicine, this is the quickest in its operation, and ought always to be given in cases which require an immediate evacuation of the stomach: these cases are generally those in which poisons have been swallowed.—The dose is from twenty to thirty grains in a cup of warm water: this medicine is called by physicians sulphat of zink.

The connexion of the stomach with every part of the

body, and the great power it exercises over all portions of the system, and particularly over the brain, have been fully explained to you: the fact is as I have before stated, that I consider the brain as the *father*, and the stomach as the *mother* of the system. In consequence of the very close connexion between the stomach and the head, emetics or pukes act as powerful and valuable remedies, in all diseases connected with the brain and its dependencies. They not only relieve the stomach, by discharging its acrid, vitiated, and sometimes oppressive contents; but they at the same time, promote the secretion and evacuation of bile. They also, and that powerfully, promote a determination to the surface, by which I mean perspiration or sweating; the fact is, that a moisture can be produced on the skin, either by vomiting or puking, or by the mere nausea or sickness of the stomach, arising from emetics given in proper doses. I have not space here to enumerate all the advantages arising from emetics: they will be found under the different heads of diseases, as treated in this work.

I will now give you some directions as to the administration of emetics, in particular cases and states of the system. If the person to whom you wish to give a puke, is of a full and fat habit of body, with a short neck, and a great determination of blood to the head you should draw some blood from the arm before giving the puke. By doing this you will render the puking easy and copious, and prevent all danger of apoplexy from too great a determination of blood to the head of the patient. Doctor Chapman one of the Professors of the Medical School of Philadelphia, states explicitly, and in strong terms, that many lives have been endangered, and some actually sacrificed for want of this necessary precaution of bleeding. In all cases where the necessity for a puke is urgent, and especially where poisons have been swallowed, give a full dose of emetic medicine at once; but in common cases you may give an emetic in broken doses as I have directed; this will prevent too great violence in the operation.

You should if convenient, always give an emetic on an

empty stomach, and in the morning; because at this time, it will always act with greater certainty and effect, and with much less distress to the patient. When you find that an emetic acts too severely, and you wish to check the operation, give from twenty to thirty drops of laudanum in a little toddy, and apply cloths wrung out of warm water to the pit of the stomach: or you may apply stewed garden mint to the stomach; or drink thin chicken soup, with some salt in it, so as to turn the operation downward. If these measures fail, give a glyster, in which you are to put double the quantity of laudanum usually given by the mouth; and if this also fails, put a large blister over the pit of the stomach, and poultices to the feet, made of pounded mustard seed, corn meal, and vinegar. The quantity of laudanum I have mentioned, has reference to grown persons, and not to children. In all cases consult the table of medicines.

ACTIVE PURGATIVES.

These are such medicines as purge freely. When you use them with the intention that they shall act mildly on the bowels, and only keep them gently open, they are called *laxatives* by physicians: these medicines are usually mixed with honey, molasses, or any kind of syrup that is convenient; their operation is always promoted by mild drinks, such as thin gruel pleasantly warm, or any kind of warm tea. If at any time you take a purgative medicine, such as calomel for instance, and it should not operate in due time, it will always be proper to assist the operation by some one of the laxative medicines.

CALOMEL.—A purgative; the dose for a grown persons is from fifteen to twenty grains—and I now again, for the last time, tell you, that small doses of this medicine act more unkindly than large ones. In a reasonable dose calomel will work off without assistance, while in a small dose, it is liable to remain in the system, if not removed by the assistance of laxative medicines. I am now speaking of the calomel when given with the intention of purging.

Calomel and Jalap: purgatives; ten grains of each, mixed with honey, molases, or any kind of syrup, is a dose for a grown person. This valuable preparation was a favorite with the celebrated Doctor Rush; he generally gave it in fevers—it both purges and sweats freely. Twenty grains of each, mixed as above, is a dose for a grown person.

Calomel and Gamboge: purgative; ten grains of calomel, and three grains of gamboge, mixed with honey, molasses, or any kind of syrup, is a dose for a grown person: it is a valuable and active purge, given in bilious fevers.

Lee's Anti Bilious Pills: purgative; they are made of five grains of calomel, ten grains of Jalap, two grains of gamboge, and half a grain of Tartar emetic. This is a valuable preparation, and very easily made; and the information I have given, will enable you to prepare these pills yourself, and always to have them fresh for use. Those obtained from the stores are generally old, hard and dry, and do not operate as if fresh and newly made.

Cook's Pills: a valuable purge, particularly when the liver is diseased, and in female complaints, where obstructions and irregularities take place in the monthly discharges. These pills are made with equal quantities of rhubarb, aloes and calomel, ground fine, well mixed together, and made into pills of a common size, with a little honey or syrup. A dose of these pills for a grown person consists of three or four of them, which operates freely as a purge. These pills may be frequently taken, until the desired effect is produced.

Salts, Senna, and Manna: purgatives; take of each of these articles half an ounce, and put them into a pint of hot water: after which you are to cover the vessel in which you make the preparation. For a grown person, take of this a teacupful every hour until it operates freely.

Salts and Tartar Emetic: purgative; to a common dose of salts, and one grain of emetic tartar—this is a very valuable purge to remove bile.

May, Apple, Jalap, Rhubarb: purgatives.—The roots of these plants act in doses, from thirty to fifty grains each, taken separately, as an effective purge. If either of these roots are given with calomel, the dose should be from five to ten or fifteen grains of calomel, mixed with about twenty grains of the May Apple, Jalap, or Rhubarb root well pounded.

LAXATIVES.

These are medicines which gently open the bowels.

Castor Oil, an innocent and valuable medicine; the dose for a grown person, is from two to three table-spoonfuls. The most agreeable way of taking this laxative oil, is in coffee, or a little spirits of any kind.

Sweet Oil—generally called Olive Oil.—It acts on the bowels the same as castor oil. The dose for a grown person is from two to three table-spoonfuls: like castor oil, you may take it in a little spirits or coffee.

Charcoal in Powder.—This is one of the most valuable and innocent medicines we possess; particularly for persons laboring under *dyspepsia* or *indigestion.* To persons of a *costive habit* of body, the use of pounded charcoal is invaluable, from its always keeping the bowels open and regular. The dose for a grown person is one table-spoonful, mixed with honey, milk, or cold water. The preparation of charcoal as a medicine is very simple. It consists in merely burning the charcoal used by smith's over again: to do which, you are to place it in an iron vessel, and expose it to a hot fire until it becomes of a red heat; then suffer it to cool, pound it very fine, and put it into a dry bottle, which is to be tightly corked. This is the whole secret of preparing the charcoal for medical purposes. It is an excellent medicine in all depraved conditions of the stomach; and it will also check the violent vomitings, or pukings which accompany bilious and yellow fevers: and, I will now disclose to you a secret respecting the use of charcoal which is probably unknown to the physicians of the United states. Whilst I was at Havana, a city in the Island of Cuba, I discovered the secret, by which the Spanish physicians check and relieve the approaching symptoms of *Black Vomit* in *Yellow Fever*: the medicinal preparation is *charcoal* and *oil of turpentine* mixed: but I could never ascertain the quantity of each. This matter, however can easily be ascertained by experiment.

MAGNESIA CALCINED.—Two tea spoonfuls of this medicine is a dose for a grown person; it must be taken in half a tumbler of cold water. If you take *uncalcined magnesia*, a table spoonful will be required as a dose; This medicine corrects acidity of the stomach, and gently opens the bowels. It is also well adapted to women in a family way, and to persons afflicted with dyspepsia or indigestion. A dose taken at bed time, will generally afford to dyspeptic persons, a pleasant night's rest by aiding the digestive powers.

CREAM OF TARTAR. This is a cooling and innocent laxative medicine, and is remarkably well adapted to the warm season. It may be taken in cold water sweetened with sugar. The dose for a grown person, is a table-spoonful, in a tumbler of water.

MANNA.—This is the most innocent laxative medicine made use of in the practice of physic. On account of its extreme mildness in operating, it is better adapted to infants than any purgative known.—Used as a laxative, it is seldom given to grown persons alone, but generally combined, or mixed with senna: the compound is called Senna and Manna. If the manna be given alone, the dose for a grown person is from one to two ounces, dissolved in hot water. If you give it combined with senna, half an ounce of manna, and the same quantity of senna made into a a tea, with about a pint of boiling water, is the dose for a grown person. [See the heads senna and manna, in the Index.]

FLOUR OF SULPHUR.—This is nothing but *brimstone*, purifyed and powdered very fine. From one tea-spoonful to ten, or about the same quantity given in broken doses, three times a day, will moderately purge a grown person.

Whenever any of the above purgative or laxative medicines purge too much, and the patient is becoming weak, if you wish to check the operation, you are to give a dose of laudanum *from twenty to thirty drops:* or you may give a glyster, in which you are to put double the quantity of laudanum taken by the mouth, and at the same time apply hot cloths wrung out of warm water, as warm as they can be borne to the stomach of the patient; either of these measures will stop the operation of the medicines.

In some cases from the bowels being torpid, medicines of a purgative nature will not produce a passage. In such cases you are to wait a reasonable time for their operation; if they do not operate, you are next to give glysters, [For further instructions as to glystering, see under the head Clysters or Glysters.] If these means fail, which they sometimes do, instead of giving heavy doses of medicine by the mouth, give glysters of warm water, and at the same time, pour the coldest water over the belly of the patient. Sailors when at sea, and when they have no medicines on board, frequently relieve themselves from costiveness of the bowels, by merely laying with their naked bodies over the but of a cannon, the coldness of which seldom fails to produce a strong disposition to stool. In severe constipation of the bowels; when the common remedies fail to procure a passage or stool, give a mixture of castor oil and oil of turpentine, of each half an ounce at one dose—and if it does not operate in due time, you are to repeat the same. This powerful and valuable discovery has been lately used with great success in the city of New York.

STIMULANTS.

Stimulants are medicines which excite the whole system into action; the best of which are our common spirituous liquors, intended by Divine Providence as medicines, but which we abuse in their employment as luxuries of daily use, by which they are converted into poisons, pregnant with deadly mischief: destroying the reasoning faculties, and entailing upon the unfortunate devotee a train of corporeal afflictions which infallibly eventuate in his premature dissolution. They are therefore to be regarded, rather than a blessing as a curse upon posterity and a nation. It is a fact certainly known to those who are in the habit of constantly using stimulants, that they require to be frequently administered, or else they loose their power: that when the system has for any length of time been accustomed to those stimulants, it is necessary gradually to increase the quantity to produce the same action upon the system which was excited by their early or first use. The stimulants generally considered medicinal, or used in medicine are as follows:—

SULPHURIC ETHER.—This is a valuable stimulant in cases of great debility or weakness, in hysterical cases, in cramp of the stomach, in checking vomiting or puking, in allaying sea sickness, and discharging wind from the stomach. Externally applied to the head, it will greatly assist in relieving head ach. Either is to be kept well corked, or it will loose its strength; and when it is taken, it must be drank as quick as possible after it is mixed with water, or it will loose the power, or effect it is intended to produce.—Dose, from one to three tea spoonfuls mixed in a stem or wine-glass of cold water.

SPIRITS OF HARTSHORN. This is a strong and active stimulant, it is generally used in hysterical complaints, and nervous head-ache, and is also a valuable remedy in dyspepsia. [See that head.] By the alkaline property which it possesses, it neutralizes acids in the stomach, at the same time communicating strength to that organ. In all extreme cases of debility of the stomach, attended with vomiting and spasm, as is frequently the case with habitual drunkards, Hartshorn will be found a most valuable remedy.—It will relieve the sting of the bee, wasp, and other insects, by keeping the wounded part wet with it.—Dose from one to two tea-spoonfuls.

Opium, and the preparation made from opium, called **Laudanum**, when given in small doses act as stimulants—when given in larger doses, produce sleep and relieve pain. [For a full description of both these articles, see under the head of Opium—and for doses, see Table of Medicines.]

Spirit, or Oil of Turpentine, when taken internally, is one of the most active and diffusible stimulants: pervading the whole extent of the system; but with greater force to certain parts, and in cases where the bowels are obstinately constipated, or bound; in *puerperal*, or child-bed fever, [see under that head] and in epileptic fits, [see under that head] particularly where these complaints are brought on by worms, it also acts as an evacuant, or purge. The dose is from three to four tea-spoonfuls, alone, or with a small portion of water.

Spirit of Lavender.—This is a mild and pleasant stimulant, and is generally administered to females in hysterical affections. When mixed with *sulphuric ether* in equal quantities, it is valuable in debility, or weakness of the system. The dose of lavender alone is three tea-spoonfuls.

There is nothing more difficult in the practice of medicine, than to determine when it is proper to prescribe stimulants; nor is it possible for me, here to point out to you the exact time, or to give further light on the subject, than in advising you to be guided by the state of the system; avoid their application during fever, as they invariably increase it; nor never prescribe them in no case, until proper evacuations have been made. It is only in the protracted and feeble stage of diseases that they can be resorted to with any hope of advantage.—By watching their operation, you can readily perceive by the absence or presence of the following symptoms, whether their administration is proper or not: pain in the head; delirious wanderings, or in other words, the patient talks wildly; great watchfulness; stricture, or tightness of the breast; restlessness and anxiety; with a hot, dry skin, parched tongue, and a quick, small and corded pulse.—Upon the appearance of any, or all of the above symptoms you are immediately to desist in the use of stimulants.

ANODYNES.

Anodynes are those medicines which ease pain and procure sleep.

OPIUM in doses of from two to five grains. [See table of medicines, and also for a full description of Opium, see under that head.]

LAUDANUM; made by dissolving an ounce of Opium in a pint of good spirits of any kind—it is generally fit for use in five or six days. Fifty drops of laudanum are equal to two grains of Opium. [For doses of this, or any other medicine refer to the table of medicines.]

PAREGORIC; made by adding half a drachm of Opium—or one ounce of laudanum to a pint of spirits of any kind, and mixing with them half a drachm of flowers of benzoin, the same quantity of oil of ani seed, and one scruple of camphor. The dose is three or four tea-spoonfuls. [For the different ages refer to the table of medicines.]

ANTI-SPASMODICS.

Anti-Spasmodics, are medicines which are given to remove spasm or cramp, and generally used by physicians for this purpose:

OPIUM, or LAUDANUM, in doses depending on the extreme urgency or danger of the case.

HOT TODDY, made with spirits, hot water, and sweetened with sugar.

SULPHURIC ETHER, dose from two tea-spoonfuls, to a table-spoonful in half a cup of cold water.

ASSAFŒTIDA, a lump weighing; from eight to ten, or even

twenty grains; or if you use the tincture which is nothing more than assafœtida, steeped in whiskey as follows: Take of assafœtida two ounces, and put it in a pint of old whiskev, or good spirits of any kind; let it stand for ten davs, and the tincture is ready for use. Dose from one tea spoonful to four, mixed in a little cold water.

Essence of Peppermint, given in a large dose, mixed with hot toddy.

The best means for removing spasms are the warm bath, [See under that head,] bleeding freely and applying cloths wrung out of hot water, or hot salt to the skin, over the part where cramp or spasm is seated.

TONICS.

Medicines which increase the tone of the muscular Fibres, and thereby strengthen the whole body.

Peruvian Bark: this bark is obtained from South America; there are three kinds, the red, the yellow, and the pale; the red bark when pure is the best. It has however been ascertained that the medicinal properties of our common dogwood, is equal if not superior to the imported bark

The dose in substance of the peruvian bark is from two to four tea spoonfuls, in a stem or wine glass of water, taken every three or four hours when there is no fever. If it should disagree with the stomach, it may be given in decoction, by putting an ounce of the bark in a quart of hot water to which add a little Virginia Snake root, frequently called black snake root, to which add a small portion of cinnamon or ginger. When it becomes cold, you are to mix with it half a pint of the best Maderia or Teneriffe wine. [Dose a stem or wine glass full every two or three hours]

Dogwood Bark or **Wild Cherry Tree Bark**, pounded fine and taken in doses of thirty or forty grains, are equal to the Peruvian Bark. I have been in the habit of using in my practice equal quantities of the barks of Dogwood, Wild Cherry and poplar, (I allude to the poplar of the forest of which our boats are made,) these three barks steeped in good spirits of any kind, and administered in moderate doses say three or four times a day, is superior in its tonic effects to any medicines I have ever used. The bark of the poplar is one of the most valuable medicines we possess; I can assert from experience, that there is not in all the Materia Medica, a more valuable and certain remedy for dyspepsia or indigestion, than poplar bark. In hysterical complaints, this bark combined with a small quantity of laudanum, is a valuable remedy. In worms it has been prescribed to a child when convulsions or fits had taken place: after taking a few doses, several hundred dead worms were discharged with the stools. The dose of the powder, to a grown person, is from twenty grains to two drachms: or the bark may be used in tincture: that is, steeped in spirits, or as a tea; its virtues are always greatest when given in substance or powder.

Columbo Root is a mild but powerful tonic, communicating vigor to the stomach: when properly administered, it does not produce stricture, nausea, or in other words. sickness of the stomach and oppression; and is well adapted to dyspeptics, or those persons laboring under *indigestion;* for the stomach will bear this substance with advantage, while most other tonics produce disagreeable symptoms.— This medicine will also restrain or stop vomiting or puking: it is frequently substituted for Peruvian bark, in consequence of its milder action on the system. Dose from ten, twenty to thirty grains of the powder, in half a tea cupful of milk or cold water three times a day. In dyspeptic cases, or enfeebled digestion, small doses answer better than large ones. The tincture is a useful form of administering this medicine, which is prepared as follows: Take of columbo root three ounces, bruise it with a hammer, put it in a quart of good spirits of any kind, or good wine, let it stand five days, shaking it frequently, then strain it, and it is fit for use: it should be taken occasionally through the day, as pleasantly prepared as the stomach is capable of receiving it.

NITRIC ACID.—Read Diseases of the Liver where you will find a full description of this medicine.

It is a most powerful tonic, particularly in chronic affections of the liver, and where the constitution has been much injured by the use of Mercury, or the venereal disease. The best method of taking it is to make a quart of cold water pleasantly sour with the medicine, and add to it sugar or any kind of syrup, which renders it agreeable to the taste, when it may be drank through the day in such quantities as the stomach will bear. In taking this medicine, however, it is best to take it through a quill, as the acid is apt to injure the teeth.

GENTIAN ROOT.—This makes a strong and valuable bitter, and is much used in weakness of the stomach, and to increase the appetite. Take two ounces of gentian root, one ounce of orange peel, and half an ounce of canella alba, put them in a quart of spirits of any kind, or good Mederia or Teneriffe wine: after eight or ten days, shaking it frequently so as to extract their strength, it then yields a pleasant and healthful bitter, and may be used at pleasure, or as the stomach may require it.

VIRGINIA SNAKE ROOT, sometimes called black snake root, worm wood, tansy, chamomile flowers, horehound, wild centaury commonly called centry, and hops; all of which yield a pleasant and innocent bitter when made strong by boiling, and then adding to the tea an equal quantity of spirits: or as a tincture, by steeping them for several days in good spirits of any kind: these articles may be used separately or mixed together, as you may have it in your power to procure them.

ELIXIR VITRIOL. It is a very pleasant and useful tonic; it restores and strengthens the appetite, and gives tone to the digestive organs, and restrains those sweats which frequently occur after severe fevers, called by medical men *colliquative* sweats, which mean those sweats which melt down as it were, the strength of the body. Elixir vitriol is one of our most popular and highly esteemed medicines, for restraining hemorrhage, which means flooding from the uterus or womb, and in hæmoptysis, which means spitting of blood. The dose is from fifteen to twenty drops, every two or three hours, mixed in a stem or wine glass of cold water, or in as much water as will make it pleasantly sour.

Iron in its operation on the system, evinces all the effects of a powerful and permanent tonic; no medicine perhaps, leaving behind it such lasting impressions. It increases the activity and volume of the pulse, corrects the state of the blood and its secretions, and invigorates or strengthens the whole system. The numerous advantages arising from the use of Iron as a medicine, are embraced within the sphere of chronic debility.

The chalybeate waters with which the western country abounds, are springs impregnated with iron, and are found upon almost every branch and creek. The water of these valuable springs should be used by persons laboring under the following complaints:—*Chlorosis*, which means green sickness, [see under that head:] in *Hypochondriasis*, commonly called vapors or low spirits; in *Hysterical affections;* the *whites*, a disease to which women are subject; [see under that head] *paralysis*, or palsy, [see under that head:] in *scrofula* or king's evil; rickets in children; and in dyspepsia, or indigestion, [see under that head.] I have now enumerated the various cases in which the chalybeate waters are beneficial, as well as the principle complaints in which iron is employed. When this medicine is used in substance, it is generally obtained from the Apothecary or Doctor's shops, in the form of rust or iron, and given in doses of five or ten grains, three times a day mixed in syrup of any kind. By putting a few grains of the rust of iron in a bottle filled with common *soda water*, it makes as valuable a chalybeate drink as the water of any the springs which are impregnated with iron. I again for the last time, tell you that tonics, must not be given when they produce fever.

SUDORIFICS.

Sudorifics are medicines which produce free and copious sweating. Diaphoretics are those which occasion only gentle perspiration, or moisture of the skin.

TARTAR EMETIC, called by physicians *Tartarized Antimony*, when given in small doses, so as to produce slight sickness at the stomach, is most generally attended with perspiration, and is proper in *Nervous* and *Bilious fevers*.

NITROUS POWDERS.—To sixty grains of nitre—which is nothing more than Saltpetre—pounded very fine, add sixteen grains of calomel, and one grain of tartar emetic: mix them well together, and then divide the compound into eight equal portions, one of which you are to give every two or threc hours, in a little syrup of any kind. If these powders should purge which they sometimes do, you should omit or leave out the calomel —The nitrous powders are considered a valuable medicine in bilious fevers.

DOVER'S POWDER—This powder is one of the most certain sudorific, where it is often difficult, by other means, to produce a copious sweat. The dose is from five to twenty grains, according as the person's stomach and strength can bear it. It is proper to avoid much drinking immediately after taking this medicine; for by so doing it is apt to be vomited or puked up, before it has had due time to operate as a sweat. The manner of preparing them are as follows: if you cannot obtain them already prepared at any apothecary or doctor's shop. Of ipecacuanha in powder, and opium in fine powder, each one drachm, vitriolated tartar, or saltpetre, (either will do) one ounce finely powdered; you are to be very particular to grind all these articles together, into the finest powder; when thus ground, as fine as it is possible, you have prepared and ready for use, this valuable medicine. Opium intended to make these powders, ought to be pounded perfectly fine in a mortar, during the coldest weather, and kept for this purpose in a bottle. In warm weather, the opium becomes too soft to admit of being reduced to powder. Dover's powder is one of the most valuable remedies we have, for quieting the bowels in dysentery or flux, after proper evacuations have been made.

ANTIMONIAL WINE and SPIRITS OF NITRE.—Take equal quantities of each, and mix them together: the dose is one, two, and three tea-spoonfuls: if it inclines to vomit, or puke, you are to lessen the quantity of antimonial wine one half to two of the spirits of nitre. This is valuable in fevers to promote perspiration.

IPECACUANHA, given in small doses—say one or two grains, every two or three hours, mixed with a little warm water or syrup, will excite perspiration.

SENEKA SNAKE Root, Virginia Snake Root, Butterfly Weed sometimes called pleurisy root, dittany, boneset, called by some thoroughwort. These roots or herbs are all valuable for their sweating powers. [For a full description of each refer to their different heads.]

OINTMENTS FOR SORES.

SIMPLE OINTMENT.—This, as its name expresses, is innocent, and merely intended to keep the parts soft and from exposure to cold: made by melting four ounces of bees wax with half a pint of sweet oil; or in a less quantity, observing the proportions. Suet and clear hog's lard will answer if the oil cannot be conveniently had.

BASILICUM OINTMENT.—Healing, and exciting; used in dressing sores. It is made by melting one ounce of bees wax, one ounce of resin, and an ounce and a half of clean hog's lard together.

LEAD OINTMENT.—For dressing sores of an inflammatory nature: pound very fine one drameh of sugar of lead, and mix it well with six ounces of hog's lard.

RED PRECIPITATE OINTMENT.—This ointment is generally used for curing the itch; it is also valuable for old sores on the legs, when applied in dry powder, after cleansing them well with castile soap: it will also destroy what is called proud flesh. The way to make this ointment is, to mix one drachm of the powdered precipitate with an ounce of hog,s lard, and rub them well together.

Tar Ointment.—Used in diseases of the skin, particularly Scald Head: made by melting together equal quantities of tar and the best mutton suet.

Jamestown Weed.—This valuable plant, of which I have given a full description, [For further information see under the head Jamestown Weed.] forms one of the best ointments for piles and old sores: made by first bruising, and then stewing the leaves in hog's lard, and then strained; the proportions in which the leaves and lard are to be mixed are about one part of the leaf to one of lard.

Turner's Cerate.—This ointment which is so celebrated in burns [for a full description of its extraordinary virtues refer to the head Turner's Cerate,] is prepared as follows: take of calamine in fine powder, half a pound; bees-wax the same quantity; hog's lard one pound; melt the wax with the lard and put it out in the air; when it begins to thicken, which it will do as it gets cool, mix with it the calamine, and stir it well until cold.

When you enquire for this article in an Apothecary or Doctor,s shop, ask for calamine in powder; it is a mineral imported from England and Germany, and found in mines intemingled with the ores of different metals.

Blistering Ointment.—Take of Spanish flies—called, medically speaking, *cantharides*—bees. wax, resin, and tallow, equal quantities of each: melt first the wax, resin and tallow together the flies are to be taken and pounded very fine, and mixed with the composition a little before it gets entirely cold, or firm.

Tartar Emetic ointment—called by physicians *Ointment of Tartarized Antimony.*—This is a valuable external or outward stimulant, and forms a most beneficial application in all deep seated inflammations, of the chest especially. It occasions a pustular eruption on the skin, or in other words, numerous pimples, which discharge in a short time; these discharges, or runnings may be kept up by the occasional application of the ointment, as expressed under that head. the method of making this ointment is as follows:—take of tartar emetic one drachm—or two, if you wish to make it strong—mixed well with one ounce of hog's lard, and it is fit for use: or if you prefer it, sprinkle it on a piece of leather, on which an adhesive—commonly called a strengthening plaster, has been previously spread, taking care not to cover the edges of the adhesive plaster with the ointment so as to prevent it from touching and adhering, or sticking to the skin.

Volatile Liniment.—This is a valuable preparation to be rubbed on the skin as an external stimulant in sore throats, rheumatism, spasms, pains, &c. After rubbing it well in, which should be continued from twenty minutes to half an hour, flannel should be wrapped round the afflicted part. Volatile liniment is made by mixing equal quantities of spirits of hartshorn and sweet oil: by adding to this mixture, a tea-spoonful or two of laudanum, the preparation will be much improved in its efficacy in removing pain.

MERCURY.

I shall mention only such mercurial medicines as are daily and commonly used.

Calomel is considered the most valuable of the mercurial medicines, in every disease in which I have directed its use. Full, plain, and explicit directions have been given as to the doses, and the effect intended to be produced by this mineral, and the injuries which frequently result from its improper use.

Blue Pill.—There is scarcely an indication to be fulfilled—says Dr. Chapman—by mercury the purgative effect excepted, to which this preparation is not adequate. It is much prescribed in cases where salivation is demanded, and as an alterative which you will see fully described in Diseases of the Liver, [see under that head.] The Blue Pill is made by triturating, or rubbing quicksilver with the conserve of roses till the globules, or little balls of mercury are entirely extinguished, or destroyed: the pills should be so prepared as to contain about a grain of the metal: the dose in general is, a pill in the morning, and one at night. This is the mildest preparation of mercury, but it is by no means an inactive medicine.—The dose may be increased, if necessary, to as high as six pills.

Mercurial Ointment, generally known by the people in the country as *oil of Bayse*. The old plan of preparing this ointment required great labor. The following is a quick and effectual method of preparing this article; take an ounce and a half of balsam of Peru, to every pound of mercury; triturate for ten minutes, and the mercury will be, not only extinguished, but apparently oxydized. Then add the proper proportions of suet and lard to make an ointment. As soon as the whole is well mixed, which may be done in three minutes, the ointment has a fine blue color, and possesses full activity.

SWAIM,S PANACEA.

This medicine, on its first appearance before the public, excited great hopes of its being an invaluable remedy for several complaints supposed to be incurable, particularly scrofula. The high recommendations which accompanied it, by some of the most distinguished Phisicians of Philadelphia, entitled it to some confidence, and so much were its virtues appreciated, that this medicine sold at the extravagant price of five dollars per bottle; its immediate and successful sales, realized to Mr. Swaim a large fortune. In due time, however, like all *patent medicines*, it sunk into dignified retirement, being nothing more than an old friend with a new face: its principal and component part being the same as the French medicine called Rob Syphilitique, which is *Corrosive Sublimate*—one of the most active preparations of mercury.

Swaim's Medicine is made from sarsaparilla, marsh reed

grass, borage flowers, senna, rose leaves, sassafras and winter green; these articles are boiled together in water, and strained off: sugar and honey are then added, so as to form the consistence of syrup, when the most active mercurial preparation, *corrosive sublimate* is mixed with it.

The Rob, in its effects, is similar to Swaim's medicine; its preparation, however, is more simple, and the addition of the former, adds nothing to its virtues. Both these medicines are only valuable in the secondary stages of that dreadful disease which I have so plainly described under the head venereal disease.

LIVERWORT.

This plant grows so abundantly, and is so well known in the western country, that a description would be unnecessary. The excitement produced throughout the United States in sonsequence of its being a supposed remedy, or cure for consumption, led to a full investigation of its virtues, when like thousands of its predecessors, it has only proved to be an innocent pallative remedy. By using it as a tea, it assists expectoration, or a discharge from the lungs; allays the irritation of the cough: and in some instances, lessens the frequency of the hectic symptoms. [See under the head *Consumption.*]

"SCROFULA OR KING'S EVIL.

This disease is most frequently among the children of the poor, and negroes, who are ill-fed, ill-lodged and ill-clothed; it is also hereditary, but never contagious. It most commonly occurs in children from the third to the seventh year; frequently however it discovers itself at a later period in habits peculiarly disposed to it.

SYMPTOMS.—It is known by indolent hard tumors of the lymphatic glands, particularly those of the neck, behind the ears or under the chin. The upper lip and division of the nostrils are swelled, with a smooth skin and hard belly. In the progress of the disease, these tumors degenerate into ulcers of bad digestion; the discharge of which consists of a white curdled matter, resembling somewhat the coagulum of milk; and previous to their breaking, they acquire a sort of purple redness, and a softness to the touch.

TREATMENT.—As soon as these tumors are discovered, endeavor to disperse by sea-bathing, or bathing in salt and water, one pound to three gallons of water, or cold water alone, or by frequent application of lead water. Warm fomentations and poultices of every kind, do harm, as they seem only to hurry on a suppuration, which, if possible, should be prevented —A large draught of sea- water every morning will be found a useful drink. Peruvian bark and steel used alternately every two weeks, will be of infinite service by giving tone to the system. The remedy however, most to be depended upon in this disease, is the muriate of lime, given in doses of ten to eighty drops, gradually increased three or four times a day, diluted with water or tea. When a suppuration takes place, the solution of arsenic should be given twice or thrice a day. The best application to scrofulous ulcers, is a powder composed of one pound of finely powdered bark, and one ounce of white lead, in powder, mixed well together; or a fine powder of calamine stone alone, and the ulcers covered with it daily, keeping it on by brown paper and a bandage. Where these are not to be obtained, the constant application of linen rags, moistened with a solution of one ounce of sugar of lead, in a pint of water, may answer every purpose.

With respect to the diet, it should be nourishing and easily digestible, avoiding all viscid food. Moderate exercise in a dry warm air is exceedingly beneficial."

"WHITE SWELLING.

Is distinguished by an acute pain, without any external inflammation of a joint, attended with a gradual increase of its size: Though all the joints are occasionally subject to it, yet its most useful seat is in the knee.

White swellings are generally of a scrofulous nature, but sometimes they are produced by rheumatic affections, and sometimes follow strains that have been neglected, or badly treated.

Treatment.—As soon as an affection of this kind is discovered, the patient should remain in bed, and the limb kept perfectly at rest; without which, remedies cannot produce any good effect.

The great object is to prevent the formation of matter, by the immediate application of leeches, or scarifications to the part affected, and by which eight or ten ounces of blood may be taken away, every other day, or oftener according to circumstances. The whole joint should then be kept continually wet and cold with the solution of crude sal ammoniac, by means of four or five folds of old linen. After the local affections is somewhat abated, frictions with the volatile liniment, or a mixture of soft soap and spirits of camphor, to which may be added some tincture of cantharides, will have a good effect. With one or other of these liniments, the joint is to be rubbed well twice a day, and afterwards covered with a piece of flannel that has been soaked in the same. If this should not produce good effects, the part must be rubbed night and morning with mercurial ointment, in the quantity of two drachms at a time, and continued until the mouth is gently affected.—The cure may then be completed by small blisters on each side of the joint, which should be kept for a length of time.

If the disease in spite of these remedies continue to advance, emollient poultices must be applied often, until various abscesses appear, and these should be opened as soon as they seem to point, and afterwards to be treated as ulcers.

In cases where the white swelling is evidently scrofulous, tonic medicines, such as bark, steel, &c. and a nourishing diet, to correct the constitutional affection, with stimulating applications to the joint, form the best remedies."

"MILK SICK.

For this complaint I do not know the technical name; because I have never seen a single word in print on the subject, from any man but myself.

A great portion of the people in the western country are subject to this dreadful malady. It is caused by the vapors which arise from poisonous minerals in the earth, and settle on the grass and other vegetables that cattle eat. This fact is clearly proven by many circumstances: Frst, by the very appearance of the water, and the rocks, particularly in the lower parts of Indiana, and other sections where it is prevalent. Second, the very dogs are affected with it, from using the water. Third, it seldom makes its attacks till in the summer or fall, after the waters are all very low, at which time, we know that they contain the greatest proportion of *mineral* or other *impure* substances; also that vegetable substances at this time become tough, and contain much less juice, in proportion to the vapor which settles on them. Fourth, if it had been a vegetable which produced the Milk Sick, it would have been found long ago; for to my own knowledge, it has been deligently searched for in many places, by numerous people and not found. Fifth, the scope of land on which it is taken by the cattle, has frequently been ascertained to be very small; and by enclosing it so that they could not get in, the malady was prevented. In this case if it had been a vegetable of any kind, its growth certainly would have extended over the enclosure in 30 or 40 years; for I am acquainted with a place in East Tennessee of nearly that age. A sixth proof is, that you may let the place remain unenclosed, and cattle will always be liable to the complaint as long as there is vegetable matter enough of any kind, to induce them to feed on it; unless it is possible that the richness or chemical properties of some vegetable might counteract the poison. It any thing will, I should think red clover might. People take it from using the milk of cows that are affected with it. Cattle may have the poison in them for weeks, or even months; and so may people before they show it. But whenever any person or animal is overheated, the disease makes an attack, except on cows that gives milk; they seldom die with it, owing to the poison being carried off with the milk.

SYMPTOMS.—If attacked immediately after supping the milk, you have a weak trembling feeling all over you: and sometimes a dizziness in the head, and a burning at the stomach, with vomiting and thirst; and in all cases, the breath has a peculiar smell; by which you will know it from any other poison, both in man and beast. If it is brought on by heat, the vomiting is not so sudden.

TREATMENT.—The instant you feel the symptoms, bruise or beat to pieces, a handful of wild ipecac root, [for further information see the head *American Ipecacuanha*] put it into spirits, and give a table spoonful every few minutes, which will empty the stomach, and make the puking ligther in a short time, and the stimulons of the spirits will brace the nervous system at the same time. For this reason, or some peculiar effect produced by their combined influence, this seems to be much the best mode of administering this medicine.

After the patient has puked sufficiently to cleanse the stomach, the vomiting will cease. Whether it does or not, give a table spoonful of fine sulphur, and if thrown up repeat the dose again and again. A little of the *vegetable caustic* dissolved in water week enough to be drank, may be taken occasionally. After the puking has entirely ceased, give from one to two or three table-spoonfuls of castor oil, with one of sulphur. If the bowels are the least bound, injections must be used at the beginning, of warm milk and sweet oil or castor oil, or thin gruel with soap suds in it. But the wild ipecac must be depended on, more than any thing else; for it certainly possesses a specific efficacy in this complaint if taken in time. As a proof of this, you never find any section of country subject to this malady, without a bountiful supply of this plant in the same region. If there be any other successful remedy for this disease, I do not know it. No mineral should ever be used but the sulphur; and it, not till the Ipecac has had its full influence. Calomel, Tartar Emetic, and all such articles are death! because wherever they have been administered in this complaint they appear to exert a united and deadly influence with the poison which is already in the system. *Diets* for a few days must be light, without any salt."

REMARKS.

In making an addition to this medical work; I feel sensible of the insufficiency of space, to write as fully and as plainly as I could wish, on such important and useful subjects, as might be communicated to my countrymen. The rapid sale of my book, and the great patronage I have received in my humble efforts to be useful to my fellow creatures, fills my heart with joy and gratitude, and language is inadequate to express to my fellow citizens, how much I estimate their goodness, or how willing I feel still to continue my feeble efforts through the assistance of Almighty God, to do them good, and to unfold to them such things in plain language, as may soothe their bodily infirmities, and perhaps the means of relieving them from pain and sickness. To the profession of medicine the life of man stands greatly indebted through all its ages, from the cradle to the grave, and that the use of second means was intended by the Deity, cannot be controverted. Behold the spontaneous gifts of nature, yield in almost every fragrant herb and flower, medicine to heal and relieve our maladies, recalling to our minds the splendid proofs of the *Divine Majesty* showing the incomparable superiority of nature over the most elegant works of human contrivance. Behold for a moment, the forms and colors that embellish the vegetable world, and see how many thousands of the human race like the grazing cattle, without reflection trample on the flowery meads, and forget that those plants are the works of God, and intended by our Heavenly Father, in infinite mercy, for the use of his creatures; wander not then, that so many constitutions are destroyed in this country by the daily and constant use of mineral poisons, which if properly treated by the medical plants, would have been otherwise preserved, leaving the system free from the effects of such medicines as I consider worse than the original disease. But the time is not fare distant, when the reflecting part of this community will be fully satisfied, that the medicinal herbs and roots of the United States, are better adapted to our constitutions and diseases than the mineral poisons, so constantly and freely used in the present day. I have ever loved and cherished an exalted opinion of the vegetable kingdom, and I never have prescribed a single mineral, without feeling sensible there was something defective in my medical education. And although I have prescribed them throughout my work, in the spirit of truth, and according to the practice of medicine at this time, I still deplore, and conscientiously acknowledge, that there is not a substitute for this *Herculean* remedy *calomel*, in which any confidence can be placed, notwithstanding the many boasted substitutes daily advertised by quacks and pretenders, in the healing art, nor has this invaluable remedy, or boasted panacea of our profession, developed its powers so as to be perfectly and fully understood by even the most learned and observing practitioners. That it has done much good to mankind, I acknowledge, by its affording relief in many diseases which would otherwise have proved incurable, or perhaps terminated fatally, but whether the effects of this powerful medicine is left lurking in the system for years, and perhaps never eradicated, is quite doubtful; the occular demonstration of my daily practice, and intercourse with my fellow men, proves beyond the possibility of doubt, as to the injurious effects produced in many cases by the indiscriminate use of calomel, particularly to those whose constitutions and inherent disorders subject them to the most awful effects from this medicine.

Then let me, as a parent bestowing his parting counsel and benediction on his children, advise you to avoid as much as possible, *this*, as well as all other *active* medicines, remembering to administer it with due caution and judgment, and when required to use, let it be administered in active doses, by which I mean it is to be removed from the system; and for this purpose, an active dose is by far the best, by enabling it not only to be beneficial, but work itself off. You will find in the practice of medicine, that in nine cases out of ten, active purging will relieve; you are also to remember, that the mind has powerful influence not only over diseases, but particularly over the digestive organs. Thus when the mind is intensely occupied; the digestive powers of the stomach are suspended, mental activity controls the functions of the stomach to an equal extent. During the period of deep thought, the vital energy of the body is so entirely directed to the brain, that not only the stomach, but the extremities experience a diminution of excitement as is proved by their coldness and insensibility. This condition of the brain, will affect the stomach and intestines, as even to suspend the operation of active medicines.—Doctor Rush states that during the Revolutionary war, he knew Officers who were unexpectedly drawn into battle after having taken drastic cathartics, and yet suffer no inconvenience from them until the excitement of it had passed away. I have seen two distressing sea-sickness promptly relieved by the mental anxiety produced by an engagement between vessels of war. The stimulation caused by this sublime spectacle, produced a revulsion from the stomach to the brain, and thus relieved the one of the irritation accompanying this distressing disease, and the other from that depressed state indicated by languid feelings and obtuseness of intellect. The mind having such full and powerful effects over the whole system, should be a sufficient evidence to guard you in many complaints, particularly, in diseases of the stomach, against the use of too much medicine, depending generally upon diet, moderate exercise, rest, temperance in all things, particularly in eating; change of climate, in sea-bathing, and the use of the tepid or warm bath, mineral springs, foot exercise in all chronic complaints, and in assisting nature, by innocent remedies, to throw off disease. Your good sense will suggest to you the importance of time; and the remedies mentioned in chronic disorders, by which I mean diseases of long standing, rather than destroying the coats of the stomach, and paralyzing the last glimmering of hope, by a farago of medicines. Physicians prescribe much, but use but few medicines themselves. Let then, this hint suffice, by showing you, that much is to be expected by simple remedies, discriminating judgment, and the influence of the mind upon the corporeal body, but do not understand me, that I wish you to discard medicine *altogether*, but by its limited use, and depending much on the *simple*, yet efficient directions I have here recommended to you, you will have but little use for physicians or their prescriptions.

ACCIDENTS.

When an accident takes place by a fall from a horse, or height, or being thrown from a carriage, or receiving a blow from a stick, or any similar injury to those I have mentioned, it will be poper, if possible, to bleed from the arm, but from any other part, if these parts are injured so as to prevent it. The loss of blood must be regulated according to the situation and circumstances of the case: for frequently the injury has been so severe as to deprive *apparently*, the patient of life: in this situation you must wait for the returning symptoms of animation, using friction; or in other words rubbing so as to restore the circulation; this will be proper over the region of the heart and stomach, temples, and the extremities, and bathing the temples with the spirit in which camphor has been dissolved, or spirit of hartshorn, or strong vinegar, at the same time applying it occasionally to the nose; and should the person be able to swallow, or so soon as they may be a little restored, it will be proper to give a little wine and water, or water and spirits of any kind, or any other gentle stimulant that may be convenient. In all cases of suspendid animation, it is highly essential to continue for any length of time, friction, and in many difficult cases, you will find the tepid bath of great service in restoring life; for I have frequently witnessed the person restored, when all, and even the most distant hope seemed at an end; therefore let me implore you in such cases, to use gentle and continued friction on the body, for some vital spark may yet linger, and be warmed into animation—Providence may bless your kind efforts, and what heart-felt gratification will it afford you to be the humble instrument of restoring the life of a fellow creature, who, perhaps, in an unexpected and unprepared state, has been thus situated with the last glimmering hope sinking fast into eternity. If I had space—and I regret I have not—I could give you several interesting cases that have fallen under my care, and many I have witnessed, particularly in the cases of drowing, in which the most happy effects have been produced by perseverance. But on this highly important subject, let me refer you to the head *suspended animation.*

In all cases where the patient is unable from severe injury to walk, it is necessary immediately to prepare a conveyance—and for this purpose, take two boards sufficiently long and broad, and then nail two cross pieces with the ends projecting about a foot for handles—or make, if the plank is not convenient, a litter formed of the branches of trees. On either of these convey your patient to the nearest house. If the person should be bleeding, you must stop the blood before moving him or her. In removing him on, and from this litter to the bed, be extremely careful as many serious accidents occur by being in too great a hurry and alarm; frequently there is considerable pain inflicted unnecessarily, by awkwardly stripping off the coat or pantaloons; therefore rip up the seams, by which you prevent very often much unnecessary pain: recollect never to use the least force. When the patient is stripped, and the room cleared of *all* unnecessary lookers on, which is generally the case, much to the annoyance of the patient and his physician, *particularly if a female,* then proceed to ascertain the injury. If a male, with calmness and firmness—if a female, with tenderness and delicacy, yet with certainty, as to the nature of the injury. I would here remark in plain language, as I have always done in my advice and writings, that *false delicacy* has in many instances destroyed the lives of many females, that might have otherwise been easily preserved. With these remarks and directions I shall in as few words as possible, and in plain language, proceed to give such directions in Surgery as may be easily performed by the most humble person who will but attend to the directions.

Injuries may be simple or compound; that is it may be a contusion or bruise, a wound, a fracture, or dislocation, or it may be two or all of them united, in one or several parts.

A Contusion is of course the consequence of every

blow, and is known by the swelling and the skin being bruised and discolored—wounds require of course no explanation.

FRACTURES, in other words, broken bones, are known by the sudden and severe pain, and by the appearance of the limb being out of shape—sometimes by its being shortened, and by the person being unable to remove it without great pain. But the most certain way to ascertain it, is to grasp the limb above and below the spot supposed to be fractured, and by moving it gently different ways, you hear a grating noise occasioned by the broken ends of the bone rubbing against each other. Very often, however before you can arrive to render assistance, the limb becomes swollen. In such a case always reduce first the swelling, as by twisting the limb or other experiment, it will give the most excruciating pain to the afflicted person.

DISLOCATION, or in other words, bones being out of joint, are easily perceived by the deformity of the joint which you can compare with its fellow, and plainly observe the difference, and from the person being in great pain and unable to move the limb; and by its being longer or shorter than common, and from the impossibility of moving it in any direction, without great misery.

CONTUSION OR BLOW.

If slight, you must bathe the part frequently with cold applications, such as vinegar and water, ice water, or cold spring water; this will reduce or keep down inflammation or fever; this must be occasionally used for five or eight hours; but if fever should come on, then bleed and purge well with salts, and diet the person on the lightest food and cooling drinks. If the fevers should still continue, you must repeat the bleeding and purging; perhaps a good active dose of calomel followed by a dose of salts, in this event would cut short the fever. Be particular as to the patient passing his water, as it frequently happens from a blow, that the nerves of the bladder becomes palsied, and the patient feels no desire to make water, although the bladder is full. In this case it is highly important to attend to drawing off the water by a catheter, an instrument for this purpose, for directions how it is used, [see under the head directions for passing the catheter.]

The most serious effects, however, resulting from coutusion, is when the blow is on the head, producing either concussion or compression of the brain. [See those heads.]

SPRAINS.

Sprains are to be treated with the coldest applications: and for this purpose Nature's remedy is by far the best: *cold water*. Plunge the sprained part into cold water, and hold it there as long as you can bear it; after which, dry it with a coarse towel, and rub on it spirits of camphor: by which I mean, spirits that camphor has been dissolved in, rub this well in and bind it with flannel, and every morning and evening, pour cold water on it from the spout of a tea-kettle, held up at a considerable height. This simple remedy will relieve you in a short time, and to a weak joint of any kind, this is an invaluable prescription. I have removed the weakness of an ancle of long standing, by it, when all other applications failed.

CONCUSSION OF THE BRAIN.

Symptoms.—The person is stunned—the breathing is slow—great drowsiness and stupidity—the pupil of the eye rather contracted, or drawn up—frequent vomiting, or puking. After a time he recovers.

REMEDIES.

Apply cloths dipped in cold vinegar and water, to the head; and if you have ice its application will be greatly beneficial. So soon as the stupor is off, bleed and open the bowels with epsom salts, or any cooling purge; by all means, confine him to the bed, and the lowest and most cooling diet and drinks—the room kept dark but cool, and no noise whatever. In this quiet situation you are to endeavor to prevent inflammation of the brain, which, if it comes on must be met by *free* and *copious* bleeding, blisters and purging.

COMPRESSION OF THE BRAIN.

Symptoms—Loss of sense and motion.—slow, noisy, and difficult breathing—the pulse is quite slow and irregular—the muscles relaxed, as in a person just dead—the pupil of the eye enlarged, and will not contract, even for a strong light—the person cannot be roused, and bears a resemblance to one afflicted with an apoplectic fit.

REMEDIES.

Bleed freely, and shave the head, and apply cold applications to it until you can procure a good surgeon, and *this must be done immediately* or it will be too late, as there is nothing but an operation in this case that will save life.

WOUNDS.

Wounds are of three kinds: first incised wounds, which means a clean cut—secondly, a punctured wound, which means a wound produced by sharp pointed instruments, as needles, awls, nails, &c.—contused wounds, which means wounds accasioned by round or blunt bodies, as musket balls, club, stones, and all gun-shot wounds, are included in this last mentioned term.

REMEDIES.

In all wounds, the first thing to be done, is to endeavor to stop the flow of blood; should this be but trifling, draw the edges of the wound together with your hand, and hold them in that position some time, when the blood will frequently stop. If it still continue, and the quantity large, or of a bright red color, flowing in spirits, or with a sudden jerk, then clap your finger on the spot it springs from, and press it with firmness while you request some other person to pass a handkerchief round the limb, (supposing the wound to be in one,) above the cut, and to tie its two ends together in a hard knot. A stick of any kind, must now be passed under the knot, (between the upper surface of the limb and the handkerchief,) and turned round and round until the stick is brought down to the thigh, so as to make the handkerchief encircle it with considerable tightness; you may then take off your finger; if the blood still flows, tighten the handkerchief by a turn or two of the stick, until the blood ceases. The patient may now be removed (taking great care to seenre the stick in its position) without running any risk of bleeding to death by the way. As this apparatus must not be left on for any length of time without destroying the life of the parts, endeavor as quick as you conveniently can, to secure the bleeding vessels; for I shall give you such ample and plain directions, that any person of common sense may take them up and secure them in a proper manner, and perfectly safe. In the first place, wax together three or four threads of a sufficient length, cut it into as many pieces as you think there are vessels to be taken up each piece, being about a foot long. Now wash the part with warm water, and then with a sharp hook, similar to a crooked awl, or a slender pair of pincers in your hand, fix your eye steadfastly upon the wound, and direct the handkerchief to be gently loosed by a turn or two of the sick; you will now see the mouth of the artery, from which the blood springs; seize it with your hook or pincers, draw it a little out while the person who assists you, passes the wax thread) called by medical men, a ligature) round the artery or bleeding vessel; now tie it up tight with a double knot. In this way, take up one after the other, each bleeding vessel you can see or get hold of.

Should the wound be too high up in a limb to apply the handkerchief don't be alarmed, for the bleeding can still be commanded. If it is the thigh, press firmly in the groin, or if in the arm, with the hand-end or ring of a common door key, make pressure above the collar bone, and about its middle, against the first rib which lies under it. The pressure is to be continued until you can obtain assistance, and then tie up the bleeding vessels as before directed. If the wound is on the head, you must press your finger firmly on it until a compress (which means several folds of linen) is furnished; this is to be bound firmly over the artery by a bandage. If the wound is in the face; or so situated that pressure cannont be effectually made, or you cannot get hold of the vessel, and the blood flows fast, put a piece of ice; or a cloth wet with tanner's ooze, or flour, and let it remain on until the blood coagulates, you can then remove it and apply a compress or bandage. It is important that this simple method I have described should be practiced so as to enable any one to compress the great arteries in these situations, thereby preserving many a man who would for the want of this simple assistance, bleed to death before a surgeon or medical aid could be procured.

INCISED WOUND.

The meaning of an incised wound, is a clean or fresh cut. Wash away all the dirt that may be in the wound with a sponge or linen rag and warm water: when the blood is stopped, draw the sides of the wound nicely together, then confine it in this situation by narrow strips of sticking plaster, placed at short distances apart, and directly across the wound. Now a fold (or soft compress of cold linen or lint,) is to be laid over and confined by a bandage.

In many cases you will find inflammation follow. If this should be the case, then remove the strips, and bleed and purge the patient, and keep him on very low diet, and as quiet and cool as possible: in other more plain language, endeavor to keep down fever—and now recollect, that matter must form before the wound can heal; therefore it is best to encourage it by applying a soft poultice of any kind, until the matter is produced; after which you may use any simple ointment in its place. The usual or common method of narrow strips of linen, spread with sticking plaster, called by physicians adhesive plaster, form the best means of keeping the sides of the wound together when they can be applied; yet if the wound is in the ear, nose, tongue, lips, bag, by which I mean the privates, or the eyelids, then use stichos, which are made in the following manner: thread a common needle with a double waxed thread, pass the point of it through the skin at a little distance from the edge of the cut, and bring it out of the opposite one to the same distance. Should the wound be so large, as to require more than one stich, cut off the needle, thread it again, and proceed on to make as many stiches as necessary; leave all the threads loose until all the stiches are passed, when the ends of each tread must be tied in a hard double knot, drawing the thread in such away that it bears a little on the side of the cut. When the edges of the wound are partly united by inflammation, cut then the knots, and draw out carefully all the threads. From the plain manner in which I have written and explained to you, you will easily perceive, that in all wounds after stopping the flow of blood and cleansing the parts, the important point is to bring the sides of the wound even, and together, so that it may grow together as quick as possible, without producing any matter: this is called by physicians, healing by the first intention. Now to produce this desirable effeet, in addition to what I have already mentioned, you must recollect two things necessary to be attended to; first, the position of the patient; and secondly, the application to the bandage. Let the position be such as will relax as much as possible, the skin and muscles of the part wounded; by attending to this strictly, you will prevent, or in a great measure lessen the tendency to separate or open. My method in such cases, is as follows: take a common bandage of proper width and length, and pass it over the compress moderately tight, so as to keep them in their proper place, and by its pressure, the wound will heal immediately and keep it from separating or opening. In many cases; the wound is so large and so severely painful that the limb or body of the patient cannot be raised or moved, for the purpose of removing or applying it: then spread the ends of one or two strips of linen or leather with sticking plaster, which may be applied in place of the bandage, in the following way: stick one end of the strip to the sound skin, at a short distance from the edge of the compress, over which it is to be drawn with moderate firmness, and secured in the same manner on the opposite side; if you see that it is necessary to secure it more fully apply a second or third, or until properly secured. As I have before told you, if violent inflammation come on, in all wounds, the proper practice is to reduce it by bleeding, purging, &c. but if you see any symptoms of approaching locked jaw, give your patient wine, brandy, opium, porter, &c. in other words stimulate him freely, and give a generous diet.

PUNCTURED WOUNDS.

These wounds called by physicians punctured wounds, are produced by any sharp pointed instrument, as nails, awls, &c.

TREATMENT.—First stop the bleeding, then with-draw the needle, splinters, glass, or any thing that may be in a wound of this nature, provided it can be done easily; and if enlarging the wound a little will enable you to get any foreign body out, it is best to do so. Though it is not always necessary to enlarge wounds of this nature; yet when the weather is very warm, I advise you not to neglect doing so because it is a precaution against locked-jaw, which occurs frequently in wounds of this description. I recollect a case in 1816, that occurred at Savannah, Georgia, A Miss.—— D. L——, a most amiable and accomplished lady in making preparation for a ball, by accident, stuck a needle slightly in her heel. The puncture being slight, she attended the ball. On the following day, symptoms of locked jaw commenced and the second day notwithstanding the skill afforded her by several eminent professional gentlemen, she died. So soon as you enlarge a wound of this description as directed, pour a little turpentine into the wound, or touch it with caustic, and then cover it with a poultice moistened with laudanum; the object of the poultice is to form matter. When this is done, you must then treat it as a common sore, with mild ointment of any kind. Frequently in such cases, there is a great deal of pain; if so, give laudanum in large doses,—you need not fear giving laudanum in broken doses, until the patient gets ease; for I have often given it as high as two hundred drops, say, thirty at each dose, before partial ease could be afforded. In warm weather, inflammation often occurs, in such a case bleed in moderation, and purge freely—recollect here to use the lancet with care and discretion.

CONTUSED WOUNDS.

Wounds of this description are made by round or blunt bodies, as musket balls, clubs, stones, &c. In such wounds, you may have little to fear of loss of blood, as they are attended generally by little bleeding; if any it must be stopped.

If the wound is produced by a ball and the ball can be felt, or easily got at, it is proper to extract,—it is proper to do so, or any piece of the wad or cloth, or clothing should be withdrawn—for instance, if the ball can be plainly felt immediately under the skin, then make an incision across it and take it out. But remember well, this salutary counsel—never allow any poking in the wound to search for a ball or any articles differently situated from what I have plainly described, for many deaths occur, which if properly managed, or in other words, so much unnecessary science dispensed with, would have been entirely cured. The best extracter in such cases is a soft bread and milk poultice. In fact, by long experience and reflection, I should say that gun-shot wounds, that have formed a lodgment must not be opened either lightly or wantonly; nor under the idea of hunting for extraneous substances; for the parts themselves will bring these to the surface, and such as cannot thus be extracted, give little trouble, nor do they prevent the healing of a wound, It is particularly vain to hunt balls, because they take a wayward course and often take a lodgment where the surgeon or physician would be the least inclined to look for them. Even if the ball can be felt, and yet the skin is sound, some eminent surgeons think it will not be prudent to extract it before the original wound is healed. because, where it rests it can do no harm, and it is better to have only one wound at a time than two. When a ball has wounded a cavity, as for example, the abdomen, which means the belly; if the ball has passed with little velocity, the parts will heal by the first intention. [You will recollect I explained plainly, to you the meaning of healing by the first intention.] If, however, it has passed with such velocity or quickness, as to produce a slough, meaning an inward huse, the *adhesive inflammation* will take place on the peritonæum, meaning the skin which lines the belly, and covers the abdominal viscera, in other words, the bowels, and the organs in the belly and chest. The adhesive inflammation, as remarked will take place on this peritonæum all around the wound, which will prevent the general cavity from taking part in the inflammation, although the ball shall have not only penetrated, but wounded, those parts not immediately essential to life, in its passage through the body; for whatever solid viscus has been pierced, the surfaces in contact surrounding every orifice, will unite by the adhesive inflammation, so as to form one continued canal, with which the general cavity has no communication. If any extraneous or outward body has been carried in by the ball, it will be included in these adhesions, and with the *slough*, will be conducted by one of the orifices to the outward surface.

If the ball has wounded the liver or the surface, these may soon acquire the healing disposition; if the stomach, intestines, kidneys, ureters, or bladder, such injuries are generally mortal; for their contents escape into the cavity of the abdomen or belly, and universal inflammation of the peritonæum takes place, attended by great pain and tension or swelling, which terminates in death. But if the wound is small and the bowels are not full, adhesions may take place all round the wound, which will confine the matter, and make it go on in its right channel. When the ball has not penetrated any of the viscera of the abdomen, but only by contusion produced death in a part, whenever the slough comes away, the matter contained in that viscus will escape, but as the adhesive inflammation takes place between the surface in contact, the new channel will be preserved entire, and cut off the communication between the external air and the cavity of the abdomen. This channel may however, in time be closed, and the contents may pass by their accustomed course. A young gentleman was shot through the body, the balls three in number, entered on the left side of the navel, and came out behind, just above the superior vertebræ of the loins. The first water he made was bloody—in less than a fortnight, John Hunter, the most eminent Surgeon of London, pronounced him out of danger, being persuaded, that whatever cavities the balls had entered, were united by the adhesive inflammation, so as to form one complete canal, and that neither, the extraneous matters carried in with the balls, nor any slough, which might separate from the sides of the canal, nor matter formed in it, could get into the cavity of the abdomen, but must be conducted to the external surface of the body, either through the wounds or from an abscess forming for itself, which would work its own exite somewhere. Soon after this conclusion, some Fæces, (meaning that which should pass from the fundament,) coming through the wound, confirmed him in his opinion respecting the efforts of nature; which are great on such occasions to secure the cavity of the abdomen; yet he feared this wound might in future perform the functions of the fundament. He saw clearly, that an intestine had received a bruise sufficient to kill the part, and that till a separation of the slough had taken place, both the intestines and the canal were still complete, and therefore did not communicate with each other; but that when the slough was thrown off; the two were laid into one at this part, and that therefore, the contents of the intestines got into this wound. This symptom, however, gradually decreased by the contraction of this opening, till an entire stop to the passage of the fæces by it took place, and the wounds were healed, and the gentleman entirely restored to health.

Having fully described to you the effects of gun shot wounds, and their general effects, I shall conclude by directing you in such cases, should the inflammation be great, bleed and purge.—If your patient labors under great pain, give laudanum, and if the parts assume a dark look, threatening a mortification, cover them with a blister. Where the wound is much torn, wash the parts very nicely with warm water, and then, (having secured every bleeding vessel,) lay them all down in as natural a position as possible, drawing their edges gently together, or as much so as possible, by strips of sticking plaster, or stiches, if necessary. Now apply a soft bread and milk poultice over the whole.

WOUNDS OF THE EAR, NOSE, &c.

Treatment.—Wash the parts well, so as to cleanse them from all dirt, &c. and then draw the edges of the wound together by as many stiches as are necessary. If the part is even completely separated, and has been trodden under foot, by washing it in warm water, and placing it even, and accurately, in its proper place, by the same means it may still adhere or grow on.

WOUNDS OF THE SCALP.

Treatment.—In wounds of the scalp, it is necessary to shave off the hair.—After this operation is performed, wash the parts well, and draw the edges of the wound together with a sticking plaster. If it has been torn up in several places, wash and lay them all down on the skull again, drawing their edges together as nearly as possible, by a sticking plaster, or if necessary, by stiches. Then cover the whole with a soft fold or bandage smeared with some simple ointment of any kind.

WOUNDS OF THE THROAT.

Treatment.—Seize and tie up every bleeding vessel you can get hold of.—If the wind pipe is cut only partly through, secure it with sticking plaster. If it is completely divided, bring its edges together by stiches, taking care to pass the needle through the loose membrane that covers the wind pipe, and not through the wind pipe itself. The head should be bent on the breast during this operation, and secured by boulsters and bandages in that position, to favor the approximation of the wound.

WOUNDS OF THE CHEST.

Treatment.—If the wound in the chest is a simple incised wound, draw the edges of it together by sticking plaster, cover it by a fold or compress of linen, and pass a bandage round the chest. The patient is to be confined to his bed, kept on very low diet, and bled and purged, in order to prevent inflammation. If, however, inflammation should come on, you must reduce it by copious and frequent bleeding. Should this wound be occasioned by a bullet, extract it, and any pieces of cloth, &c that may be lodged in it, if possible, and cover the wound with a piece of linen smeard with some simple ointment, taking great care that it is not drawn into the chest. If a portion of the lung protrudes or projects out, return it to its proper place immediately, but be as gentle and cautious as possible.

WOUNDS OF THE BELLY.

In wounds of the belly, close it by strips of sticking plaster, and stiches passed through the skin, about half an inch from the edge of the wound, and cover the whole with a soft compress of linen, secured by a bandage.—Any inflammation that may arise is to be reduced by bleeding, purging, and a blister over the whole belly. Should any part of the bowels come out at the wound, if clean and uninjured, return it as quickly as possible; if covered with dirt, clots of blood &c., wash it in warm water previous to returning it. If the gut is wounded, and only cut partly through, draw the two edges of it together by a stich, and return it; if completely divided, you must connect the edges by four stiches of equal distances, and replace it in the belly; always leaving the end of the ligature or thread projected from the external wound, which must be closed by sticking plaster. In five or six days, if the threads are loose, withdraw them very gently, and carefully.

WOUNDS OF THE JOINTS.

In wounds of this description, you are to bring the edges of the wound together by sticking plaster, without any delay;

keep the part perfectly at rest, bleed, purge, and live very low, so as to prevent inflammation. But should it come on, it must be met at the first approach of bleeding to as great an extent as the condition of the patient will warrant, and by plaster covering the whole joint. If the joint seems like it would be a stiff one, keep the limb in that position which will prove most useful; that is, the legs should be extended, and the arm bent at the elbow. Wounds of the jointsare always highly dangerous, and frequently terminate fatally.

WOUNDS OF TENDONS.

Tendons or *sinews* are frequently wounded and ruptured. They are to be treated precisely like any other wound, by keeping their divided parts together. The tendon which connects the great muscle forming the calf of the leg with the heel, called the tendon of *Achilles*, is frequently cut with the adze, and ruptured in jumping from heights. This accident is to be remedied by drawing up the heel, extending the foot and placing a splint on the fore part of the leg, extending from the knee to beyond the toes, which being secured in that position by a bandage, keep the foot in that positiou just mentioned. The hollows under the splint must be filled with tow or cotton. If the skin falls into the space between the ends of the tendon, apply a piece of sticking plaster, so as to draw it out of the way. It usually takes five or six weeks to unite, but no weight should be laid on the limb for several months.

OF FRACTURES.

As I have before plainly pointed out to you, how *fractures* may be known, it will be unnecessary for me to dwell on this subject.—It will however, be advisable, for you to recollect this general rule. In cases, where, from the accompanying circumstances, and symptoms, a strong suspicion exists that a bone is fractured, it will be proper for you to act as though it were positively ascertained to be so.

FRACTURES OF THE BONE OF THE NOSE.

Treatment.—From the exposed situation of the bones of the nose, they are frequently forced in. When this is the case, any smooth article that will pass into the nostril should be immediately introduced with one hand, so as to raise the depressed portions to the proper level, while the other is employed in moulding them into the required shape. If violent inflammation follows, bleed, purge, and live on the lowest kind of diet.

FRACTURES OF THE LOWER JAW.

Treatment.—There is no difficulty in discovering this accident by looking into the mouth: and it is to be relieved by keeping the lower jaw firmly pressed against the upper one, by means of a bandage passed under the chin and over the head. If it is broken near the angle, or that part nearest the ear, place a cushion or roll of linen behind it, over which the bandage must pass, so as to make it push that part of the bone forward. The parts are then to be confined in this way for twenty or twenty-five days; during which time all the nourishment that is taken by the patient: should be sucked between the teeth. If in consequence of the blow, a tooth is loosened, do not meddle with it, for if let alone, it will grow fast again.

FRACTURES OF THE COLLAR BONE.

A fracture of the collar bone is of very common occurrence, and is known at once, by passing the finger along it, and by the swelling &c.

Treatment.—To reduce it seat your patient on a chair, with his shirt off, and place a stout compress of linen, made in the shape of a wedge, under his arm; the thick end of which should press against the arm-pit. His arm bent to a right angle at the elbow, is now to be brought down to his side, and secured in that position, by a long bandage, which passes over the arm of the affected side, and round the body. The (fore-arm meaning that which reaches from the elbow to the wrist,) is to be supported across the breast by a sling. It then takes from four to five weeks to re-unite.

FRACTURES OF THE ARM.

Treatment—Seat your patient on a chair on the side of a bed, let some one assist you to hold the sound arm, while another person grasps the wrist of the broken one, and steadily extending it in an opposite direction bending the fore-arm a little to serve as a lever. You must now place the bones in their proper situation. Two splints made of shingle or stout pasteboard, long enough to reach from below the shoulder to near the elbow, must then be well covered with tow or cotton, and laid along each side of the arm, and kept in that position by a bandage. The fore-arm is to be supported in a sling. Two smaller splints may for better security, be laid between the first ones, that is one on top, and the other underneath the arm to be secured by the bandage, in the same way as the others.

FRACTURES OF THE BONES OF THE FORE-ARM.

As I have before, and I again tell you, it is that part which reaches from the elbow to the wrist, that is designated or called the *fore-arm*. When this is fractured, they are to be reduced precisely in the same way, with the exception of the mode of keeping the upper portion of it steady: which is done by grasping the arm above the elbow. When the splints and bandage which I have directed you how to make are applied, support it in a sling.

FRACTURES OF THE WRIST.

Fractures of the wrist very seldom take place. When this accident does happen, the injury is generally so great as to require amputation or taking it off. If it is possible to save the hand, lay it on a splint, well covered with tow or cotton. This is to extend beyond the fingers—place then another splint opposite to it, lined with the same materials, and secure them by a bandage. The hand is then to be carried in a sling. The bones of the hand are frequently broken. In such a case fill the palms of the hands with a soft compress or folds of linen, or domestic cloth, or tow or cotton, and then lay a splint on it long enough to extend from the elbow to beyond the ends of the fingers, and then to be secured by a bandage. If the finger is broken extend the end of it until it becomes straight. Place the fracture or broken bone in its place, and apply two small pasteboard splints, one below and the other above, which you must secure by a narrow bandage. The upper splint ought to extend from the end of the finger over the back of the hand. It may sometimes be proper to add two additional splints for the sides of the finger.

FRACTURES OF THE RIBS.

When after a fall or blow, the patient complains of a pricking pain in his side, we may suspect a rib is broken. The way to discover it, is by placing the ends of two or three of your fingers on the spot where the pain is, and desiring the patient to cough, when the grating sensation will be felt. All that is necessary, is to pass a broad bandage round the chest, so tight as to prevent the motion of the ribs in breathing, and to live on a light diet.

FRACTURES OF THE THIGH.

The thigh is perhaps the most difficult fracture to manage; and the inginuity of one amongst the best men who ever lived (Doctor Heartshorn of the city of Philadelphia,) the world is indebted for an apparatus which does away the greatest impediments that have been found to exist in treating it so as to leave a straight limb, without lameness or deformity, nor is it the least of its merits, that any man of common sense can apply it nearly as well as a surgeon or physician.

It consists of two splints, made of half or three-quarter inch well seasoned stuff; from eight to ten inches wide, one of which should reach from a little above the hip, to fifteen or sixteen inches beyond the foot, while the other extends the same length from the groin. The upper end of the inner splint is hollowed out, and well padded or stuffed. Their lower ends are held together by a cross-piece, having two tenons which enter two verticle mortices, one on each splint, and secured there by pins. In the centre of this cross piece (which should be very solid) is a female screw. Immediately above the verticle mortices, are two horizontal ones, of considerable length, in which slide the tenons of the second cross-piece of the upper side of which, is fastened a foot block, shaped like the sole of a shoe, while in the other, is a round hole for the reception of the head of the male screw, which passes through the female one just mentioned. On the top of this cross piece to which the foot block is attached, are two pins which fall into the goovs at the head of the screw; thereby firmly connecting them. The foot block as before observed, is shaped like the sole of a shoe. Near the toe is a slit through which passes a strip and a buckle. Near the heel are a couple of strips with two rings, arranged precisely like those of a skate; of which, infact, the whole foot block is an exact resemblance. A long male screw of wood, or other material, completes the apparatus. To apply it, put a slipper on the foot of the broken limb, and lay the apparatus over the leg. By turning the screw, the foot block will be forced up to the foot by the slipper, which is to be firmly strapped to it, as boys fasten their skates. By turning the screw the contrary way, the padded extremity of the inner splint, presses against the groin, and the foot is gradually drawn down until the broken-limb becomes of its natural length and appearance; when any projection or any quality that remains, can be felt and reduced by a gentle pressure of the hand.

The great advantages of this valuable apparatus I again tell you, are the ease with which it is applied and the certainty with which it acts. The foot once secured to the block, in a way that any man of common sense understands, nothing more is required than to turn the screw until the broken limb is found to be of the same length of the sound one. It is proper to remark that this should not be affected at once, it being better to turn the screw a little every day until the limb is extended. As this apparatus may not always be at hand, it is proper to mention the next best plan of treating the accident. It is found in the splints of Desaults, improved by Dr. Physic of the city of Philadelphia consisting of four pieces. The first has a crutch head, and extends from the arm-pit to six or eight inches beyond the foot. A little below the crutch are two holes; and near the lower end on the inside, there is a block, below which there is also a hole. The second reaches from the groin, the same length with the first, being about three inches wide above and two below. Two pieces of stout pasteboard, as many handkerchiefs or bands of muslin, with some tow and a few pieces of tape, from the catalogue of the apparatus—which is to be applied as follows.

four or five pieces of tape are to be laid across the bed,

at equal distances from each other. Over the upper two is placed one of the short paste-board splints, well covered with tow. Then the patient is to be carefully and very gently placed on his back, so that his thigh may rest on the splints. One of the handkerchiefs, or a strong, soft band, is to be passed between the testicle and thigh of the affected side, and its ends held by some person standing near the head of the bed. The second handkerchief is to be passed around the ancle, crossed on the instep and tied under the sole of the foot. By steadily pulling these two handkerchiefs, the limb is to be extended, while with the hand, the broken bones are replaced in their natural form. Then the long splint is to be placed by the side of the patient, the crutch in the arm pit, (which must be defended by tow or cotton) while the short one is laid along inside of the thigh or leg. The ends of the first handkerchief being passed through the upper holes; are to be drawn tight and secured by a knot, while the ends of the second one pass over the block before mentioned, to be fastened in like manner at the lower one. All that remains is the short paste board splint, which being well covered with tow, is to be laid on top of the thigh. The tapes being tied so as to keep the four splints together, completes the operation. Cotton or tow is to be every where stuffed between the splints and the limb, and a large handful of it placed in the groin, to prevent irritation from the upper or counter extending band. You must be careful while tying the two handkerchiefs, that they are not relaxed, so that if the operation is properly perfomed, the two limbs will be nearly of an equal length.

The superior advantages of heartshorn,s apparatus over this, as well as all others, must be evident to every one acquainted with the difficulty of keeping up that constant extension which is so absolutely necessary to avoid deformity and lameness, and which is so completely effected by the screw. Next to that, however, stands Dr. Physic's, which can be made by any carpenter in a few minutes, and which, if carefully applied, will be found to answer a good purpose. Fractured thighs and legs generally re-unite in from six to eight weeks, depending, however, much on the age of the patient. Old persons frequently require three or four months. You must recollect in such cases a strawbed is the best for your patient, or a mattrass, or any bed that will not yield, so as to keep the limb in its proper position.

FRACTURES OF THE BONES OF THE FOOT.

This accident seldom occurs—the bone of the heel is sometimes, though rarely broken. It is known by a crack at the moment of the accident, a difficulty in standing, by the quick swelling, and by the grating noise on moving the heel. To reduce it, take a long bandage, lay the end of it to the top of the foot, convey it over the toes under the sole of the foot, and then by several turns secure it in that position. The foot being extended as much as possible, carry the bandage along the back of the leg above the knee, where it is to be secured by several turns, and then brought down on the front of the leg, to which it is seeured by circular turns. In this manner the broken pieces will be kept in contact, and in the course of a month or six weeks will be united.

All fractures of the foot, toes, &c. are to be treated like those of the hand and fingers.

OF DISLOCATIONS.

The signs by which a dislocation may be known, have been already explained to you. But remember the sooner the attempt is made to place it in its proper place, the easier it will be done. The strength of one man, properly applied at the moment of the accident, will often succeed in restoring the head of a bone to its place, which in a few days or even hours, would have required the combined efforts of men and pullies. After you have made several trials, with the best apparatus that can be obtained, and you find that you cannot succeed, make the patient stand up having all things in readiness, and bleed him in that position until he faints; the moment this occurs the muscle will relax; and slight force often will be sufficint, when more powerful ones have been used without effect. Also recollect to vary the direction of the extending force. A slight pull in one way, will often affect what has been in vain attempted by great force in another.

DISLOCATION OF THE LOWER JAW.

Dislocation of the lower jaw is produced by blows, or yawning, usually called gaping. It is known by an inability to shut the mouth, and the projection of the chin. To reduce it is quite simple; seat the patient in a chair, with his head supported by the breast of an assistant, who must stand behind him. Your thumb being covered with *leather* (or a glove) is then to be pushed between the jaws, as far back as possible, while with the fingers outside, you grasp the bone, which must be pressed downward, at the same time that the chin is raised. If this is properly done, the bone will be found moving, when the chin is to be pushed backwards; and the thumbs slipped between the jaws and the cheeks. If this is not done they will be bitten by the sudden snap of the teeth as they come together. The jaws should be kept closed by a bandage for a few days and the patient live upon soup.

DISLOCATION OF THE SHOULDER.

This accident is quite common, (and the most so, of all the dislocations mentioned.) You can easily discover it, by the deformity of the joint, and the head of the bone being found in some unnatural position. To reduce it to its proper place, seat your patient in a chair, place one hand on the prominent part of the shoulder blade, just above the spot where the head of the bone should be, while with the other, you grasp the arm above the elbow and then pull it outwards. Sometimes this will not succeed; if so, then lay the patient on the ground, place your heel in his arm pit, and then steadily and forcibly extend the arm by grasping it at the wrist.

DISLOCATION OF THE COLLAR BONE.

The collar bone is seldom dislocated; but should it take place, the treatment is to apply the bandages, &c. as you have been already directed for a fracture of the same part.

DISLOCATION OF THE ELBOW.

If this dislocation has occurred by falling on the hands, which is most common, or holds his arm bent at the elbow, and every endeavor to straighten it gives him great pain, it is dislocated backward. Seat the patient in a chair, let some one grasp the arm near the shoulder, and another the wrist, and forcibly extend it, while you interlock the fingers of both hands just above the elbow, and pull it backwards, remembering that under those circumstances, whatever degree of force is required, should be applied in this direction. The elbow is sometimes dislocated sideways, or latterally. To reduce it, make extensions by pulling at the wrist, while some one secures the arm above; then push the bone into its place, either inward or outward, as may be required. After the reduction of a dislocated elbow, keep the joint at a perfect rest for five or six days, and then move it gently. If inflammation should come on, treat it as I have before told you in all inflammations—bleed freely, purge, &c.

DISLOCATION OF THE WRIST, FINGERS &c.

Dislocations of this nature are common, and easily known, by the least examination; they are all to be reduced by forcibly extending the lower extremity of the part, and pushing the bones into their place. If necessary, small bands may be secured to the fingers by a narrow bandage, to assist the extension. These accidents should be attended to without delay; for if they are neglected for a little time, they become irremediable or incurable.

DISLOCATION OF THE THIGH.

Notwithstanding the hip joint is the strongest one in the whole body, it is sometimes dislocated. The method of ascertaining this accident is by a careful examination of the part. Comparing the length and appearance of the limb with its fellow, &c. sufficiently mark the nature of the accident. I will proceed to state the remedy.

Place the patient on his back, upon a table covered with a blanket. Two sheets, folded like cravats, are then to be passed between the thigh and the testicle, of each side; and their ends (one half of each sheet passing obliquely over the belly to the opposite shoulder, while the other half pass under the back in the same direction;) given to several assistants, or what is much better, tied very firmly to a hook, staple, post or some immoveable body. A large and very strong towel, folded as before mentioned, like a cravat, is now to be laid along the top of the thigh, so that its middle will be just above the knee, where it is to be well secured by many turns of a bandage. The two ends are then to be knotted. If you have no pullies, a twisted sheet or rope may be passed through the loop formed by the towels. If you can obtain the former, it is better. Cast the loop over the hook of the lower block, and secure the upper one to the wall, directly opposite to the hooks or men that hold the sheets which pass between the thighs. A steadily increasing and forcible extension of the thigh, is then to be made by the men who are stationed at the pullies or sheet, while you are turning and twisting the limb to assist in dislodging it from its unnatural situation. By these means properly applied, the head of the bone will frequently slip into the socket with considerable noise.

Should you be unable to succeed, change the direction of the extended force, recollecting always, that it is not by sudden and violent jerks that it can be put in place, but by a steady, increasing and continued pull. Should all your efforts prove unavailing, (I would not advise you to loose much time before you resort to it;) make your patient, as before directed, submit in such cases to loss of blood, by which means in those difficult cases you are to succeed.

DISLOCATION OF THE KNEE PAN.

If this small bone is dislocated, you will perceive it at once by the slightest glance. Now to reduce it; lay your patient on his back, straighten the leg, lift it up to a right angle with his body, and in that position push the bone back to its proper place. Then keep the knee at perfect rest on a pillow for a few days.

DISLOCATION OF THE LEG.

Accidents of this kind cannot happen without tearing and lacerating the soft parts, but little force is required to place the bones in their proper situation. Should the parts be so much torn that the bones slide again out of place, you had better apply Heartshorn's or Desault's apparatus, which I fully described to you for fractured thigh.

DISLOCATION OF THE FOOT.

Dislocation of the foot seldom takes place. It however may occur; therefore I will give you the treatment. Let one secure the leg, and another draw the foot, while you push the bone in the contrary way to that in which it was forced out. Then you are to cover it with folds of linen dip-ed in water in which sugar of lead has been dissolved, and apply a splint on each side of the leg, so that it reaches be-low the foot. An accident of this nature is highly danger-ous, requiring the immediate assistance of a skilful physi-cian; as, (even then,) all that can be done to remedy them is in the speedy, reduction of the bone, keeping the parts on a pillow at rest, and subduing inflammation by bleeding, low diet, and all such directions as already given to subdue fever.

OF COMPOUND ACCIDENTS.

I have fully, and as plainly as I could, before told you how to treat accidents of this kind, and what plan you are to pursue when single; it now remains for me to state to you what are to be done when they are united.

For instance. an accident happens by which a man is thrown from a height. On examination, a wound is found in his thigh—is bleeding profusely; his ancle on examina-tion is out of joint; with a wound communicating with a cav-ity, and his leg broken. In the first place stop the bleeding from the wound, then reduce the dislocation next, then draw the edges of the wound together with sticking plaster, and lastly apply to the fracture Heartshorn's or Desault's appa-ratus, which I have so fully explained before, that any car-penter can construct it for you.

OF AMPUTATION.

This means the cutting off a limb, or other part of the body. How often do those accidents happen where there is no physician or regular surgical instruments (often at sea,) at a distance in the country, and the limb requiring immediate amputation, or cutting off. The only difficulty which I confess to you, is to know when the operation *ought to be performed;* for it is sometimes the case, that the most skilful surgeon is mistaken, or at a stand whether he shall operate or not. I do know several cases that have been preserved by the obstinacy of the patient, refused to have the operation performed. But this was running a great hazard of life, and should be in all such cases, ventured upon with due caution: and the operation ought not to be performed unless under the most *careful and sound judgment.* Now to perform this operation, require nothing but firmness and common dexteriy, for any man, and that too to perform it well. Although as I have told you, there are many doubts whether an amputation should take place or not, yet in others, all difficulty vanishes; as for instance when a ball has carried away an arm; or during a storm, a tree happens to fall and mash the knee, the leg or ancle, so that those parts are greatly lacerated or torn, and the blood vessels are severely lacerated, also nerves and tendons; or the crushing or splintering of the bones almost necessarily resulting from such accidents, render immediate amputation an unavoidable and imperious duty. Now you will ask, what shall I do for instruments to perform this operation? If it is difficult to obtain surgical instruments, which is often the case in this country, or at sea. It is of no consequence. The instruments for this purpose, are few and easily obtained, which, in all cases, will answer as valuable a substitute. First, get a large carving knife, with a straight handle—have the knife as sharp and smooth as possible—a pen knife—a carpenter's tenon, or mitre saw—a slip of leather or linen, three inches wide, and twenty inches long, slit up the middle to half of its length, a dozen or more of ligatures, each about a foot long, made of waxed thread or fine twine—a hook with a sharp point, (or a shoemaker's crooked awl will answer,) a pair of slender pincers, several narrow strips of sticking plaster, called by physicians or surgeons, adhesive plaster, or adhesive strip, some dry lint, a piece of old linen, large enough to cover the end of the stump, spread with simple ointment or lard, a bandage three or four yards long, about the width of your hand, a piece of sponge, and some warm water. You are now prepared fully to perform amputation; which I will so plainly explain that any man, unless he is an idiot or absolute fool, can perform this operation.

AMPUTATION OF THE ARM.

HOW TO PERFORM THE OPERATION.

Give the patient, about half an hour before you intend operating, sixty drops of laudanum; now having all things in readiness, seat him on a narrow and firm table or chest, of a convenient height, he is now to be supported by an assistant, clasping him round the body. If the handkerchief and stick have not been previously applied, place it as high upon the arm as possible, (the stick being very short.) and so that the knot may pass in the inner side of it. Your instruments having been placed regularly on a table, and within reach of your hand, while some one supports the lower end of the arm, and at the same time draws down the skin, take the large knife and make one straight cut all round the limb through the skin and fat only; then with a penknife separate as much of the skin from the flesh above the cut, and all round it, as will form a flap to cover the face or end of the stump; when you think there is enough separated, turn it back, where it must be held by an assistant, while with a large knife you make a second straight incision round the arm and down the bone, as close as you can to the doubled edge of the flap, but taking great care not to cut it. The bone is now to be passed through the slit in the piece of linen befor mentioned, and pressed by its edges against the upper surface of the wound by the person who holds the flap;

while you saw through the bone as near it as you can. With a hook or pincers you then seize and tie up every vessel that bleeds, the largest the first, and the smaller ones next, until they are all secured. When this is done relax the skin a little—if any artery spirts blood, tie it as before directed.

The wound is now to be gently and very carefully cleansed with a sponge and warm water, and the stick to be relaxed. If it is evident that the arteries are all tied, bring the flap over the end of the stump, draw then the edges together with strips of sticking plaster, leaving the ligatures hanging out at the angles. Lay the piece of linen, spread with simple ointment or hog's lard, over the straps, and a fold or pledget of lint over that, and secure the whole by the bandage. Then put your patient to bed & rest the stump on a pillow. The handkerchief and stick are to be left loosely round the limb so that if any bleeding happens to come on it may be tightened at once hy the person who watches by, the patient. If this accident takes place, by which I mean the bleeding, the dressings are to be taken off, the flap raised, and the bleeding vessel sought for and tied up; after which, every thing is to be placed as before. I have mentioned a handkerchief and a stick; these are substitutes for the instrument used by surgeons, called a turniquet. Remember, in sawing through a bone, a long and free stroke should be used to prevent any hitching; as an additional security against which, the teeth of the saw should be well sharpened and set wide.

It is of the greatest importance to attend to this circumstance. The ends of the divided arteries cannot at the time of operation be got hold of; or being in a diseased state, their coats give way under the hook; so that it is impossible to draw them out, and not unfrequently they are found ossified, which means turned into bone. In all such cases, having threaded a needle with a ligature well waxed, pass it through the flesh round the artery, so that when tied, there will be a portion of it included in the ligature along with the artery The needle used by surgeons for this purpose is a curved or crooked one: but a straight one will answer. When the ligature has been made to encircle the artery, cut off the needle and tie it firmly in the ordinary way.

The dressings should not be removed for several days, say from five to seven, if the weather is cool; but if warm weather, it should be removed in three days. But this you must do with great care after soaking it well with warm water, so that you can take it away without its sticking to the stump, bleeding or otherwise producing pain. Then apply a clean plaster of lint, over which put a bandage as before directed;—which dressing is to be removed and a fresh one applied every two days. In about fourteen or sixteen days the ligatures will generally come away; and in from three to five weeks, (if all goes on as might be expected, without any accident) the wound is well.

AMPUTATION OF THE THIGH.

Amputation of the *thigh* is to be performed in the same manner as that of the arm, with one exception; it being proper to put a piece of lint between the edges of the flap, to prevent them from uniting until the surface of the stump has adhered to it

---

AMPUTATION OF THE LEG.

There are two bones in the leg, which have a thin muscle between them. In such a case, you must have an additional knife to those I have before mentioned, to divide it. The knife required for this purpose must have a long narrow blade, with a double cutting edge, and a sharp point, You can grind down a carving or case knife to answer every purpose, the blade however, must be reduced to less than half an inch in width.

The linen or leather strips should also have two slits in it instead of one. Having all your preparations in order near you, your patient is to be laid on his back, on a table covered with a blanket, or on a hard bed, with as many persons as may be necessary to hold him. The handkerchief and stick are then to be applied on the upper part of the thigh. One person holds the knee, and another the thigh and leg as firmly as possible, while with the large knife the operator makes an oblique incision round the limb, through the skin, and beginning at five or six inches below the knee pan, and carrying it regularly round in such a manner that the cut will be lower down on the calf than in the front of the leg. As much of the skin is then to be separated by the pen-knife as will cover the stump. (It is here important for you to take the principal part of the flap from the hinder part of the leg, for the cut being made as directed, it should require only one inch of skin to be raised in front, and of course you must take enough from behind to meet it.) When this is turned back, a second cut must be made all round the limb and down to the bones; when with the narrow bladed knife before mentioned, the flesh between them is to be divided. The middle piece of the leather strip is now to be pulled through between the bones, the whole being held back by an assistant who supports the flap while the bones are sawed, which should be so managed that the smaller one is cut through by the time the other is only half off. The arteries are then to be taken up, the flap brought down, and secured by adhesive plaster with bandages as I have before plainly explained to you.

AMPUTATION OF THE FORE-ARM

The fore-arm has two bones in it; therefore you require in this operation the narrow bladed knife, and the strip of linen with three tails. Let the incision be made, straight round the part, as in the arm; with this exception complete it as I gave you directions in the case before this.

AMPUTATION OF THE FINGERS AND TOES.

When amputations of this kind are made, you must draw the skin back and make an incision round the finger; a little below the joint it is intended to remove; turn back a little flap to cover the stump, then cut down to the joint, bending it so that you can cut through the ligament that connect the two bones—the under one first, then that on the side.

The head of the bone is to be turned out, while you cut through the remaining soft parts. Should you see an artery spirt out the blood, immediately tie it up; if not, bring down the flap, and secure it by a strip of sticking plaster. And then put a narrow bandage over the whole.

CONCLUDING REMARKS ON AMPUTATION.

It often happens in cases of amputation, that the wound is apt to bleed, after you have dressed it—thereby giving you considerable trouble.] This is called by surgeons secondary bleeding.] Therefore, to prevent this, if necessary, before the strips of plaster are applied to the edges of the flap, give a little wine and water, or a little spirit and water, and wait a few minutes to see whether the increased force it gives to the circulation, will occasion a flow of blood, if it does, secure the vessel it comes from. But should there be a considerable flow of blood from the hollow of the bone, make use of a small plug of cedar; and if violent spasm of the stump take place, hold it carefully by your assistants; and immediately administer large doses of laudanum, it may be understood as a general rule, that after every operation of the kind, laudanum ought and must be given according to the sufferings of the patient.

MORTIFICATION.

In the general treatment of wounds and in *surgery;* remember always to stop excessive inflammation; which if allowed to go to a certain point, frequently produce mortification, or the death of the parts. Therefore always be on your guard against fever—which you may easily know, by heat, pain, redness and swelling. Now I again repeat that you must bleed and purge as much as you think your patient may be able to bear, from his situation, constitution, &c. &c. These matters are to be entirely regulated by the appearances at the same time. If the fever and pain should suddenly cease, and the part which before was red, swollen and hard, becomes of a purple color and is soft, *you are to stop at once all reducing measures*, put a large blister over the parts, and give good wine, porter, barks, and wine or quinine, or other generous stimulants so sa to support the *sinking* condition of the patient, for mortification has or is about to commence; and should you find the blisters should fail to put a stop to the disease, and the parts look dead and become offensive, cover them with charcoal or firmenting poultices, until nature separates the dead parts from the living; during which time give a free generous and strengthening diet and good wine.

In mortification of the fore arm, it frequently becomes necessary to *amputate*. This ought never to be done until after blisters have been fairlv tried to the sound parts, (*above the mortified;*) as they often separate, you should be careful to examine strictly the parts, so as to discover in time, that which may be necessary.

DIRECTIONS FOR CATHETER.

A catheter is an instrument made use of for drawing the water from the bladder. There are two kinds the male and the female. The difference between them is very little; the male has but one hole in the end that enters the bladder; the female has several; this is the only difference in the instruments. By this simple operation which every person of common sense can perform, the lives of thousands have been preserved—and this is one among the reasons I could advance for having explained the outward parts of female generation so plainly. Now many fools say that I ought to have let out an explanation of *these parts.* And why do they do so? Because they do not read the book so as to see the necessity of writing so plain. Are we ashamed of the parts which the diseases of our nature require to be explained, so as to obtain relief in case of diseases? I am writing a book not for the learned but for the unlearned; not for amusement, but to explain, in plain language, the diseases to which we are subjected, and the method to obtain relief from pain and sickness. With these remarks I shall prescribe the method of using the *Catheter*.

Holding the private member near its head, between the finger and thumb of the left hand; (standing at his side,) now with your right hand introduce the point of the instrument into the passage (out of which flows the urine:) the convex side of the catheter towards the patient's knees; and then gently, by no means using force, push the instrument down the urethra, at the same time endeavor to draw the penis on it. When you first introduce the catheter, the handle will of course be near the belly of the patient; and as it goes down the canal it will be thrown farther from it, until it enters the bladder which you will know by the water immediately flowing through the tube into the basin or pot. It sometimes occurs that you cannot succeed while the patient is on his back; if this is the case, make him stand up, or you may place him with his shoulders and back on the ground, while his thighs and legs are held up by assistants. In difficult cases I have been compelled to place the patient on his back, and when the catheter was as far drawn as it would go, I introduced the forefinger well oiled, into the fundament, and endeavored to push the point upwards while still pressing forwards with the other hand by which means I have often succeeded, when all other methods failed. You must recollect, *force* is never, on any account to be used. Vary the position of the instrument as often as you think proper, even permit the patient himself to try, but by all means use no force or violence; but humor the instrument, take your time and be cautious, and you will at least succeed. I will state to you a case. During my practice in Virginia, Botetour County, near the town of Salem, Mr. T., a young man in the prime of life, was engaged in raising a large barne, when a part of the building gave away, and he was dreadfully mashed, with a fall of thirty feet. I was immediately called into his case; it was such as to leave *but little if any hopes of his recovery*. One of the logs having fallen across his privates, placed him in such a situation as to be entirely helpless. In this critical, and I may add wretched situation, he continued five days without passing a drop of water. I had made daily unsuccessful efforts to introduce the catheter, but without success, his fever and thirst very great. I had bled him very copiously every day, and endeavored by all means to reduce inflammation. His misery was excruciating from being unable to pass his water. All my efforts to pass the instrument, from the bruised state of the parts were unsuccessful.—I then determined previous to an operation to make the last trial; when I introduced my finger as before described, into the rectum. Feeling distinctly the point of the instrument, I passed it gently into the neck of the bladder, when immediately the water flowed. So great and instantaneous was the relief afforded him, that he exclaimed, "I thank thee merciful God!". By this operation upwards of a gallon of water was drawn off. From this time his recovery gradually commenced. The instrument which I learned him to introduce, is continued, I am informed until this time, being unable to pass his water without it. He is still living in Virginia, but poor fellow, entirely deprived of the use of his lower extremities. I will now relate to you a second case—with which I shall close my remarks on the subject of this small, but valuable instrument. Two years since, I was called upon at night to visit a young lady of the most respectable family residing about ten miles from Knoxville, said by the messenger to be dying. On my arrival, I found her in great misery. She desired the room might be cleared of all save her sister, when she with the greatest delicacy declared her misery was from being unable to pass her water. In this horrible situation she had been for four days; during which time, the whole catalogue, of teas had been prescribed from water melon tea to the full extent of twenty different kinds. All had been poured down the throat of this poor innocent girl, until she declared she had rather die, than drink another draught. On examination I found I had forgotten my catheter, but as I have often done before, made a temporary instrument. I took a common goose quill, cut it off at both ends, made one of the ends perfectly smooth, passed it into the small hole which I have so plainly described in the outward parts of the female generation, and in less than five minutes this amiable and innocent girl was entirely relieved, by an operation which any old woman might have performed—saving me of a very disagreeable ride of a very cold night, and the family an expense of ten dollars.—This lady is now married, and the mother of a fine family. I have often since laughed with, about the quality and quantity of the teas administered. I have mentioned this last case to show you the actual importance and indeed the necessity of explaining these parts, which otherwise I should have veiled in different language or omitted them altogether.

DIRECTIONS FOR PASSING BOUGIES.

Bougies are made of gum elastic, about the size of a goose quill and varying in proportion to suit the urethra. They intended for removing strictures in the canal or urethra. To introduce them, take the private member between your finger and thumb, and pass the point of the instrument (after being well oiled) down the urethra as I have directed you for the catheter; when it has entered three or four inches, depress the member a little and by humoring the bougie with one hand, and the penis or member with the other, endeavor *without force* to pass it as far as may be wished. I have frequently seen the patient succeed, when every one else failed. In removing strictures, it is best to pass the *Bougie* once a day, and let it remain in from ten to fifteen minutes, so as to gradually distend the parts. When strictures are so difficult as to require an armed Bougie, which means the point that enters the urethra pointed with caustic for the purpose of removing it by burning. In such difficult cases it would be prudent to apply to a physician.

CONSUMPTION.

Remarks of Dr. Cooper upon Chronic Bronchitis taken from the New York commercial advertiser. The late lamented death of Dr. Rush from that form of consumption, known as Chronic Bronchitis, painfully reminds me, of a duty, the subscriber owes to his profession, and to society, of making known a simple form of treatment, that has never failed him in curing this form of consumption, so destructive to the Clerical and literary professions, the mode of treatment is of equal efficacy, in Carbal Phthisic, and is a valuable remedy for consumption in all its forms.—When in its chronic stages, and free from inflammatory symptoms.

This treatment is based on the pathology of consumption, as the generic name for disease. Sulphate of copper combined with gum amoniac given so as to nauseate, but not toproduce full vomiting. The usual dose for this purpose is half agrain of the sulphate and five grains of gum amoniac taken in a tea-spoonful of water. At first, twice a day, and in the convolescing state once a day.

A gargle of the sulphate is superceded when the case is properly chronic.—This alone is an abridgment of Dr. Cooper's Remarks on Consumption.

RECIPIE.

The celebrated Dr. Freelin's Recipie, with which he is said to have cured many desperate cases of consumption.

1 Quart French brandy or old rye whiskey.

1 Pint Honey.

1 Half pint new tar.

1 Pint spring water, boiled down to one quart,—a wine glass full taken every morning.

Sulphate of copper is verdigris.

DROPSY.

Take a ten gallon pot fill it with sour wood leaves or inside bark fill it up with water, boil slowly 3 hours, strain the liquor, add a lump of Allum big as half a hen egg, and a small branch of cedar bush, boil down to a quart, and bottle it tight take a table spoonful or more, if the patient can bear it three times a day, it is best before using this to puke with tartar and Ipecacuanha, and purging freely for 2 or three days before. I have known this do wonders. It is an Indian Medicine for Dropsy.

APERIENT PILLS.

Take of	Aloes	120 grs.
"	Rhubarb	120 do.
"	Ipecacuanha	60 do.
"	Jalap	60 do.
"	Gamboge	60 do.

Kayanne Capsecum, or red pepper 30 do.

Grind them fine in a mortar, wet with spirits, and work it like making biscuit dough, and then roll out into pills of common size.—Dose from two to six taken at any time—these pills are anti-dyspeptic; the persons using these pills, can eat and drink what they please, and if the pills dont work them, they wont hurt,—they are best taken at night.

DISEASES OF CHILDREN.

Not commonly noticed, yet common, 1st. Looseness of the bowels, accompanied with griping, and green stools, frequently followed with emaciation. **Treatment.**—Take 4 grains of calomel 16 grains of prepared chalk mix them well together, give four grains of the mixture every 30 minutes until the bowels shall have been freely purged; about every third night afterward, give a dose 4 grains of the mixture fc about a week.—See Dr. Dewees on diseases of children.

Another excellent preparation for worms or, cases resembling the above disease, take a tea spoonful of honey, put about as much Allum scraped fine as will lie on the point of a pocket knife give this for a few mornings on an empty stomach not suffering the child to eat or drink for half an hour afterwards.

SORE MOUTH AND THROAT.

For the Throat fry a handful of Rue (is best) wormwood or other better herbs will do, in hogs fat, slowly for half an hour, then add bees wax and tallow, untill you can spread it on a cloth, apply this round the throat extending up nearly to the ears, this plaster has done wonders.

For the mouth take Golden seal some call it yellow puccoon root dry and powder it, mixing a little Borax, put the powders in the mouth, I have known this cure desperate cases in one night.

FOR CANCERS.

Fill the sore with arsenic, put over this a poultice of onions, let it remain 48 hours, then take off the poultices, and clean out the arsenic and wash the sore three times a day with strong copperas water anointing it with the oil of hogs feet, a desperate disease treat with desperate Medicine.—Cancer warts, and even when sores begins to run, having become painful; are cured by dissolving a lump of blue stone in 3 or 4 spoonfuls of Rum applying it several times a day. Some burn the blue stone.

GRAVEL.

Make a tea of the prickly pear and drink it freely or take what is called Devils shoe string and use the tea, an old Gentleman told me he was cured of this distressing malady by using a tea made of the little kind of smart grass.

SCARLET FEVER.

This complaint is now raging violently through Virginia: and within a short time, has made its appearance throughout the Western States, with considerable severity in its symptoms, and requiring active and prompt treatment—otherwise it generally proves fatal. I have no doubt, by early attention to those symptoms and remedies which follow, you will at once cut short and easily control this *contagion*, (for it certainly is a contagious disease) similar to measles—distinguished or known from them, by the spots making their appearance on the second day of the fever: when, in measles, they usually make their appearance on the fourth day. The spots in *scarlet fever* being of a light flaming red, while those of the measles are of a dark red color. From this plain and different appearance, you can certainly distinguish at once the difference in the diseases; thereby enabling you to take at once, such prompt steps as to arrest this disorder; which, if suffered to proceed, generally, and I may add almost always, ends fatally.

Symptoms.—Cold and sudden chills stealing gradually over the whole body—while flushes of heat, great thirst, the head aches, the skin is covered with large red or scarlet patches, which after a short time unite or come together; then in a few days they disappear or go off in a kind of scurf, like bran, and the throat becomes quite hoarse or sore.

Remedies.—As you value the life of your patient, depend on emetics. or pukes, of ipecacuanha; which are to be given on the first appearance of the disease, to be followed by a dose of salts or eight grains of calomel and eight of rhubarb: and half of this dose for children. If the pulse is full and strong, and the head aches, it will be proper to draw blood, and dash cold water over the body freely and frequently. (Do not be alarmed at this last remedy, for it will be the certain one in this complaint to relieve your patient, for I have often used it with great success.) There is no disease in which the advantages of cold water have been more successful than in *scarlet fever:* but to receive the full benefit of it, it must be often used and that freely. *That is,* as often as the *heat,* &c. seem to require the use of it, which perhaps may be the case eight or nine times in the twenty-four hours.

A fine remedy in this disorder is the *Saline Mixture* made as follows:—Salt of tartar one drachm, water seven ounces, essence of peppermint five drops. When the salt of tartar is dissolved. add very gradually lemon juice, or vinegar, until the effervescence ceases. This mixture is to be taken every hour—and to children, such quantities as you can get them to take. It is a cooling mixture, produces gentle moisture on the skin, and keeps down inflammation, &c. When there is a sore throat, use any innocent gargle, such as sage and honey. with a little alum or borax in it, so as to wash or cleanse the throat *frequently;* and apply a mustard poultice to the throat.

In *scarlet fever* in the latter stage, it will be prudent for you to guard against putrescency, which symptoms I will plainly describe to you, so that you may know them; having fully the marks of *typhus fever*—difficulty in swallowing—breathing hurried—breath hot—skin dry, and burning to the touch—a quick, weak, and irregular pulse—scarlet patches break out about the lips; and the inside of the mouth and throat are of a firey red color. About the third day, blotches of a dark red color make their appearance about the face and neck, which soon extend over the whole body. If you will examine the throat, you will find a number of specks between an ash, and a dark brown color, particularly on the palate &c.—a brown fur covers the tongue—the lips are covered with little pimples containing acrid matter, which burst and produce ulceration wherever they touch. If the case is a bad one, the inside of the mouth and throat become black, and are covered with running sores, called ulcers. When these symptoms take place, it is a well marked case of *putrid fever,* and contagious. Be therefore careful, but not afraid. We cannot die in a better cause than in discharging a duty which we owe to God and our fellow creatures —the last and most solemn injunction of our blessed Redeemer, "*Love ye one another*" and the beautiful inculation of Divine Revelation. "*Do unto all mankind as ye would they should do unto you.*"

For the treatment of these last symptoms, read under the head *remedies for putrid sore throat.*

YY

EPIDEMIC CHOLERA.

This pestilence has swept from life one hundred and forty millions of the human race according to the most authentic reports of interments since August, 1817.

Sharers of the same nature, warmed with the same hopes, and as fondly attached to life as ourselves, all have been prematurely swept into eternity in quick succession, overwhelming the heart with sorrow of some affectionate parent, some tender companion, or some dear friend; and how many thousands, no doubt, unprepared for so sudden a change from life to the presence of the Supreme Judge of the Universe! It is impossible to commence writing on this awful and important subject without reflecting on the rapid extinction of human life, the excruciating miseries so many human beings must have suffered, without shuddering at the great sum of human misery inflicted by this complaint; nor can we but be sensible of the insufficiency of human efforts, against the decrees of an over-ruling *Providence.* Now are we not warned by this sad and affecting scene, in language not to be mistaken, "*Be ye also ready.*"

This destroying angel whom the *Eternal* has employed to sacrifice so great a portion of the human family has since, August 1817, been advanced over the whole field of Europe: nor have oceans, mountains, climate or distance, preserved us from its ravages. Mysterious and uncertain in its course, having no regulated or physical agents by which its location could be certainly determined, save that of its selection of the vicious, the uncleanly and the intemperate. Nothing, in my opinion can change the condition of the atmosphere which is essentially connected with this complaint. In other words the disease is in the atmosphere: and although no preventive can be taken against this complaint, yet much may be done towards staying its progress, and towards alleviating the force of the attack. The two best preventives for cholera from experience, are *Temperance* and *great cleanliness;* for experience throughout this disease, proves clearly and without any doubt, that cholera spreads itself with the most deadly effects amongst those who are negligent in personal cleanliness, and dissipated in their habits. But notwithstanding the cholera in a great measure was supposed at first to limit its ravages principally to this unfortunate part of the community, and such as were greatly exposed, yet, time and daily experience prove that many thousands have died of our most respectable citizens who were certainly of the opposite character to those I have mentioned. Yet the fact is, that all who are within the atmosphere of cholera are liable more or less to suffer from this complaint; but what are the real and physical causes that produce cholera is as yet very uncertain, even to those medical men who have had great experience in it. All that can be said is that it is in the atmosphere; nor can any thing change the condition of the atmosphere which is so essentially connected with this disorder. The persons most liable to this infection, says the French Royal Academy of Medicine, in their report, are those physically and morally debilitated; those weakened by excesses of whatever kind they may be; gluttons, drunkards, and gamesters, and women of imprudent habits, *and all persons* suffering under the pernicious effects of uncleanliness. To this testimony may be added that of all physicians and others who have watched this complaint, and the progress of the disease in India, England, France, Canada, and our own country. In all these countries the intemperate, the vicious and the lewed, when attacked, have universally fallen victims—and are the first to fall prostrate before the cholera and the most difficult to cure: and as an able physician expressed himself, generally beyond the reach of medicine. The unhappy inmates of the houses of ill-fame, and those of immoral uncleanliness in Persia, have been universally the first to be conveyed to the Cholera Hospitals.

SYMPTOMS OF CHOLERA.

I shall commence by giving you what is termed the *Premonitory Symptoms* of *Cholera*—by which is meant symptoms of the first or forming stage of this disease—and on your paying strict attention to these symptoms, will greatly depend the favorable issue of the case, and *if you do not,* in nine cases in twelve the person will die.

The person attacked with cholera, complains of weakness as if he had undergone fatigue; he feels frequently for a few moments uneasiness in the region of the stomach—but not so severe as to create alarm. Frequent evacuations or stools from the bowels, being obliged to go to stool from two to a dozen times a day—and not much griped in passing them. The countenance or features look unusually sharp, sometimes a little sick at the stomach, but this last symptom is not very common. This early evidence of the approach of the cholera is not often attended to, and seldom noticed but by those experienced in the complaints. The symptoms I have just mentioned may continue, varying sometimess better and then worse from one to ten days, before the second stage of the disorder commences. The stools at the first, are generally of a dark brown or blackish color. As the looseness continue, they gradually become less and less of a natural appearance; until they look like dirty water. Some head-ache, cramp of the fingers and toes. and belly, and almost always a swimming of the head and ringing in the ears, accompany these symptoms. Very frequently the bowels, for two or three days are costive or bound, and then looseness will again come on, and in a few hours collapse superyenes, and, in general, sickness at the stomach and vomiting or puking. Now remember that on an early attention to this looseness of the bowels will generally depend the cure, by timely application of such means as I shall advise; or if it is convenient, and you fear to trust your own judgment, make on the first appearance of these symptoms early application to a physician. Dr. Kirk, a distinguished medical gentleman, says it was found, from regular records of upwards of four thousand patients, that this looseness of the bowels prevailed in every case.

SYMPTOMS OF MARKED CHOLERA.

Having attentively perused all the numerous accounts which have been published, of the various symptoms by which the Epidemic Cholera is accompanied, I have thought it only, necessary to give you all the *general and well marked symptoms of the complaint*, without noticing every trifling deviation from the ordinary course of the disease. All you wish to be informed of is, when you are about to take it, and lastly when it has certainly attacked, I have therefore selected for you the description of the *Madris Report*, founded on extensive experience in the country which I enumerated to you its awful ravages.

This complaint generally takes place in the night or towards morning. You are taken sick at the stomach, and vomit or puke —the bowels are at once evacuated, that is in other words, you go to stool, and you seem to discharge or empty all their solid contents, and feel after you have done, great exhaustion, sinking and emptiness—after a short time you feel faintness, your skin becomes cold, and very often giddiness or swimming in the head and ringing in the ears; the power of moving your limbs seems impossible—twitchings of the muscles of the fingers and toes are felt, and these affections gradually extend along the limbs to the trunk of the body. The pulse from the first is small, weak, quick, and after a certain interval, but particularly on the commencement of spasms or of severe puking, it sinks suddenly, so as to be quickly lost in all the external parts. The skin, which from the commencement of the disease is below the natural heat, becomes colder and colder; it is seldom dry, generally covered with profuse cold sweat, or with a clammy moisture. In Europeans the skin often assumes a living hue, the whole surface becomes collapsed; the lips become blue, the nails present a similar appearance, and the skin of the feet and hands becomes corrugated and exhibits a sodden appearance; in this state the skin is insensible, even the action of the strongest medicines, such as warm spirits, or spirit in which camphor has been dissolved, or infact even the action of the most powerful stimulants; yet the patient generally complains of oppressive heat on the surface, and wishes to throw off the bed clothes.—The eyes sink in their orbits, and are surrounded with a livid or dark circle; the eye becomes heavy, and frequently the whites of the eye diffused with blood, or in other words blood shot. The feature of the face look sharp and dead, and indeed the whole countenance assumes a cadaverous aspect, and its appearance so uncommon that it is easily observed by all to be strangely and peculiarly unnatural. There is almost always urgent thirst, & a desire for cold drink, although the mouth be not usually parched. The tongue is moist, whitish and cold: a distressing sense of pain, and a burning heat at the epigastrium or pit of the stomach, are very common in this disease. Very little water is passed, bile, or saliva or spittle, is secreted; the voice becomes quite feeble and hollow, having an unnatural sound; the breathing is oppressed and generally slow, and the breath of the patient is quite cold or deficient in heat.

While these symptoms are going on, the stomach and bowels are very much affected in different ways. After the first vomiting and stool, however severe these symptoms may be, the matter passed by stool is always of a watery nature; and in some cases it is entirely destitute of color. The stools often resemble muddy water; and in others it is of a yellowish or greenish color. A very common appearance is that which is called in the East Indies "*congee stools*," resembling water in which rice had been washed, or having the appearance of various little slimy flakes, floating in the colorless water. The discharge from the stomach by puking, and those from the bowels by stool, do not appear to differ much, except that the former, or that which is puked up, has mixed with it portions of food which may have been eaten and not digested. Neither the vomiting or purging are symptoms of long continuance: they are either stopped by medicine, or the body becomes unable from weakness to puke or purge any longer: and they, together, with spasms, suddenly disappear a considerable time before death. If blood be drawn, it looks of a dark or black color, ropy, and flows slowly and with difficulty. Toward the close of the scene, great restlessness comes on, and constant anxiety and distress; and death takes place often in ten or twelve hours, and generally within seventeen or twenty hours from the commencement of the attack. During all this mortal struggle and commotion in the body, the mind remains clear, and its functions undisturbed, almost at the last moment of existence. The patient, though sunk and overwhelmed, and almost lifeless, dislikes to speak, and is greatly distressed if the least disturbed—still, however, retaining the power of thinking, and of expressing his thoughts, as long as his organs are obedient to his will, such symptoms are the most common of the *Epidemic Cholera*, where its tendency to death is not checked by medicine. Cholera, however, like other diseases, has presented considerable variety in its symptoms; thus, it may on one occasion be distinguished throughout by the absence of vomiting, and by the prevalence of purging, on another, by the excess of vomiting; and tho' more rarely, by the absence of purging. Spasm may be generally present in one instance; in another, it may not be observed. Of all, the most difficult is, that which is marked by a very slight commotion in the system—in which there is no vomiting, hardly any purging, perhaps one or two loose stools, no perceptible spasm, no pain of any kind, a marble coldness, with arrest or stoppage of circulation which comes on from the beginning, and the patient dies without a struggle.

Vomiting or puking, (as I have before told you) if entirely absent, or if it has taken place for a time, it soon stops, from the stomach being paralyzed, or in other words, as if it were really dead, or without any feeling or sensibility. Purging is a more constant symptom than vomiting in this disease, and in all cases of Cholera, *or most generally*, it is as I have before said the first symptoms of the disorder. Purging has been very rarely, and absent altogether—and when it is absent, is quite a bad symptom, for it denotes or shows plainly the attack is very dangerous—There is seldom much griping or tenesmus, which means a great and constant desire to go to stool, without doing much, and sometimes these desires are so sudden as to be irresistable. They also frequently take place at the same time, both puking and purging with spasm, and the pulse stops for a time at the wrist; as if all these symptoms originated at the instant, from one common cause. In advanced stages of the disease, purging generally ceases but in many cases a discharge of watery fluid takes place on every change of posture. The matters evacuated after the first emptying of the bowels have been occasionally observed to be greenish or of a yellowish appearance, torpid, of a frothy appearance, like yeast, and quite frequently bloody; but by far the most common appearances is, that of pure serum (which means the appearance of whey,) so thin and colorless as not to leave a stain on the patient's linen. The next in order of frequency is the *congee-like fluid;* (I have before explained to you what the congee stools meant:) the mucus is at times so thoroughly mixed, however, with the serum, as to give the whole the appearance of milk. The quantity of clear watery fluid which is sometimes discharged, is very great, and were these discharges to continue constantly, it would afford a perfect knowledge of the cause of the debility or weakness, thirst, thickness of the blood and other symptoms, but it is reduced to a positive certainty, that the most fatal and rapid cases, are by no means those which are distinguished by excessive discharges. Death on the contrary, has ensued in innumerable instances after one or two watery stools, without the development of any other symptom affecting the natural functions. Collapse has even come on before any evacuation by stool had taken place.

The peculiarly calm and undisturbed state of the mind in this disorder, has been the subject of great surprise: instances have been known of patients being able to walk, and to perform many of their usual avocations in business, even after the circulation has been so much arrested, that the pulse has not been discerned at the wrist; the cases I allude to, are those chiefly in which it has begun by an insidious watery purging; and many lives have been lost in consequence of the patient, under these false appearances, not having taken early alarm, and applied for medical aid. In other cases again, the animal functions appear to have been early impaired, and the prostration of strength to have preceded most of the symptoms. The voice in general sounds very weak, partaking of the debility prevailing in the other functions; it is commonly noticed as being remarkably feeble, often almost unable to be heard. Deafness has also been remarked in some instances to have been completely established. Coma does occasionally occur, especially towards the termination of the case, when it is fatal; but delirium has seldom been observed in this complaint.

Spasm has been held as one of the most essential features or certain accompanyments of the Epidemic Cholera, and owing to which circumstances it has received this specific name; so far however, as relates the muscles of the voluntary motion, and it is that description of spasm only to which I refer, *no symptom* is more frequently wanting. Spasms of the muscles chiefly accompany those cases in which there is a sensible and violent commotion of the system; hence they are more frequently found in cases where Europeans are the subjects of the disease, than when it attacks the natives of India, and in robust patients, more frequently than in the weakly. In the lower or more dangerous form of cholera, whether in the European or Indian, spasm is generally wanting or is present in a very slight degree. The muscles most commonly affected are those of the toes and feet, and of the calves of the legs; next to these the corresponding muscles of the superior extremities, then those of the thighs and arms—and lastly those of the trunk—producing the most distressing feelings to the affected person. It is deserving of remark, says Dr. Craigie in his account of the disease; that in seveaal instances, the first indications of the cholera are the twitchings of the fingers and toes: and a great many persons who resisted all the other symptoms of the disease were attacked by this twitching. Of all the symptoms of cholera, none are so universally present, nor indeed so important and fatal, as the immediate sinking of the circulation. It must nevertheless be admitted, that where instant remedial medicines have been successfully practiced, this symptom may not have developed itself, and that there are even cases where an excited vascular action has been observed to accompany the first preterbation of the system in cholera. Some intelligent medical gentleman have entertained doubts whether such cases belong indeed to this disease; it is, however to be remembered, that these are precisely the cases which yield most certainly and readily to appropriate remedies, and it consequently follows that a physician can seldom have an opportunity of observing whether or not this form of cholera will pass into a more aggravated stage. Cases, however have occurred, in which such degeneration has taken place, and it has been followed by death. The symptoms of excitement have likewise principally occurred among soldiers, in whom an effect upon the circulation may have been produced by the quantity of ardent spirits they are in the habit of drinking daily. The period at which a marked diminution of vascular action takes place, is somewhat various. The pulse sometimes keeps up tolerably for some hours, though very rarely: it more generally becomes small and accelerated at an early stage, and on the accession of spasm or vomiting, suddenly ceases to be distinguishable in the extremities. The length of time during which a patient sometimes live in a pulseless state, is extraordinary.

That remarkable shrinking of the features of the face, which has acquired the emphatic term of the "true cholera countenance," appears in every case, unless quickly stopped in the forming stage by medicine. This expression of countenance which conveys so truly, that of death itself, cannot be mistaken; and by an attentive observer, it will be perceived, that a similar shrinking takes place, throughout the limbs, and all the projecting parts of the body. No symptoms of cholera are so uniform in their appearance and progress, as those connected with the blood and its circulation. It is fully established, that the blood of patients attacked with cholera, is of an unnaturally dark color, and of a very thick consistence. In the great majority of the reports of the physicians of India, it is stated unequivocally, or without doubt, that after a certain quantity, of dark and thick blood has been drawn, it is common for its color to change, becoming much lighter.—When this was the case, it was considered favorably as to the termination of the case. In India, when medical aid was early administered, and the constitution of the patient otherwise healthy, the recovery from an attack of the cholera was generally very quick, owing to the peculiar constitutions of these people, in whom there is ordinarily very little tendency to inflammation or fever. But in Europeans, in whom there is much greater tendency to inflammation or fever, and a determination to some of the internal organs; consequently, the recovery from the disease by them is not so sudden or perfect. When cholera however, is of long continuance, and when the congestions appear to have been thoroughly established, few, either Europeans, or natives, who out-live the attack, are restored to health without considerable difficulty.

I have now described to you as fully and as minutely as the space allotted to me in this werk would permit; giving you the general symptoms of cholera, as it presented itself in the different districts of India, and they agree in every respect with those observed in the disease during its prevalence in Russia, Poland, North of Europe, the Canadas, &c. &c. This is proved by the history of the disease: by the most able and distinguished physicians throughout Europe and India: particularly the able report made by Dr. Keir of Moscow, to the British Government, and in the accounts transmitted from Montreal and Quebec. And all the reports made in this fatal disease, agree as to the principal cystem; that in the generality of cases there were the same excessive or constant evacuations by puking and purging a watery torpid fluid—the same collaps of the skin—coldness of the surface—sinking of the pulse—failure of strength—lividity of the face, or purple cast—shrinking of the features—spasms of the muscles, &c. all of which symptoms usually take place more or less, with some few variations (perhaps very few,) owing to the peculiarity of the constitution, or the state of the system at the time of taking the disaese. For cholera in its severity or duration, by which I mean the length of time it exists, depends much upon the local or predisposing causes. Therefore, if any decided difference has been observed between the character of cholera, as it prevailed in India, and after its extension into Europe, the Canadas and the United States, it consists merely in the gradual amelioration, of the complaint: by which I mean that it sometimes gradually loses its severity; owing as I have before told you, to the peculiarity of the climate, the predisposing causes, inviting more or less the disease wherever the disorder which is in the air, may locate or settle itself. And this is the reason why the cholera rages more violently at one place than it does at another: because the predisposing causes are greater.

Therefore, let cleanliness and temperance *in all things*, be the watch word; for experience has taught the people of the United States, that by due caution, and early attention to the proper remedies, which are simple and easily understood, this pestilence may be, and has been perfectly within the control of medicine—and that this disease is the same as the European Cholera, is fully established by the evidence of various physicians of eminence, who have witnessed the cholera both in India and Europe; and (as I have before stated to you,) its virulence and mitigation entirely depending upon local causes, or the constitution and the predisposition to an attack of this complaint.

Treatment.—The cholera has not been found to be less under the control of proper treatment than any other disease equally rapid in its course. When remedies of a proper kind, have been administered in the early stage of the complaint, and judiciously managed, a favorable termination, has in the majority of cases, been the result The difficulty is, to induce patients, or those attacked with this disorder, to apply sufficiently early for medical assistance. With the loss of a very few hours the chances of recovery are greatly diminished. "If the disease," says Dr. Annesley, whose experience in the treatment of the *Epidemic Cholera*, during its prevalence in India, was considerable, "be taken at its first commencement, or within an hour after the disorder attacks you, it is as manageable as any other acute disease; but the rapidity with which it runs through its course, requires the most active exertion before it can be checked, and the loss of an hour may cause the loss of life.

The remedies *most successfully used* in India, *throughout Europe generally*, will be noticed. The variety of different means used, and the peculiar opinions of different medical writers, many of which have proved unsuccessful, I do not think necessary to mention in a book of this kind. My object in writing so fully on this subject, has been to give you a perfect and general knowledge of this complaint, as to its violence and progress in India, and the principal remedies which proved to be the most successful in the cure of Cholera; selecting from the experience of the most distinguished physicians, such remedies as may be relied on in this epidemic.

The remedy, the good effects of which, in the treatment of Cholera, appears to have been most generally acknowledged, and the early employment of which is most insisted upon, is blood letting.

Bleeding from the arm in the first stage, when the pulse is full, and the temperature not reduced, is often sufficient to cut short the disease. The patient always feels immediate relief, particularly, where the head has been much affected. The bleeding should be performed in a horizontal position; or in other words, the patient should lie on a bed while bleeding him. Doctor Drysen, who has had great experience in this complaint, directs to increase the flow of the blood from the arm, by frictions or rubbing to the surface of the body, with flannel cloths wrung out of hot water or by bleeding while the patient is in the warm bath. [To see how to prepare and use the warm bath, see that head.]

According to Mr. Bell, "in no case in which it has been possible to persevere in blood letting, until the blood flows freely from the veins, and its color is recovered, and the oppressed chest relieved, will the patient die from that attack of the disease." He directs that when the blood has once begun to flow it ought to be allowed to bleed until these changes are observed. It is the opinion of Doctor Kenedy, that in ninety-nine instances out of a hundred, where patients are said to have died "despite of blood letting, it will be found on examination, either that no blood flowed from the incision or opening, made by the lancet, or that it came away in drops, or in a small broken stream, rarely exceeding a few ounces in quantity. "On the contrary," he adds "where blood was freely obtained to the extent of twenty ounces, and where the depletion is followed by proper auxiliaries, or other assistant remedies, the patients have usually recovered."

The testimony of the German, Russian, and Polish physicians, has all been given in favor of the beneficial effects of blood letting, when early resorted to in cholera.

The absence of the pulse, is no reason why he should not use the lancet, unless it be accompanied by other symptoms of great debility, and the system has been exhausted by previous evacuation or purging, and the surface is covered with a cold clammy sweat. Even under such circumstances, many attest the advantages of blood letting, especially when preceded by sinapisms, or in other words stimulating plasters of mustard to the belly, feet, ankles, &c.—The applications of dry heat and frictions to the surface, by which is meant bags of hot sand, bags of hot mush, bags of hot oats, bottles of hot water rolled in blankets, &c. (this is dry heat.)—frictions or rubbing as before explained, and diffusible stimulants internally, either spirits of hartshorn, brandy, wine and liquors of all kinds, given inwardly, so as to excite or rouse the circulation of the blood.

In some cases of cholera, says the able and experienced physician, Dr. Lefevre, the pulse ceases to beat very early, but upon opening a vein the blood flows slowly at first, gradually the current becomes fuller and stronger, the pulse beats very sensibly, and *the heat thus relieved*, is enabled to continue its circulation. The only cases in which bleeding would appear of doubtful propriety, during the first stage, are those occurring in old debilitated or weak persons, and in constitutions completely broke down by intemperance.

When blood cannot be drawn from the arm, and spasms continue—when severe pain and heat are felt at the epigastrium, when the skin is cold, and deluged with a cold clammy sweat, and when there is oppression of the chest and difficulty of breathing, excessive pain and confusion of the head, with great intolerance and dislike of light, no pules, or a very indistinct one, and a cadaverous or offensive smell from the body, cupping is advised over the region of the belly, with frictions of turpentine externally or outwardly, and calomel given internally. In the advanced stages of the disease, an opportunity is sometims afforded for the drawing of blood. This, according to Dr. Annesly, is marked by a struggle or effort of the circulation to overcome some resisting power, and is a most auspicious or favorable symptom which should never be over-looked. As soon as it occurs, bleeding directed with great judgment, should be resorted to.

The patient after bleeding, should be warmly covered with bed clothes, and allowed to remain perfectly still for a short period.

Sinapisms and rubefacients, or in other words, in plain English, meaning mustard poultices, mixed with strong vinegar and applied to the calves of the legs, inside the ankles, soles of the feet. &c. to act as a stimulant employed in low states of fever, and other diseases; and in cholera the object is to rouse the circulation of the blood, and to supercede the use of blisters, which are in this disorder too slow. Rubefacients means the substance which, when applied to the body or skin a certain time, makes a redness without blistering. Sinapisms and rubefacients are among the most efficacious or best means adapted to the cholera. "It may be said of them, that they are indispensable, and there is hardly any stage of the disease in which they may be employed with advantage: so long as the disease endures, so long will their use be proper, and they should be repeated continually." The pain in the bowels, and even the sickness, are often instantaneously relieved by the application of a large mustard poultice mixed with vinegar and applied over the region of the belly, and much pain is saved the patient if it be applied early. In violent cases of the disease the application of the mustard poultice mixed with strong vinegar as before directed, and applied to the ankles, wrists, calves of the legs, inside of the arms and thighs, and along the spine, is recommended in the strongest terms, in various treaties by the best informed physicians, of India, and Europe, on the cholera: and from the beneficial effects which we have seen result from the practice throughout this complaint, that it is one which should never be neglected; it would be as well probably to defer, however the sinapisms or poultices until the full effect of dry friction have been tested. When the skin has been excoriated or inflamed by the use of sinapims, anodyne fomentations, or in other words laudanum or opium steam, applied to the body, or even pulverized opium sprinkled over the tender surface, will be useful in relieving pain and sickness at the stomach.

Dry frictions are recommended as remedies of great importance and efficacy in all cases of cholera. By dry friction is meant rubbing well the whole body with your hands; hence it can only be recommended in those cases where there are plenty of attendants to wait upon the sick. Dry frictions are best adapted to, and have been found most beneficial in the early period of the attack. "The object of friction is two fold. First to restore the circulation in the part, and the heat that is dependant on it. Second to introduce remedies into the system by absorption. The first may be effected by mere dry rubbing with the hand or a warm flannel, or the flesh brush; and if persisted in, will often restore the circulation of the extremities, which were previously cold and senseless; but it requires great perseverance and long continuance; for it is necessary to keep up the circulation after it is restored; and as I have before told you, require considerable attendants or assistance to wait upon the sick. Various liniments have been proposed to assist the efforts of friction; but they may be superceded by steady rubbing with the hand, which should be sprinkled occasionally with a little powdered starch, or a little camphorated oil. Where proper and effectual rubbing cannot be maintained, stimulating liniments should be employed; because little rubbing will suffice, and the effect will be more permanent. The liniment composed of camphorated spirits and ammonia, (meaning hartshorn) will answer every purpose. When the spasms are, severe, the spirits of turpentine are the best for rubbing with. Rubbing the body with spirits is improper, as their rapid evaporation will have a tendency to increase the coldness of the surface.

Medicine may be introduced into the circulation by frictions and thus certain indications fulfilled, when the stomach is in too irritable a condition to retain the proper remedies. Especially may local pain and spasm be alleviated by frictions which opium *hyoseimus* and other narcotics, in form of liniments or other ointments.

DRY HEAT.—This remedy is strongly recommended by many of the practitioners who have witnessed cholera in the north of Europe. Mr. Keneday, a distinguished physician, recommends it in the first stage of the disease, after the bleeding, the warm bath, and the other remedies which are immediately demanded. He remarks, "as soon as the cramps are subdued, or have received a decided check, the patient with all possible expedition, ought to be removed from the bath. and be placed between dry heated blankets, Dry wa.mth should be further afforded by surrounding his body and limbs with bags of heated sand. Here dry heat, be it remembered, is the remedy, and not the sand which contains it. On this principle, bottles of hot water, rolled in flannel have been employed; and also hot ashes, bran, oatmeal, and mush, &c. &c. However to prevent loss of time, always take the first or the most convenient of the above articles that may come to hand, so as to produce any heat as early as possible. You will recollect the warm bath is always preferable in the first stage of the disease, from its great power; "*caution is necessary*," says Mr. Kenedy, "to prevent its being too long continued."

The following are the directions of Dr. Harnett, one of the British Medical commission, at Danizie, for the use of the warm bath. "It has been found necessary to guard against the indiscriminate use of the hot water and vapour baths, (or steam generally used by a pipe under the bed clothes.) In hot water after the perspiration has broken out; and above all, in the clammy stage of the disease; and after marked venus congestion has taken place, when it seems to increase the latter. which is particularly observable in the brain and heart. The bath should be used either in the critical moment in the beginning of the disease, or at farthest, instantly after, if admissible even then. To obviate the determination of blood to the head, cold applications ought to be occasionally applied to it, while the patient is in the bath.

The patient should be most gently and otherwise judiciously placed in the bath, with respect to the gradually inclined position of his body, and due support of the head, neck and shoulders; and the immersion or subjection should be short, merely long enough for the positive communication of heat and its effects, when he ought to be as gently and judiciously taken out, well wrapped up in hot blankets, promptly laid on a bed, and gently rubbed with warm, dry, coarse thread towels, all over, and wiped dry as fast as the clammy sweat oozes out. There is much handy and careful personal management requisite, in this essential part of the treatment.

Calomel.—This medicine has been greatly used in cholera, by a majority of English Surgeons in India, and is spoken highly of by such of them as have witnessed the disease in the north of Europe. In many instances the use of this powerful medicine has been carried or given to an enormous extent—doses of a scruple to half a drachm being considered the smallest dose adapted to the disease; others however have condemned the use of the remedy to this great extent, and recommended it to be given in smaller doses frequently repeated, and in general combined with opium. The evidence which is advanced in favor of the beneficial effects of calomel, under both modes of administration, might at first view appear perfectly conclusive, but in making up an opinion on this subject, it is necessary to recellect in almost all these cases which are adduced where the practice is supposed to have been eminently successful, other important remedies have at the same time been employed—especially bleeding; frictions, and stimulating applications to the surface—and very commonly the warm bath. Upon the early and judicious employment of the last mentioned medicines nearly all the writers agree that the cure of the disease mainly depends; by many they are themselves supposed fully sufficient—and that the various internal remedies that have been resorted to are useless or absolutely pernicious. Among the physicians of Russia, Poland and Germany, there are but few who recommend the use of calomel at all, and the majority denounce in very decided terms, its employment in the early stages of cholera, or to the extent to which it was carried by the practitioners in India. In Warsaw, the result of experience showed, according to Dr. Hille, that whether in larger doses, or in small ones frequently repeated, the calomel did more harm than good; and hence its use was either entirely abandoned, or it was given in a single dose of a few grains combined with opium. Dr. Gibbs writing from St. Petersburg, says expressly, that one and a half-scruple doses of calomel would not do there; Dr. Lefevre very properly remarks, that small doses combined with opium can be of no use in the first stage. In slight cases, he adds, where the quantity of opium is sufficient to allay the spasmodic action, while time is allowed for the calomel to act gradually, the combination however may be of service: but it must share the same fate as all the vaunted nostrums which when administered indiscriminately, lose even the merit to which they are really entitled.

In Dunaburg no calomel was administered, and of 745 cases, many of which were in the last stages of the disease when first seen by the physicians, only 75 terminated fatally.

Opium.—No remedy has been proposed in the treatment of cholera, which has so great a mass of testimony in its favor as opium. Nearly all the physicians, whatever may be their opinions as to the nature of the disease, have administered it. By some it is recommended in the largest possible doses, by others, however when given in smaller doses, it is considered much more efficacious, and less liable to produce injurious consequences.—Mr. Orton. an eminent praetitioner considers it "probable that a single dose of opium, alone, given at the very commencement of the disease would be found in a great majority of instances to put an effectual check to its progress." The Polish, and a few of the German physicians object, however, to the administrating of opium in cholera.

Internal Stimulants —The exhibition of either, brandy, ammonia (or hartshorn,) and other stimulants, I find to be very gently recommended, especially in the advanced stages of the disease. They are directed to be used or continued until re-action is fairly established, after which they are to be gradually relinquished. In the early stage of the disease, there is less evidence of their good effects than during that period in which the clammy sweat, icy coldness of the surface, scarcely perceptible pulse; and sunken countenance indicate a state of collapse, which if not speedily removed, the loss of the patient is inevitable. Many persons have employed the most powerful stimulants even from the commencement of the attack, and with no sparing hand. This practice is highly improper, and certainly by experience known to end in fatal consequences. Stimulants require at the times, much judgment and great caution in their employment, or they will most assuredly produce far more harm than good; and should be given under no other circumstances than those I have described, and even then, it is questionable whether they do not produce more evil than benefit.

PURGATIVES.—Though considered by many physicians as indispensible remedies in the treatment of cholera, they do not appear, with the *exception of calomel*, to have been very generally employed until after the more pressing and violent symptoms of the disease have been subdued. At this particular juncture it is very generally admitted that they have been productive of the best effects. They are proper so long as the bowels do not perform their functions regularly and the stools have an unusual appearance; nor is there any danger of re-producing the disease by their continuance, so long as we take these marks for our guide. It is much more likely to recur or return from neglecting to administer them; for purging by calomel is necessary, for you will find the quantity of unhealthy matter which is often evacuated by stool, remains for a long time after the complaint has been subdued. Such is the experience of Dr. Lefevre, in regard to the use of purgatives. He says, they are found indispensable, by producing copious discharges of vitiated bile. "A full dose of calomel," remarks the Doctor. "is often useful in the beginning of the convalescences as it act upon all the secretions. But the simple purging, which is so requisite after this disorder is best effected by small and repeated doses of castor oil." The virtues of the last medicine, have indeed been axtalled in a very great manner, by the physicians both in India and Europe. "The success under its use was very considerable, and there seems," says Mr. Scott, "to be sufficient evidence to warrant a more extensive trial." *It is admitted by all*, that purgatives which produce frequent watery stools, with griping are improper in this disease—are very prejudicial, and ought and must not be given.

ENEMATA.—Which means glysters, [how to prepare and give them, see that head.]—When the stomach is so irrita-ble that it will not retain any thing or constant puking, by which the exhibition of remedies by the mouth cannot be given, glysters, (called enemas,) will be proper, not only in the first attack of the complaint, but in the latter state of the disease also: especially in such cases as have been atten-ded with much spasm, and the bowels continue sore for a long time after, and every motion on the stool is productive of pain. In this case, an enema or glyster of half a pint of flax seed tea, and ten drops of laudanum, produces immediate relief—administered in this manner, the opium is less liable to produce injurious consequences than when given by the mouth. Injections, or glysters in plain English, given of hot water above blood heat, have been, highly spoken of in cases of great collapse or sinking and general coldness of the skin. After drawing up the water with a syringe (or squirt) and letting this warm water remain up a while, the water may be withdrawn by the syringe and a fresh supply of warm water introduced. Mr. Fife speaks favorably of injections of mustard—they have he says, promptly brought on a dis-charge of urine, after it had been entirely suppressed.

MURIATE OF SODA.—(Nothing in English but our com-mon salts.)—This has been spoken of by a few of the conti-nental physicians as a powerful remedy in cholera, and is rec-ommended by the eminent Mr. Searl, as an emetie in the com-mencement of the case. I cannot say that the evidence in its favor is very strong. It is true, we are told by Dr. Barry, that at St. Petersburgh, two German physicians declared in his presence at the medical council "that during the preceding eleven days they had treated at the custom house hospital, thirty cholera patients of whom they lost none. They gave him two table spoonfulls of common salt in six ounces of hot water at once, and one spoonful of the same cold, every hour afterwards." But let it be recollected, that these gentlemen, as well as the others who have recommended this remedy, always promised bleeding, that is, first bled, then used the salt and warm water, (and also, used other valuable remedies, upon the importance and good effects of which in cholera, there is but little difference in opinion. It is thus that many remedies *in this* and *other diseases,* acquire a fictitious reputation from being conjoined or mixed with others of acknowledged power—when had they been omitted, the case would in all probability, have proceeded as rapidly, or perhaps even more so, to a favorable termination.

DRINKS.—A strange diversity of opinions exist among the writers upon cholera, as the proper drinks to be allowed the patient. By some, dilutents of every kind were entirely prohibited, in consequence of a supposition that they increased the vomiting. The great desire of the patient is for cold water—he appears to labor under the most distressing thirst, the calls of which, it must be evident, cannot be disregarded, without materially increasing his suffering, and eventually the disease under which he suffers. Mr. Scott, in common with nearly all the best practitioners, admits, the propriety of allowing some bland dilutent, but maintains that it should be given of tepid warmth. He conceives that cold drinks are always dangerous, and generally fatal. This was the opinion very generally of the surgeons of India. Mr. Annesley however, gave cold water, with a slight impregnation of nitric acid—in other words, made pleasantly sour. This was the general drink at the hospital under his care, and was found to relieve the most distressing symptoms of the disease, the burning sensation of the stomach. From the experience of the European Physicians, it would appear very fully settled, that cold drinks are not more prejudicial than warm, and when desire by the patient, should be freely given.

According to Dr. Lefevre, iced lemonade has often been taken with advantage. The diluted nitric acid, he states may be added with great benefit to the common drinks. Fifty drops of the diluted acid, added to a pint of water, sweetened to the taste, is a grateful beverage. Dr. drysen of Friga, says that when the thirst is great, warm or even hot drinks are the best, and are often retained and even desired by the patient. He directs infusions of the various mild aromatic herbs, or when these are unpleasant to the patient, of common tea. But when the patient desires earnestly cold drinks they may be given in small portions at a time, without fear of any bad consequences. Fresh milk moderately cool, he states has been found very beneficial; and when diarrhœa, is considerable, a decoction of rice and barley, or thin tapica, &c. may be given, and when there is entire absence of pain or tenderness of the belly—a little port wine may be added. A cup of strong coffee, he has found very readily to stop the vomiting or puking in this disease; he advises the patient in cases of the drink being rejected by the stomach, to be allowed to swallow small portions of ice somewhat rounded into the shape of a pill by being rolled between the fingers—a practice also recommended by Brussais.

The strongest testimony in favor of warm water, is that given by Dr. Strum, a Surgeon in the polish Army: writing from the encampment near Karmienka. "The treatment which we now pursue, is probably already known to you, as Dr. Helbig has been ordered to publish an account of it by the government. It consists in nothing else than giving to the patient as much warm, nearly hot water, as he is able to drink, in the quantity of a glassfull every fifteen or twenty minutes. By the time he has taken fourteen glasses the cure is complete, with the exception of a slight diarrhœ which it is not proper too sudenly to suspend. The effects of this plan of treatment are so quiek and effectual, that in two house, or often sooner, the patient is well—particularly when it is commenced with sufficiently early.

TREATMENT OF THE SECONDARY STAGE OF CHOLERA.

After the more violent symptoms have been removed, that is, after the vomiting and purging have been suspended, the regular action of the heart established, and the circulation and heat of the stomach permanently restored, the attention of the physician must be directed to guard against or remedy local congestions, to prevent inordinate re-action, and to produce a healthy action of the bowels. Congestion is most liable to take place after the first stage or that of collapse is over, in the liver and lungs, and sometimes that of the head also. For this, moderate blood letting, local or general according to circumstances, is the most certain remedy. When febrile symptoms with determination to the brain present themselves, topical bleeding, (such as cupping &c.) near the temples, will be found very successfully to relieve it. The judicious employment of blisters, and of cold applications to the head, will also be of advantage. When that healthy condition of the bowels has not been produced by the remedies administered in the first stage, moderate doses of calomel, followed by castor oil, or other mild purgatives, will be necessary. As soon as the discharges have become healthy or well tinged with bile, (that is that you have fully roused the liver into action,) the patient may be considered out of danger, and the purgatives discontinued; but not until then. Tenderness or fixed pain in the region of the stomach; or any part of the abdomen or belly, call for the immediate application of leeches, or cupping.

I have now *fully* and as *minutely* as I conceive it necessary in a work of this kind, given you the various remedies which have been proposed, and strongly recommended, in the treatment of cholera by different writers—together with the practice of the most distinguished physicians in India, and Europe. You will after reading attentively this subject, see plainly that no *decided* or *positive* or certain method is laid down, for the treatment of this dreadful scourge of the human race. In plain language, it has commenced in the United States, and the physicians of this country have been compelled to establish a practice founded on their own experience, and to adopt or use such remedies according to the symptoms; or the effect of the disease, at the time of its location, upon the habits, constitutions, &c. and the effects of climate, together with such predisposing causes as may exist at the time this disorder is prevalent.

A TABLE OF MEDICINES

FOR

FAMILIES,

WITH THEIR

DOSES AND QUALITIES ANNEXED.

These doses must be increased, or diminished, according to the strength and habit of the patient.

A TABLE OF MEDICINES

	Adults,	*from* 20 *to* 15	*from* 15 *to* 10	*from* 10 *to* 6
	from to	from to	from to	from to
tion,	4 12 drops	5 10 drops	4 8 drops	3 6 drops
ne,	2 4 drms	2 3½ drms	2 3 drms	1¼ 2½ drops
	5 20 grs	5 18 grs	3 15 grs	3 12grs
'a,	20 80 drops	20 60 drops	15 40 drops	10 30drops
gton,	20 80 drops	20 60 drops	15 40 drops	10 30drops
a,	½ 2 dams	½ 1½ drms	25gr 1½ drms	20 60grs
	10 60 grs	10 40 grs	10 30grs	5 20grs
	6 20 grs	5 15 grs	3 10grs	2 8grs
ar,	½ 2 ozs	½ 1½ ozs	3 10drms	2 8drms
lk. liqr.	½ 2 drms	¼ 1½ drms	½ 1drm	23 40drops
	10 60 grs	10 30 grs	10 40grs	8 30grs
ed,	20 50 grs	20 40 grs	15 35grs	15 30grs
	½ 3 ozs	½ 2½ ozs	¼ 2ozs	3 8drms
rmint,	10 60 drops	10 50 drops	8 35drops	6 20drops
	10 40 drops	10 30 drops	8 25 drop	6 20drops
ic,	½ 2 drms	½ 1½ ozs	30drp 1 drm	20 60drops
	5 23 grs	5 20 grs	4 18grs	3 15grs
	5 15 grs	5 10 grs	4 10grs	3 15grs
irits,	½ 1½ drms	½ 1 drm	20 30drops	10 40drops
	15 30 grs	15 25 grs	12 20grs	10 15grs
	15 40 grs	10 30 grs	8 23grs	5 20grs
	20 60 drops	20 50 drops	15 40drops	10 30drop
	½ 2 drms	½ 1½ drms	20 60grs	15 45grs
	1 2 ozs	1 1½ ozs	1 1¼ozs	¼ 1oz
	10 30 grs	10 25 grs	8 20grs	6 15grs
	½ 3 grs	½ 2 grs	¼ 1gr	
	1 4 drs	3 drms	1 2drms	50 100drops
	15 40 grs	12 35 grs	10 35grs	8 30grs
	5 25 grs	4 20 grs	3 15grs	2¾ 13grs
	1 5 grs	1 4 grs	¾ 3grs	½ 2grs
	1 2 ozs	1 2 ozs	3 14drms.	2 12drops
r,	10 25 grs	10 20 grs	8 18grs	6 15grs
'ender,	30 100 drops	25 75 drops	20 60drops	15 50grs.
r,	2 8 drms	2 6 drms	1 4drms	1 3drms
quinine	2 8 grs	2 6 grs	1 4grs	1 3grs

rom 6 to 4	*from* 4 *to* 2	*from* 2 *to* 1	*under* I	Q
rom to	from to	from to	from to	
2 5 drops	1 4 drops	¼ 3 drops	¼ 1 drop	Tonic,
1 2 drams	1 1½ drams	I 1¼ drams	¼ 1 dram	Emetic.
2 10 grs	2 8 grains	1 6 grains	¼ 5 drops	Cathartic.
10 20 drops	8 15 drops	5 10 drops	2 5 drops	Corrobora
10 20 drops	8 15 drops	5 10 drops	2 5 drops	Corrobora
15 45 grs	10 30 grains	8 20 grains	5 15 grains	Tonic.
4 15 grs	5 10 grains	3 8 grains	1 5 grains	Cathartic.
2 4 grs	1 3 grains	1 2 grains	½ 1 grain	Stimulant
2 5 drams	1 4 drams	½ 2 drams	½ 1 dram	Aperient.
20 40 drops	15 30 drops	10 20 drops	5 10 drops	Stimulant
5 25 grs	5 20 grains	4 15 grains	2 10 grains	Tonic.
12 30 grs	10 25 grains	7 20 grains	5 15 grains	Absorben
2¼ 6 drams	2 5 drams	1½ 4 drams	1 2 drams	Purgative
4 15 drops	3 12 drops	2 10 drops	1 6 drops	Carminati
5 15 drops	3 42 drops	2 10 drops	1 4 drops	Tonic.
15 56 drops	10 40 drops	8 30 drops	5 10 drops	Stim. & a
3 12 grs	2 10 grains	2 8 drains	1 6 grains	Aromatic.
1 3 grs				Active pu
10 20 drops	5 10 drops	3 8 drops	2 6 drop	Stimulant
8 12 grs	5 10 granis	4 8 grains	1 5 grains	Emetic.
5 15 grs	4 12 grains	3 8 grains	2 5 grains	Purgative
8 20 drops	5 15 drops	3 8 drops	2 6 grains	Anodyne.
12 40 grs	10 35 grains	8 25 grains	5 20 grains	Absorben
3 6 drams	2 4 drams	1 2 drams	½ 1 dram	Aperient.
5 12 grs	2 10 grains	2 8 grains	1 4 grains	Febrifuge
				Anodyne.
30 60 drops	20 50 drops	10 40 drops	2 20 drops	Anodyne.
5 25 grs	4 20 grains	4 12 grains	2 10 grains	Purgative
2 10 grs	1 6 grains	½ 2 grains		Tonic.
½ 1¼ grain	½ 1 grain	¼ ½ grain		Astringen
2 8 drams	2 6 drams	1 4 drams	1 3 drams	Purgative
4 8 grains	3 6 grains	2 4 grains	1 3 grains	Absorben
10 35 drops	5 20 drops	4 15 drops	2 10 drops	Cordial.
½ 2 drams	20gr 1 dram	10 40 grains	5 20 grains	Aperient.
½ 2 grains	½ 1 grain	¼ ½ grain	¼ ½ grain	Tonic.
1¼ 2 grains	½ 2 grains	¼ 1 grain	¼ 1 grain	Emetic.
4 10 drops	3 8 drops	2 6 drops	1 5 drops	Tonic.
4 20 drops	3 15 drops	2 10 drops	1 5 drops	Diuretic.
4 20 drops	3 15 drops	2 10 drops	1 5 drops	Stimulant
6 15 grains	3 6 grains	1 3 grains		Emetic.

MEASURES.

8 pints } make { 1 gallon. | 8 fluid dr'ms { make | 1 flui
16 fluid ounces } make { 1 pint. | 60 drops { make | 1 flui

Spotted something that isn't quite right?

Let us know and we'll fix it for future reprints.
And as a thank you for your diligence, we'll
send you a free Sothis book of your choice.

publisher@sothis.press

This page intentionally left blank

Except of course for that line above. And this one.
And whilst we have your attention, perhaps you'd
like to follow us on Instagram @sothis.press. Go on.

Made in the USA
Monee, IL
08 November 2026

68091708R00371